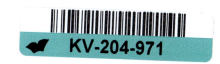

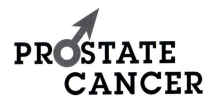

PROSTATE CANCER

Basic Mechanisms and Therapeutic Approaches

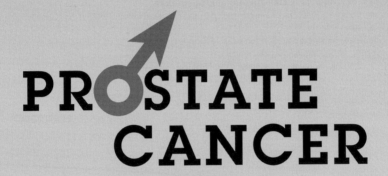

PROSTATE CANCER

Basic Mechanisms and Therapeutic Approaches

Editor

Chawnshang Chang

George H. Whipple Professor
University of Rochester, USA

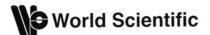 **World Scientific**

NEW JERSEY • LONDON • SINGAPORE • BEIJING • SHANGHAI • HONG KONG • TAIPEI • CHENNAI

Published by

World Scientific Publishing Co. Pte. Ltd.

5 Toh Tuck Link, Singapore 596224

USA office: 27 Warren Street, Suite 401-402, Hackensack, NJ 07601

UK office: 57 Shelton Street, Covent Garden, London WC2H 9HE

Library of Congress Cataloging-inPublication Data
Prostate cancer : basic mechanisms and therapeutic approaches / edited by Chawnshang Chang.
 p. cm.
 Includes bibliographical references and index.
 ISBN 981-256-067-X (alk. paper)
 1. Prostate--Cancer. I. Chang, Chawnshang, 1955–

 RC280.P7P75835 2005
 616.99'463--dc22

 2004062902

British Library Cataloguing-in-Publication Data
A catalogue record for this book is available from the British Library.

Typeset by Stallion Press
Email: sales@stallionpress.com

Printed in Singapore by Mainland Press

CONTENTS

LIST OF CONTRIBUTORS AND AFFILIATIONS

Bo-Ying Bao, *Departments of Pathology & Laboratory Medicine and Urology, University of Rochester Medical Center, Rochester, New York*

Elie A. Benaim, *Department of Urology, UT Southwestern Medical Center, Dallas, TX*

Ralph A. Brasacchio, *Department of Radiation Oncology and JP Wilmot Cancer Center, University of Rochester Medical Center, Rochester, New York*

Chawnshang Chang, *George H. Whipple Lab for Cancer Research, Departments of Urology, Pathology, Radiation Oncology, and the Cancer Center, University of Rochester, Rochester, New York*

Eugene Chang, *Departments of Urology and Pathology, University of Rochester Medical Center, Rochester, New York*

Philip Chang, *George H. Whipple Lab for Cancer Research, Department of Urology, Pathology, Radiation Oncology, and the Cancer Center, University of Rochester, Rochester, New York*

Ching-Shih Chen, *Division of Medicinal Chemistry and Pharmacognosy, College of Pharmacy, The Ohio State University, Columbus, Ohio*

Hong Chen, *Department of Urology, UT Southwestern Medical Center, Dallas, TX*

Kuen-Feng Chen, *Division of Medicinal Chemistry and Pharmacognosy, College of Pharmacy, The Ohio State University, Columbus, Ohio*

Ming Chen, *Departments of Urology and Pathology, University of Rochester Medical Center, Rochester, New York*

Siu-Ju Chen, *Department of Biochemistry and Molecular Biology, University of Nebraska Medical Center, Omaha, NE*

Anand Chokkalingam, *Celera Diagnostics, LLC, Alameda, California*

Sonal J. Desai, *Department of Biological Chemistry and Cancer Center, University of California at Davis, Sacramento, CA*

Noahiro Fujimoto, *Department of Urology, University of Occupational and Environmental Health, Iseigaoka, Yahatanishiku, Kitakyushu, Japan*

Thomas A. Gardner, *Urology Research Laboratory, Departments of Urology, Microbiology and Immunology, Walther Oncology Center, Indiana University Medical Center, Indianapolis, Indiana*

Kelley M. Harsch, *The Cleveland Clinic Foundation, The Lerner Research Institute, Cleveland, Ohio*

Warren D.W. Heston, *The Cleveland Clinic Foundation, The Lerner Research Institute, Cleveland, Ohio*

Jer-Tsong Hsieh, *Department of Urology, UT Southwestern Medical Center, Dallas, TX*

Ann W. Hsing, *Division of Cancer Epidemiology and Genetics, National Cancer Institute, Bethesda, Maryland*

Yueh-Chiang Hu, *George H. Whipple Lab for Cancer Research, Departments of Urology, Pathology, Radiation Oncology, and the Cancer Center, University of Rochester, Rochester, New York*

Juan Antonio Jiménez, *Urology Research Laboratory, Departments of Urology, Microbiology and Immunology, Walther Oncology Center, Indiana University Medical Center, Indianapolis, Indiana*

Chaeyong Jung, *Urology Research Laboratory, Departments of Urology, Microbiology and Immunology, Walther Oncology Center, Indiana University Medical Center, Indianapolis, Indiana*

Chinghai Kao, *Urology Research Laboratory, Departments of Urology, Microbiology, and Immunology, Walther Oncology Center, Indiana University Medical Center, Indianapolis, Indiana*

Jose A. Karam, *Department of Urology, UT Southwestern Medical Center, Dallas, TX*

Ani Khodavirdi, *Department of Pathology, Keck School of Medicine, University of Southern California, Los Angeles, California*

Samuel K. Kulp, *Division of Medicinal Chemistry and Pharmacognosy, College of Pharmacy, The Ohio State University, Columbus, Ohio*

Hsing-Jien Kung, *Department of Biological Chemistry and Cancer Center, University of California at Davis, Sacramento, CA*

Sang-Jin Lee, *Urology Research Laboratory, Departments of Urology, Microbiology and Immunology, Walther Oncology Center, Indiana University Medical Center, Indianapolis, Indiana*

Yi-Fen Lee, *Departments of Pathology & Laboratory Medicine and Urology, University of Rochester Medical Center, Rochester, New York*

Fen-Fen Lin, *Department of Biochemistry and Molecular Biology, University of Nebraska Medical Center, Omaha, NE*

Ming-Fong Lin, *Department of Biochemistry and Molecular Biology, Department of Surgery/Urology, College of Medicine and Eppley Institute for Cancer Research, University of Nebraska Medical Center, Omaha, NE*

Hiroshi Miyamoto, *Departments of Pathology & Laboratory Medicine and Urology, University of Rochester Medical Center, Rochester, New York*

Peter S. Nelson, *Fred Hutchinson Cancer Research Center, Seattle, Washington*

Jing Ni, *Departments of Urology and Pathology, University of Rochester Medical Center, Rochester, New York*

Rey-Chen Pong, *Department of Urology, UT Southwestern Medical Center, Dallas, TX*

Pradip Roy-Burman, *Department of Pathology and Department of Biochemistry and Molecular Biology, Keck School of Medicine, University of Southern California, Los Angeles, California*

Jun Shimazaki, *Department of Urology, Graduate School of Medicine, Chiba University, Chiba, Japan*

Jason E. Tasch, *The Cleveland Clinic Foundation, The Lerner Research Institute, Cleveland, Ohio*

Huei-Ju Ting, *Departments of Pathology & Laboratory Medicine and Urology, University of Rochester Medical Center, Rochester, New York*

Clifford G. Tepper, *Department of Biological Chemistry and Cancer Center, University of California at Davis, Sacramento, CA*

Suresh Veeramani, *Department of Biochemistry and Molecular Biology, University of Nebraska Medical Center, Omaha, NE*

Xingqing Wen, *Departments of Urology and Pathology, University of Rochester Medical Center, Rochester, New York*

Chun-Te Wu, *George H. Whipple Lab for Cancer Research, Departments of Urology, Pathology, Radiation Oncology, and the Cancer Center, University of Rochester, Rochester, New York*

Hong Wu, *Department of Molecular and Medical Pharmacology, University of California, Los Angeles School of Medicine, Los Angeles, California*

Qingquan Xu, *George H. Whipple Lab for Cancer Research, Departments of Urology, Pathology, Radiation Oncology, and the Cancer Center, University of Rochester, Rochester, New York*

Zhiming Yang, *George H. Whipple Lab for Cancer Research, Departments of Urology, Pathology, Radiation Oncology, and the Cancer Center, University of Rochester, Rochester, New York*

Shuyuan Yeh, *Departments of Urology and Pathology, University of Rochester Medical Center, Rochester, New York*

Yi Yin, *Departments of Urology and Pathology, University of Rochester Medical Center, Rochester, New York*

Ta-Chun Yuan, *Department of Biochemistry and Molecular Biology, University of Nebraska Medical Center, Omaha, NE*

Min Zhang, *Departments of Urology and Pathology, University of Rochester Medical Center, Rochester, New York*

PREFACE

Prostate cancer is the second leading cause of death in men. Charles Huggins first found that metastatic prostate cancer responds to androgen-ablation therapy, which heralded the beginning of a new era of prostate cancer therapy. Later, Andrew Schally and others showed that advanced prostate cancer responded to the LHRH agonist as decreased serum testosterone level to 25% and marked reduction in cancer-associated bone pain. The discovery of androgen receptor (AR) led to the screening of chemical libraries for AR blockers. Since then, antiandrogens, including flutamide and casodex, have been in continual use as therapeutic agents. Yet, with either androgen ablation via surgical or medical castration, with or without additional combination of various antiandrogens, eventually most of, if not all, prostate cancers still progress into the Hormone Refractory stage and the detailed reasons for this remain unclear. Cloning of the AR, generation of AR antibodies, finding of AR coregulators and their applications to prostate cancer progression reveals the essential roles of AR in the prostate cancer progression and opened a new approach for AR ablation therapy by targeting the AR, instead of androgens, to battle the prostate cancer.

Chapters 1 to 6 discuss current effective hormonal therapy, immunotherapy, chemotherapy, radiation therapy, and gene therapy, as well as androgen ablation therapy. Chapters 7 to 15 discuss the recent advances in the field of study of the basic mechanisms behind the growth of prostate cancer and how some of these mechanisms can be used to treat prostate cancer. Chapters 16 and 17 include recent research in the study of prostate cancer in newly developed mouse model systems. Many of these studies have distinct potential advantages as they lead toward advances in the clinical treatments of and drug therapies for these androgen-related diseases. We feel our book should be of interest as both a study guide and research reference for students, basic scientists, and clinicians.

I would like to dedicate this book to my PhD advisor Dr. Liao, whose research philosophy and Taiwanese dignity deeply influences my continued academic career. I would also like to thank Drs. Carbone, Wilding, Messing, Lardy, and Gorski for their help in establishing my independent academic research career at the University of Wisconsin and the University of Rochester. Finally, I thank my copyeditors, Mrs. Karen Wolf and Dr. Loretta Collins, for their invaluable editorial and proofreading assistance.

Chawnshang Chang, PhD
University of Rochester, New York, USA

EDITOR — CHAWNSHANG CHANG, PH.D.

Chawnshang Chang was born and raised in Taiwan. In 1997 he became the George Hoyt Whipple Distinguished Professor at the University of Rochester in Rochester, New York.

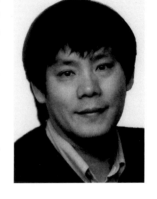

He received his B.S. from the National Taiwan University and Ph.D. from the University of Chicago in 1985. In 1990, at the University of Wisconsin-Madison he began his independent research career and was promoted to full professor in 1996.

Dr. Chang has published more than 250 peer-reviewed articles related to AR and TR2/TR4 orphan receptors. His landmark discovery, the first cloning of the androgen receptor (AR) cDNAs (*Science*, 240: 324–326, 1988), provided the framework for the subsequent studies of basic androgen mechanisms and their clinical applications. Several androgen-related diseases, such as prostate cancer, Testicular Feminization Syndrome, and Kennedy's Neuron Disease were linked to mutations of the AR. In recent years several new androgens or anti-androgens were developed based on the targets of the AR.

In 1996, Dr. Chang's Lab isolated the first AR coregulator and within a few years identified and isolated another 10 AR coregulators (*Endocrine Review*, 23: 155–200, 2000), which modulate AR functions, and enable AR to cross-talk to many signal transduction pathways. Generation of the first floxed AR mouse (*PNAS*, 2002) further provided the first tissue-specific AR knockout mouse, as well as the first female mouse without functional AR. These mice allow the *in vivo* study of androgen actions in selective tissues, including prostate, testis, liver, muscle, bone, and the female breast and ovary.

Many Universities have presented Dr. Chang with various awards and honorary professorships. His generosity is well known in the academic community and Taiwanese society and more than 700 labs throughout the world have benefited by collaborations using his AR reagents.

1

HORMONAL THERAPY FOR PROSTATE CANCER: CLINICAL AND EXPERIMENTAL EVIDENCE

Hiroshi Miyamoto and Chawnshang Chang

Departments of Pathology & Laboratory Medicine and Urology
University of Rochester Medical Center
Rochester, New York, USA

Introduction

The role and mechanism of androgen function have been studied in a variety of androgen target organs, including the prostate. As is the case with normal prostate development, the growth of prostatic neoplasms is generally dependent on androgens, especially on 5α-dihydrotestosterone (DHT). Since 1941 when Huggins and Hodges[1] published their Nobel Prize-winning study on the effects of hormone manipulation in patients with metastatic prostate cancer (PCa), hormonal therapy remains the critical therapeutic option for advanced disease. Multiple strategies have been used to reduce serum levels of androgens or interfere with their function via the androgen receptor (AR) (Fig. 1). However, considerable uncertainty remains as to the appropriate choice/timing and actual benefits of hormonal therapy in various situations. Indeed, PCa is still the second leading cause of cancer-related death among men in the United States.[2] In this chapter, we systematically review clinical and experimental evidence supporting current strategies of hormonal therapy in PCa.

The AR and Androgens

The AR, a member of the nuclear receptor superfamily, functions as a ligand-inducible transcription factor that regulates the expression of target

1

H. Miyamoto & C. Chang

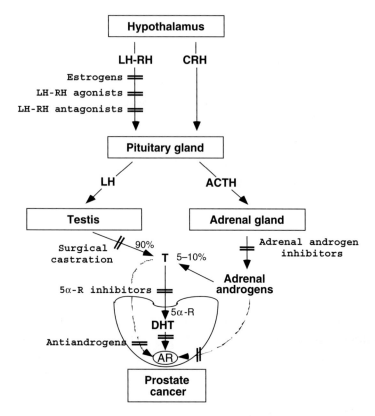

Fig. 1. Strategies for hormonal therapy. LH-RH=Luteinizing hormone-releasing hormone; CRH=corticotropin-releasing hormone; LH=luteinizing hormone; ACTH=adrenocorticotropic hormone; T=testosterone; 5α-R=5α-reductase; DHT=5α-dihydrotestosterone; AR=androgen receptor.

genes in response to ligands in target cells.[3,4] Recent studies have also revealed that the AR modulates transcription by recruitment of coregulators that influence a number of functional properties of the receptor, including ligand selectivity and DNA binding capacity (reviewed in Ref. 5).

Testosterone is secreted by Leydig cells in the testis and is the major sex hormone circulating within the blood of males. In a variety of androgensensitive tissues like the prostate, testosterone is irreversibly converted by 5α-reductases to the more potent androgen, DHT.[4,6] Upon binding of androgens, the androgen-AR complexes form homodimers, and they translocate into the nucleus and bind to androgen responsive elements located on target genes, such as prostate-specific antigen (PSA), which is clinically used for the detection and monitoring of PCa recurrence and progression. Besides testosterone and DHT, several precursors of testosterone mainly secreted by adrenal glands, dehydroepiandrosterone (DHEA), DHEA sulfate, Δ^4-androstenedione, and Δ^5-androstenediol, can also stimulate the AR through their conversion to testosterone/DHT in peripheral tissues, including the prostate, or by directly binding to the AR.[7–10]

Strategies of Androgen Deprivation

Multiple approaches at androgen deprivation have been used for the treatment of PCa (Fig. 1). The agents and strategies used for androgen deprivation therapies are listed in Table 1.

Surgical Castration

Surgical castration by bilateral orchiectomy is the most immediate method to reduce circulating testosterone by >90% within 24 hours,[11] and there is no risk of a paradoxical flare of the disease. Since the 1960s, the Veterans Administration Cooperative Urological Research Group (VACURG) trials, the earliest large-scale randomized studies of hormonal therapy, demonstrated the clinical effectiveness of surgical castration.[12,13] Compared to placebo, orchiectomy retarded cancer progression in advanced cases, but no clear survival advantage for castration over placebo was seen. Recent clinical studies (i.e. surgical *vs.* chemical castration) are discussed later. Although surgical castration may be underused, some studies suggest that many patients prefer this approach for the reasons of convenience and cost.[14] On the other hand, other studies suggest that this treatment approach is unacceptable to many patients, causing considerable psychological problems, with irreversible impairment in libido and erectile function in most cases.[15,16]

Medical Castration

Diethylstilbestrol (DES)

In the 1940s, the first reversible medical castration method was achieved by administration of DES, a semi-synthetic estrogen compound.[1] The

Table 1. Treatment Options as Hormonal Therapy for Prostate Cancer

Modality	Methodology	Mechanism/Action	Advantages	Disadvantages
Surgical castration	Bilateral orchiectomy	Orchiectomy, ↓T	Rapid ablation of testicular T; Relatively simple procedure, lower cost	Definitive castration; Associated psychological problems; Irreversible loss of libido/sexual potency; Reduced muscle mass/energy; Hot flashes; Anemia/osteoporosis; Unaffected adrenal androgens
Medical castration	Estrogens (DES)	Suppresses LH-RH secretion, ↓LH, ↓T; Direct effect via ER (?)		Cardiovascular events (estrogens); Flare phenomenon (LH-RH agonists); Reduced muscle mass/energy; Loss of libido/sexual potency; Hot flashes; Anemia/osteoporosis; Unaffected adrenal androgens
	LH-RH agonists (Leuprolide, Goserelin)	Suppresses LH-RH secretion, ↓LH, ↓T	Reversible castration; Ablation of testicular T	
	LH-RH antagonists (Abarelix)	Antagonizes LH-RH receptor, ↓LH, ↓T	More acceptable than orchiectomy	
CAB	Castration + antiandrogen	Ablation of testicular T + competitive inhibition of adrenal androgens	More effective (?)	Increased side effects; Antiandrogen withdrawal response

Table 1. (*Continued*)

Modality	Methodology	Mechanism/Action	Advantages	Disadvantages
Antiandrogen monotherapy	Non-steroidal antiandrogens (Flutamide, Nilutamide, Bicalutamide)	Antagonizes AR in target tissues, $\uparrow$T	Competitive inhibition of testicular/adrenal androgens Retaining sexual potency Less severe side effects Oral administration only	Gynecomastia Less effective (?)
	Steroidal antiandrogens (CPA, Megestrol acetate)	Antagonizes AR in target tissues, Suppresses LH-RH secretion, LH, $\downarrow$T	CAB effect Oral administration only	Cardiovascular events Side effects due to lowering of serum T Gynecomastia
IAB	Intermittent hormonal therapy		Longer androgen-sensitive period(?) Reduced side effects/costs	Investigational May achieve continuous androgen ablation
TrAB	Intermittent CAB + 5α-R inhibitor (Finasteride, Benzoquinoline)		Superior to IAB or CAB (?)	Investigational
SAB	5α-R inhibitor + antiandrogen or LH-RH agonist		Superior to monotherapy (?)	Investigational

T = Testosterone; DES = diethylstilbestrol; LH-RH = luteinizing hormone-releasing hormone; LH = luteinizing hormone; ER = estrogen receptor; CAB = combined androgen blockade; AR = androgen receptor; CPA = cyproterone acetate; IAB = intermittent androgen blockade; TrAB = triple androgen blockade; 5α-R = 5α-reductase; SAB = sequential androgen blockade.

VACURG studies identified equivalent overall survival rate in the DES group (5 mg/day) to the orchiectomy group, but non-cancer-related deaths, most of which were cardiovascular events, were noted.[12,13] Subsequent trials have shown that DES at 3 mg/day is equivalent to other treatment options in overall survival rates.[17–21] However, cardiovascular toxicity with events including myocardial infarction, deep vein thrombosis, edema, and transient ischemic attack was observed in 8%–33% of patients. Gynecomastia was also significantly seen in patients with 3 mg/day DES. A low-dose of DES (1 mg/day) was also evaluated,[13,22] but whether DES at 1 mg/day is as effective and safe as other treatment options is still controversial. After the development of luteinizing hormone-releasing hormone (LH-RH) agonists, with fewer cardiovascular events and no resulting gynecomastia, DES is now only rarely used as a first-line hormonal treatment in North America. Instead, several studies have evaluated the efficacy of DES as a salvage therapy after failure of first-line androgen deprivation. Recent studies, using 1–3 mg/day DES with or without anti-thrombotic agents, including warfarin and aspirin,[23,24] identified response rates by PSA measurement to be 43%–79% with median durations of progression of 6–7.5 months and with 2.8%–28% cardiovascular events.

It was generally believed that the primary mechanism of action of DES was to decrease androgen levels through hypothalamic-pituitary suppression, but recent evidence indicates that the mechanism is probably more complex. Kitahara *et al.* reported stronger suppression of testosterone by DES than by surgical castration or other means of chemical castration, such as the administration of a LH-RH agonist.[25] The same group also suggested that DES might reduce serum DHEA sulfate.[26] A direct cytotoxic effect of estrogens has also been suggested in PCa *in vitro*, presumably through both estrogen receptor (ER)-dependent and ER-independent pathways.[27–29] This is consistent with the finding that phytoestrogens, which have steroidal structures similar to estrogens and are found in a variety of plant foods, inhibit PCa cell proliferation.[49] Indeed, ERβ has been detected in human PCa cell lines, including LNCaP, PC-3 and DU145, and in normal and malignant prostate tissues, whereas ERα is expressed in PC-3 cells and in stromal (not epithelial) cells of the prostate.[30–32] Furthermore, it is suggested that loss of ERβ in PCa tissues is associated with tumor progression.[32,33] These findings might be able to explain the evidence that administration of DES could be more effective than other androgen ablation therapies in suppressing PCa growth if unfavorable side effects of DES are not considered.[12,13] On the other hand, we previously showed that a natural estrogen, 17β-estradiol, but not DES, increased AR transcriptional activity in PCa cells.[34]

LH-RH Agonists and Antagonists

The introduction of LH-RH analogues, obtaining medical castration, has lead to a dramatic change in the treatment of advanced PCa.[35] In the United States, two LH-RH agonists are commercially available: leuprolide acetate and goserelin acetate.

LH-RH is generally secreted by the hypothalamus in pulses, leading to pulsatile secretion of LH by the pituitary. This in turn promotes testosterone secretion by the Leydig cells of the testes. However, constantly high levels of LH-RH that occur with agonist administration down-regulate the receptors in the pituitary, inhibit LH secretion, and thereby reduce testosterone production. In addition, some studies have suggested a direct inhibitory effect of LH-RH via LH-RH receptors in PCa cells.[36,37]

Several randomized studies showed the equivalent effectiveness between surgical castration and LH-RH agonist administration.[38,39] Recently, depot LH-RH agonist preparations have been developed, which last 3 to 4 months and have the same efficacy as classical preparations.[40] Thus, the depot preparations have now become the most widely used form of androgen deprivation. Side effects of LH-RH agonists include hot flashes, reduced libido, and osteoporosis.[41] In addition, LH-RH agonists often cause an initial surge of LH release, with a corresponding increase in serum testosterone and DHT lasting 1 to 2 weeks. This surge may stimulate PCa growth with a worsening of related symptoms, which is known as the flare phenomenon.[42] Therefore, administration of an antiandrogen or estrogen for a week before and during the first few weeks of LH-RH agonist therapy is often used in an attempt to limit the clinical sequelae caused by this hormonal surge.[42,43]

LH-RH receptor antagonists recently have been developed for androgen deprivation.[44] Since abarelix, the first peptide antagonist, directly blocks the binding of LH-RH to its receptor without agonist activity, there is no initial flare phenomenon as occurs with LH-RH agonists.[44,45] Recent clinical studies have demonstrated that abarelix monotherapy achieves medical castration and a reduction of serum PSA levels to the same extent achieved by LH-RH agonists.[46–48] However, long-term follow-up studies are necessary to determine whether LH-RH antagonists can be routinely used for advanced prostate cancer.

Combined Androgen Blockade (CAB)

Monotherapy with surgical or medical castration results in marginal or no decline of adrenal androgens that not only can be converted to testosterone/DHT but are likely to possess intrinsic androgenic activity.[9,10,49] Thus, men who undergo castration still have relatively high levels (up to 40%) of DHT and 5%–10% of testosterone.[7,50] The basis of CAB (also called maximal androgen blockade) is concomitant neutralization of both testicular and adrenal sources of androgens. CAB consists of treatment with a LH-RH agonist or surgical castration combined with a non-steroidal antiandrogen. Antiandrogens include a number of compounds that interfere with the binding of androgens to the AR in the target cell, which ultimately prevents the activation of AR pathways in those cells. CAB has been advocated as the most effective hormonal treatment for patients with advanced PCa. However, this approach implies increased side effects and cost, and there are few supportive data showing a meaningful improvement in survival associated with the addition of antiandrogen.[51,52]

Several early, randomized trials demonstrated a significant survival advantage of CAB in patients with advanced PCa, compared to castration alone.[53–56] In 1998, however, Eisenberger *et al.*[57] reported a trial of 1387 patients with metastatic PCa who were randomized to surgical castration and placebo *vs.* flutamide. There were no differences in progression-free or overall survival between the two arms. Several factors were hypothesized to explain the discrepancy between the results of this study and earlier reports. First, patients in this study might have had less aggressive disease. Second, castration with a LH-RH agonist, especially a daily regimen of leuprolide injections in the first study,[53] might not have been as complete as surgical castration. Third, the LH-RH agonist plus placebo group may have experienced initial flare leading to worsening the disease. In 2000, the Prostate Cancer Trialists' Collaborative Group[52] published a meta-analysis of 27 trials of CAB *vs.* monotherapy involving 8275 patients with advanced PCa. The difference in the 5-year survival rate was not statistically significant (25.4% with CAB *vs.* 23.6% with castration alone). However, a statistically significant difference ($p < 0.02$) in favor of castration plus a non-steroidal antiandrogen was observed. More recently, another meta-analysis of 20 randomized trials concluded that there was a 5% improvement in 5-year survival (30% *vs.* 25%) with CAB.[58] However, only 7 of the 20 studies might be considered as high-quality trials and no significant improvement with CAB was seen in the meta-analysis of these 7 studies. In summary, recent data show that CAB provides a minimal advantage (up to 5% improvement in 5-year survival) over castration monotherapy. It is generally recommended to use an antiandrogen before and during the first several weeks of LH-RH agonist therapy to prevent possible symptoms of the flare. With these data, prolonged treatment beyond 1 month with CAB may not be the first choice of hormonal therapy for advanced PCa.

Antiandrogen Monotherapy

There are two types of antiandrogens, steroidal, such as cyproterone acetate (CPA) and megestrol acetate, and non-steroidal, such as flutamide, nilutamide, and bicalutamide. As noted, antiandrogens are generally used in conjunction with castration as CAB. However, castration based approaches are usually associated with side effects, which have a negative impact on quality of life (QOL). Monotherapy with a (non-steroidal) antiandrogen is becoming an increasingly attractive alternative therapeutic approach. Most of non-steroidal antiandrogens increase within normal physiological range the serum levels of androgens due to the suppression of the pituitary feed-back. Thus, this means of androgen blockade can preserve gonadal function and therefore provide potential QOL benefits, particularly in terms of retained potency and libido, no muscle weakness, and less bone demineralization.

Flutamide

Flutamide was the first non-steroidal antiandrogen that was widely used as a component of CAB. However, the use of flutamide monotherapy for advanced PCa has not been extensively studied in phase III trials.[59] Initial open studies assessing the clinical efficacy of flutamide as monotherapy were reviewed by Delaere and Van Thillo.[60] Among approximately 500 previously untreated patients with advanced PCa, 68% achieved at least a partial response. But most studies were relatively small, and there seemed to be differences in the criteria of response. Several trials have compared the efficacy of flutamide as monotherapy with that of DES, orchiectomy, or CAB. Boccardo reviewed these studies and found no significant differences in response rates/duration among these groups.[52] In a double-blind randomized study to compare the efficacy of flutamide with 3 mg/day DES,[21] however, DES produced significantly longer overall survival than flutamide (43.2 months *vs.* 28.5 months). Because some adverse effects, such as hepatotoxicity, were noted, the rate of treatment withdrawal for any drug-related adverse events was highest with flutamide among 3 nonsteroidal antiandrogens.[59] There have been no comparative studies of the efficacy of different non-steroidal antiandrogens as monotherapy.

Nilutamide

No randomized studies of monotherapy with nilutamide or comparative studies with any other hormonal therapy have been reported. One small study (26 patients) evaluated the efficacy of nilutamide as monotherapy, demonstrating that 21 (91%) of the 23 evaluable previously untreated patients with metastatic PCa had a response, with a median overall survival of 23 months.[61] The survival rate in this study might be less than that achieved by CAB with nilutamide.[62] In addition, nilutamide was associated with a high incidence (31%) of visual problems (light-dark adaptation disorders).[61] Other unique adverse effects of nilutamide, when used as either monotherapy or a component of CAB, include alcohol intolerance and interstitial pneumonitis.[61,62] Nilutamide has been reported to cause a higher incidence of nausea and vomiting than the other nonsteroidal antiandrogens, whereas the incidence of diarrhea and gynecomastia is lower with nilutamide than flutamide.[59,62] These results may discourage conducting larger trials with nilutamide monotherapy.

Bicalutamide

Of available non-steroidal antiandrogens, bicalutamide as monotherapy has been most extensively studied. In early comparative trials using bicalutamide at 50 mg/day, castration was shown to be superior to bicalutamide monotherapy, in terms of survival rate in patients with metastatic disease.[63] However, subsequent trials with bicalutamide at 100 or 150 mg/day have revealed equivalent efficacy between bicalutamide monotherapy and surgical or medical castration.[52,64,65] Other comparative studies also showed no statistically significant differences in survival between bicalutamide at 150 mg/day monotherapy and CAB (castration with flutamide or nilutamide) with better tolerability in the bicalutamide monotherapy group.[66,67] Bicalutamide at 150 mg/day has been shown to have a more favorable side effect profile than flutamide and nilutamide,[59] although there was still a high risk of gynecomastia and breast pain. Since bicalutamide has a longer elimination half-life of approximately 6 days than flutamide (6 hours) or nilutamide (56 hours), it can be given once daily *vs.* flutamide (or nilutamide in many studies) dosed 3 times daily.[62,68,69] The most recent and largest trials involving 8113 patients confirmed these observations (clinical efficacy, QOL benefit, and tolerability).[70] Thus, bicalutamide at 150 mg/day is thought to be an appropriate dosage, and this treatment, either alone, referred to as peripheral androgen blockade, or as adjuvant therapy, could be a standard option in patients with localized or locally advanced PCa.

CPA

CPA, a progestational antiandrogen, was the first antiandrogen used for the treatment of advanced PCa in Europe. It acts as an AR antagonist, as well as causes partial suppression of pituitary gonadotropins, which results in a rapid and sustained 70% decrease in testosterone levels.[71] Therefore, CPA, as a single agent, may yield CAB. In clinical studies, there were no significant differences in tumor response rates or disease specific survival between CPA and any other forms of androgen deprivation, such as surgical castration, estrogens, LH-RH agonists, and nonsteroidal antiandrogens.[59,72] Unfortunately, CPA has been reported to induce severe cardiovascular complications in about 10% of patients, although the rate is lower than those of DES (up to 33%).[18] Other complications include gynecomastia, loss of libido, erectile dysfunction, and central nervous system effects such as headache, fatigue, and weakness that are possibly attributable to the lowering of serum testosterone levels. Therefore, the use of CPA as monotherapy might be limited to those who find surgical castration unacceptable. In addition, CPA can be used to block LH-RH induced flare reactions and to suppress surgical or medical castration-related hot flashes.[71,72]

Neoadjuvant/Adjuvant Hormonal Therapy with Radical Prostatectomy

Neoadjuvant Hormonal Therapy

Radical prostatectomy is a treatment modality which can offer the possibility of PCa cure if surgical margins are negative. However, surgical attempts for a cure in patients with apparently localized PCa often fail because the cancer is incompletely resected possibly due to clinical understaging before the surgery or micrometastases existing at the time of surgery. The theoretical purposes of neoadjuvant treatment are to lower the pathological stage, reduce the likelihood of positive margins, eliminate micrometastases, and ultimately increase patient survival.

Laboratory experiments using the Shionogi tumor model support this rationale.[73] Pathologically positive surgical margins were detected in 66% of mice undergoing wide tumor excision (group 1) and in 33% of mice treated with neoadjuvant castration 10 days before wide excision of progressed tumor (group 2). Subsequent androgen-independent tumor recurrences were seen in 92% of group 1 and in 44% of group 2. There were statistically significant differences in overall tumor-free survival rates (group 1: 20% *vs.* group 2: 56%, $p < 0.05$).

Several prospective randomized trials have been performed to investigate the significance of neoadjuvant androgen deprivation for 3 months before radical prostatectomy.[74-77] Most studies demonstrated a significant reduction in prostate volume and margin-positive rates in the patient groups with neoadjuvant androgen deprivation. Unfortunately, these studies failed to show a significant improvement in seminal vesicle invasion, lymph node involvement, or PSA recurrence. None showed an advantage of neoadjuvant treatment in overall survival. Possible reasons for this discrepancy include an insufficient duration of neoadjuvant hormonal therapy. Gleave *et al.*[78] observed 547 patients who were randomized to receive neoadjuvant CAB for 3 or 8 months prior to radical prostatectomy. Positive margin rates were significantly lower in the 8-month than 3-month group (12% *vs.* 23%, p = 0.0106), and the authors concluded that the optimal duration of neoadjuvant androgen deprivation is longer than 3 months. However, rates of local or biochemical recurrence and long-term survival were not reported in this study. In addition, an 8-month delay of surgery might carry a high risk for patients with androgen-independent tumor. Neoadjuvant hormonal therapy should therefore remain under investigation.

Adjuvant Hormonal Therapy

There are a few retrospective studies showing a significantly positive effect of adjuvant hormonal therapy following radical prostatectomy on disease-free survival.[79,80] In a large retrospective, non-randomized series from the Mayo Clinic, continuous hormonal therapy prolonged overall survival in patients with nodal metastases who underwent radical prosta-tectomy. However, in earlier analyses, the benefits of this treatment were seen only in men with DNA diploid cancers.[80] Zincke *et al.* also retro-spectively reviewed 707 patients with stage pT3b disease, including 157 patients who received adjuvant hormonal therapy, and found that adjuvant hormonal therapy significantly improved the mean 10-year survival rates.[81] The Eastern Cooperative Oncology Group (ECOG),[82] in a prospective randomized clinical trial, investigated the effect of adjuvant hormonal therapy in 98 patients with clinically localized PCa and lymph node metastases. Androgen deprivation (goserelin or surgical castration) was initiated within 12 weeks of radical prostatectomy and pelvic lymphadenectomy in the adjuvant group, whereas, in the observation group, androgen deprivation was delayed until disease progression (almost always initiated at diagnosis of metastases). After 7.1 years of median follow-up, immediate treatment was associated with significant advantages in overall (85% *vs.* 64%; p = 0.02) and cause-specific (93% *vs.* 68%; p = 0,001) survival rates. The ECOG study has been criti-cized because of its relatively small number of patients and lack of central pathological review to determine Gleason grades.[83] However, a recent reanalysis of Gleason grades by central pathology review reveals no significant changes in outcomes, including survival.[84] With mean follow-up of 10 years highly significant differences in overall (72% *vs.* 49%; p = 0.025) and cause-specific (87% *vs.* 57%; p = 0.001) survival rates were observed.[84] Adjuvant therapy with antiandrogen, such as flutamide[85] or bicalutamide,[70] has also been reported to reduce biochemical recurrence in a broad spectrum of post-prostatectomy patients. However, these studies are too premature to evaluate survival or other meaningful outcomes.

Hormonal Therapy with Radiation Therapy/ Brachytherapy/ Chemotherapy

Radiation Therapy

Zietman *et al.*[86] demonstrated that prior androgen deprivation enhanced the effect of radiation on eradicating androgen-sensitive Shionogi mouse mammary tumors. An additive effect of androgen deprivation and radiation on apoptosis was also observed in both Dunning rat prostate tumors and LNCaP human PCa cells.[87,88] Also a recent study using a xenograft model demonstrated a synergistic inhibitory effect of castration and radiotherapy.[89] LNCaP-bearing mice treated with castration prior to radiation had significantly decreased mean tumor volume and serum PSA levels, compared to those treated with castration or radiation alone, throughout the observation period up to 11 weeks after initiation of treatment. Interestingly, in an androgen-sensitive Dunning rat prostate tumor model, testosterone treatment after castration and radiotherapy failed to stimulate tumor growth, suggesting cancer cells lost their androgen sensitivity through irradiation.[90,91] Moreover, in this model, castration 14 days prior to radiation was found to be superior in suppressing tumor growth, compared to androgen deprivation alone, radiation alone, or androgen deprivation 3 days after radiation.[91]

Three prospective studies revealed statistically significant improvements in overall survival in favor of early hormonal therapy in the radiotherapy setting. The European Organization for Research and Treatment of Cancer Genitourinary Group conducted a randomized phase III trial comparing external irradiation alone with combined therapy, with concomitant plus adjuvant androgen deprivation plus radiation, in locally advanced PCa patients.[92] From 1987 to 1995, 415 patients with WHO grade 3, stage T1-2 cancers, or stage T3-4 tumors of any grade were randomized to (1) radiotherapy plus goserelin, starting on the first day of irradiation and continuing monthly for 3 years (CPA was also given during the first month to prevent flare phenomena), *vs.* (2) radiotherapy alone followed by the same hormonal therapy upon clinical progression. With median follow-up of 66 months, 5-year clinical disease-free survival was 74% in the early hormonal therapy group and 40% in the control group (p = 0.0001), and 5-year overall survival was 78% and 62%, respectively (p = 0.0002).[92] Five-year local disease control was particularly impressive (although biopsies were not done), with 98% in the combined treatment group *vs.* 74% in the control arm being clinically free of local recurrence.

The Radiation Therapy Oncology Group (RTOG) has conducted several large, prospective randomized trials to assess the potential benefit of early *vs.* late and of short-term *vs.* long-term hormonal therapy in PCa patients treated with radiotherapy. In the RTOG protocol 85-31, 977 patients with T1-2 N1 or T3 non-metastatic disease, including post-prostatectomy cases, were randomized to receive goserelin starting at the last week of radiotherapy, and continuing indefinitely, or radiotherapy with deferred androgen deprivation at relapse. While initial publication of results at a median follow-up of 4.5 years reported that immediate goserelin treatment significantly improved local and distant disease control as well as disease-free survival (all p < 0.0001), there was no difference in overall survival.[93] However, a recent update of data at a 7.3-year mean follow-up demonstrated significant improvement in overall survival with estimated 10-year survivals being 53% and 38% in the immediate and deferred treatment groups, respectively.[94]

A parallel trial (RTOG 86-10) was performed to evaluate the efficacy of short-term hormonal therapy in PCa patients receiving definitive radiation therapy.[95] A total of 456 patients with T2-4 tumors were randomized to receive CAB with goserelin and flutamide for 4 months (2 months before and 2 months during radiotherapy) with radiotherapy *vs.* radiotherapy alone, with salvage hormonal therapy with orchiectomy, LH-RH agonist, or antiandrogen to be initiated when clinically indicated for relapse or progression of disease. At median follow-up of 6.7 years, early hormonal therapy was associated with a significant improvement in local and distant disease control and disease-free survival. Fewer patients in the combination arm (45%) received salvage hormonal therapy than those in the control arm (63%) (p < 0.001). However, no significant differences between the two arms were apparent for either overall survival at 5 years (71% *vs.* 69%) or at 8 years (53% *vs.* 43%).

Horwitz *et al.*[96] compared the above two studies and concluded that statistically significant improvements in biochemical disease-free status, distant metastases failure, and cause-specific failure rates were observed for adjuvant long-term hormonal therapy compared with short-term adjuvant hormonal therapy or radiotherapy alone in patients with locally advanced non-metastatic PCa.

Hanks *et al.*[97] reported the results of another randomized RTOG study (protocol 92-02) comparing short-term and long-term hormonal therapy involving 1554 men with T2c-4 disease and a PSA <150 ng/ml who received goserelin and flutamide 2 months before and 2 months during radiotherapy plus either no further therapy or 24 months of additional goserelin alone. With median follow-up of 4.8 years, long-term androgen deprivation led to significantly improved local (p = 0.0001) and distant (p = 0.001) disease control and a trend in longer disease-free survival (92% *vs.* 87%, p = 0.07). However, there was no significant difference in 5-year overall survival between the two arms (78% *vs.* 79%). A subset analysis comparing the results from centrally reviewed Gleason scores 8–10 patients from the RTOG 85-31 also showed a statistically significant advantage in patients receiving long-term androgen deprivation in estimated 5-year overall survival (80% *vs.* 69%; p = 0.02) and disease-free survival (90% *vs.* 78%; p = 0.007) rates.

Brachytherapy

Brachytherapy is increasingly used in patients with localized, low- to intermediate-grade PCa. Neoadjuvant androgen deprivation therapy is commonly given to patients who have a large prostate, to downsize the prostate, making the brachytherapy procedure easier and more feasible. Indeed, it has been reported that prostate volume was reduced by up to 40% after 3 months of androgen deprivation therapy.[78] Thus, combining hormonal therapy with prostate brachytherapy may reduce brachytherapy-related morbidity and improve patient outcome. However, no additional benefits of adjuvant hormonal therapy over the prostate brachytherapy on survival were apparent.[98] Because no prospective, randomized studies have been published, the impact of hormonal therapy in conjunction with brachytherapy remains unclear.

Chemotherapy

Previous studies have established the role of chemotherapy in the palliation of symptoms in patients with PCa after failure of hormonal therapy,[99,100] although its clear survival benefit is not reported. Among a variety of drugs, mitoxantrone- and estramustine-based regimens have been extensively studied and shown to have a significant palliative benefit.[100] Estramustine has an estradiol moiety and has been used in PCa patients for several decades. Estramustine, as a single agent, decreases serum testosterone to castration levels, with significant cardiovascular toxicity. Combination regimens of chemotherapy with other hormonal therapies have also been investigated for locally advanced, presumably androgen-sensitive, PCa. In a study by Pettaway *et al.*,[101] 33 high-risk patients (either clinical stage T3 or Gleason score >7) were treated with ketoconazole, doxorubicin, vinblastine and estramustine plus a LH-RH agonist and an antiandrogen for 12 weeks before radical prostatectomy. Thirty-three percent of them were found to have prostate-confined disease at the time of surgery. In another multicenter study, 50 locally advanced patients were treated with paclitaxel, estramustine, and carboplatin plus a LH-RH agonist for 4–6 months. Of the 23 patients who underwent radical prostatectomy, 45% of them attained organ-confined disease.[100] There were no comparisons of combination regimen to hormonal therapy alone.

Several *in vitro* studies investigated combinations of chemotherapy and hormonal therapy. Kreis *et al.*[102] showed synergistic effects on growth inhibition of either androgen-sensitive LNCaP, androgen-insensitive DU145 and PC-3, or all cell lines, using combinations of estramustine plus flutamide or PSC833 (Sandoz) plus bicalutamide. Other studies demonstrated that androgen deprivation could trigger apoptosis of androgen-sensitive cancer cells via a transient increase in cytosolic calcium, resulting in activation of Ca^{2+}- and Mg^{2+}-dependent endonucleases.[103,104]

Therefore, chemotherapy may become more effective when combined with androgen deprivation. In contrast, androgen deprivation was also shown to promote androgen-dependent cells to enter the G0 phase of the cell cycle instead of undergoing apoptosis.[105] Therefore, these cells might be more difficult to eradicate with subsequent chemotherapy.

Intermittent Androgen Deprivation

Intermittent androgen blockade (IAB) aims at delaying the onset of androgen-independent growth of PCa, as well as reducing side effects and costs. Laboratory studies have supported the hypothesis that IAB prolongs the initial androgen-sensitive period. Langeler *et al.*[106] showed that intermittent androgen suppression could delay the emergence of androgen-independent clones induced in LNCaP after long-term culture with androgen deprivation. Akakura *et al.*[107] and Sato *et al.*[108] studied IAB in castrated animals bearing androgen-dependent tumors treated with intermittent exposure to androgens. The results suggest that IAB induces multiple apoptotic regressions of androgen-dependent PCa and prolongs the time to androgen-independent progression, compared to continuous androgen deprivation.

The first attempt at IAB was reported in 1986.[109] Twenty patients with advanced PCa were treated with intermittent hormonal therapy (DES in 19 cases and flutamide in one case) until subjective improvement was noted, with a mean initial treatment duration of 10 months (range 2–70 months). The therapy was then stopped, and re-started when tumors relapsed, with a mean interval time of 8 months (range 1–24 months). All relapsed patients responded to re-administration of the drug. Patients had better QOL during the break in the treatment and DES-induced erectile dysfunction was reversed in 9 of 10 patients within 3 months of treatment interruption.

The availability of agents that induce reversible medical castration, such as LH-RH agonists, and serial serum PSA measurements after the mid-1980s, made it easier to introduce IAB and to monitor disease activity. Several clinical studies of IAB have been reported.[110–113] These intermittent hormonal therapies consist of an initial androgen deprivation period using a LH-RH agonist with or without a non-steroidal antiandrogen of usually between 6 and 9 months, followed by an off-therapy interval

(6–15 months). When PSA values meet threshold criteria (>5–10 ng/ml), treatment is resumed. Most of the initial responders (57%–100%) respond to re-treatment. This cyclic treatment continues until the patient develops androgen-independent tumors. While off-treatment, many patients had improvement in libido, erection, and energy, as well as fewer hot flashes. However, retrospective comparison of survival in these patients was similar to those who were treated with continuous androgen blockade. Interestingly, in certain patients, especially in those who received androgen deprivation for longer periods, gonadal function and serum testosterone levels did not recover.[114] These findings suggest that intermittent administration of LH-RH agonists may achieve continuous androgen deprivation, resulting in reduction of cost. A recent study also showed that the median duration of castration levels of serum testosterone was 5.5 months (range 3.5–10 months) after a single injection of long-acting (3-month) depot LH-RH agonist and that the method of re-dosing LH-RH agonists based on serum testosterone levels appeared efficacious, safe, and cost-effective.[115]

The debate continues as to whether IAB improves survival. Large, randomized, phase III clinical trials, comparing intermittent *vs.* continuous androgen deprivation are currently ongoing to assess endpoints including survival, time to androgen-independent progression, and QOL. Furthermore, intermittent triple androgen blockade (TrAB), another form of IAB using a 5α-reductase inhibitor, finasteride, during off-treatment periods, is also being evaluated.[116]

5α-Reductase Inhibitors

Two 5α-reductase enzymes have been identified: type 1, the predominant enzyme in extraprostatic tissues, such as skin and liver; and type 2, predominantly expressed in the prostate.[6] The type 2 5α-reductase has been implicated in, at least partially, the regulation of early prostate growth as well as later hyperplastic growth. Therefore, finasteride, the first 5α-reductase inhibitor specific for the type 2 enzyme, which significantly decreases levels of both serum and intraprostatic DHT by 70%–80%, reduces the total size of the prostate gland.[117] Thus, finasteride treatment has been a useful form of androgen deprivation for benign prostatic hyperplasia (BPH), with fewer adverse effects than antiandrogen treatment. However, the therapeutic activity of finasteride itself on PCa has not been identified. The effect of finasteride in conjunction with other forms of hormonal therapy has been investigated. In addition to TrAB,[116] sequential androgen blockade (SAB), a combination therapy with finasteride plus an antiandrogen or an LH-RH agonist, has been evaluated and has been shown to substantially decrease the PSA levels in men with metastatic PCa while maintaining sexual potency in most patients.[118,119] However, phase III studies, comparing SAB with traditional hormonal therapy, such as CAB, have not been conducted and the survival benefit thus remains unknown.

The benzoquinoline, LY320236, is a newer and dual (type 1/2) 5α-reductase inhibitor currently in phase I trials of PCa.[120] The antitumor activity of benzoquinoline has been demonstrated in human PCa xenograft models.

Concluding Remarks

Many options involving the AR, androgens, and their antagonists are available for the treatment of PCa (Fig. 1). Numerous clinical studies have shown equivalent effects on therapeutic benefits by different hormonal treatment strategies. Each treatment strategy/hormonal agent has favorable and unfavorable effects (Table 1). Patients with advanced PCa will clearly benefit from androgen deprivation-based treatments for symptom palliation and improvement of their QOL. However, whether these therapies prolong survival when administered before there are symptoms caused by disease progression remains controversial. Thus, despite a number of previous clinical and experimental studies, finding suitable patients, timing of, and options for hormonal therapy remain problematic.[121] Data from recent studies support the premise that an earlier treatment in patients' disease course likely leads to better outcomes,[82,84,92] but it is not easy to predict the best timing of hormonal therapy for patients with asymptomatic advanced disease. Observation may still be a reasonable choice for these patients.

Currently, available options for hormonal therapy almost never lead to cures in patients with advanced PCa because these patients eventually develop androgen-independent tumors. In addition, another type of failure of hormonal therapy, antiandrogen withdrawal syndrome, has been observed in a significant number (15%–80%) of patients treated with CAB. Although the exact mechanisms for androgen-independent PCa and antiandrogen withdrawal syndrome are far from being fully understood, possible mechanisms were discussed in recent review papers.[122,123] To improve overall survival of patients with advanced PCa, novel treatment strategies that prolong the androgen-dependent state, but will not induce antiandrogen withdrawal syndrome, and that are effective against androgen-independent disease, need to be identified. Furthermore, it may be necessary to explore more individualized approaches, such as selectively blocking the activated AR pathway in cancer cells. Finally, second-line hormonal therapy and PCa chemoprevention using hormonal therapy are other interesting topics that are not discussed in this chapter (please refer to Chapter 6 in this volume).

References

1. Huggins C, Hodges CV (1941) Studies on prostatic cancer. I. The effects of castration, of estrogen and of androgen injection on serum phosphatases in metastatic carcinoma of the prostate. *Cancer Res* 1:293–297.
2. Jemal A, Murray T, Samuels A, Ghafoor A, Ward E, Thun M (2003) Cancer statistics, 2003. *CA Cancer J Clin* 53:5–26.
3. Chang C, Kokontis J, Liao S (1988) Molecular cloning of human and rat complementary DNA encoding androgen receptors. *Science* 240:324–326.
4. Chang C, Saltzman A, Yeh S, Young W, Keller E, Lee H-J, Wang C, Mizokami A (1995) Androgen receptor: An overview. *Crit Rev Eukaryot Gene Expr* 5:97–125.
5. Heinlein CA, Chang C (2002) Androgen receptor (AR) coregulators: An overview. *Endocr Rev* 23:175–200.
6. Russell DW, Wilson JD (1994) Steroid 5α-reductase: Two genes/two enzymes. *Annu Rev Biochem* 63:25–61.
7. Geller J (1985) Rationale for blockade of adrenal as well as testicular androgens in the treatment of advanced prostate cancer. *Semin Oncol* 12(Suppl 1):28–35.
8. Culig Z, Hobisch A, Cronauer MV, Cato ACB, Hittmair A, Radmayr C, Eberle J, Bartsch G, Klocker H (1993) Mutant androgen receptor detected in an advanced-stage prostatic carcinoma is activated by adrenal androgens and progesterone. *Mol Endocrinol* 7:1541–1550.

9. Miyamoto H, Yeh S, Lardy H, Messing E, Chang C (1998) Δ^5-androstenediol is a natural hormone with androgenic activity in human prostate cancer cells. *Proc Natl Acad Sci USA* 95:11083–11088.

10. Miyamoto H, Chang C (2000) Antiandrogens fail to block androstenedione-mediated mutated androgen receptor transactivation in human prostate cancer cells. *Int J Urol* 7:32–34.

11. Maatman TJ, Gupta MK, Montie JE (1985) Effectiveness of castration versus intravenous estrogen therapy in producing rapid endocrine control of metastatic cancer of the prostate. *J Urol* 133:620–621.

12. Byar DP (1973) The Veterans Administration Cooperative Urological Research Group's studies of cancer of the prostate. *Cancer* 32:1126–1130.

13. Byar DP, Corle DK (1988) Hormone therapy for prostate cancer: Results of the Veterans Administration Cooperative Urological Research Group studies. *J Natl Cancer Inst Monogr (NCI Monogr)* 7:165–170.

14. Chadwick DJ, Gillatt DA, Gingell JC (1991) Medical or surgical orchiectomy: the patients' choice. *BMJ* 302:572.

15. Fosså SD, Aass N, Opjordsmoen S (1994) Assessment of quality of life in patients with prostate cancer. *Semin Oncol* 21:657–661.

16. Clark JA, Wray NP, Ashton CM (2001) Living with treatment decisions: Regrets and quality of life among men treated for metastatic prostate cancer. *J Clin Oncol* 19:72–80.

17. The Leuprolide Study Group (1984) Leuprolide versus diethylstilbestrol for metastatic prostate cancer. *N Engl J Med* 311:1281–1286.

18. deVoogt HJ, Smith PH, Pavone-Macaluso M, de Pauw M, Suciu S, and members of the European Organization for Research on Treatment of Cancer Urological Group (1986) Cardiovascular side effects of diethylstilbestrol, cyproterone acetate, medroxyprogesterone acetate and estramustine phosphate used for the treatment of advanced prostate cancer: Results from European Organization for Research on Treatment of Cancer Trials 30761 and 30762. *J Urol* 135:303–307.

19. Emtage LA, Trethowan C, Kelly K, Arkell D, Wallace DM, Hughes M, Hay A, Blacklock R, Jones M, Rouse A, Farrar D, Young C, Blackledge G (1989) A phase III open randomized study of Zoladex 3.6 mg depot *vs.* DES 3 mg per day in untreated advanced prostate cancer: A West Midlands Urological Research Group Study. *Prog Clin Biol Res* 303:47–52.

20. Citrin DL, Resnick MI, Guiman P, Al-Bussam N, Scott M, Gau TL, Kennealey GT (1991) A comparison of Zoladex® and DES in the treatment of advanced prostate cancer: Results of randomized, multicenter trial. *Prostate* 18:139–146.

21. Chang A, Yeap B, Davis T, Blum R, Hahn R, Khanna O, Fisher H, Rosenthal J, White R, Schinella R, Trump D (1996) Double-blind, randomized study of primary hormonal treatment of stage D2 prostate carcinoma: Flutamide versus diethylstilbestrol. *J Clin Oncol* 14:2250–2257.

22. Robinson MR, Smith P, Richards B, Newling DW, de Pauw M, Sylvester R (1995) The final analysis of the EORTC genito-urinary tract cancer cooperative group phase III clinical trial (protocol 30805) comparing orchiectomy, orchiectomy plus cyproterone acetate and low dose stilboestrol in the management of metastatic carcinoma of the prostate. *Eur Urol* 28:273–283.

23. Orlando M, Chacon M, Salum G, Chacon DR (2000) Low-dose continuous oral fosfestrol is highly active in 'hormone-refractory' prostate cancer. *Ann Oncol* 11:177–181.

24. Malkowicz SB (2001) The role of diethylstilbestrol in the treatment of prostate cancer. *Urology* 58(Suppl 2A):108–113.

25. Kitahara S, Yoshida K, Ishizaka K, Kageyama Y, Kawakami S, Tsuji T, Oshima H (1997) Stronger suppression of serum testosterone and FSH levels by a synthetic estrogen than by castration or an LH-RH agonist. *Endocr J* 44:527–532.

26. Kitahara S, Umeda H, Yano M, Koga F, Sumi S, Moriguchi H, Hosoya Y, Honda M, Yoshida K (1999) Effects of intravenous administration of high dose-diethylstilbestrol diphosphate on serum hormonal levels in patients with hormone-refractory prostate cancer. *Endocr J* 46:659–664.

27. Mangan FR, Neal GE, Williams DC (1967) The effects of diethylstilboestrol and castration on the nucleic acid and protein metabolism of rat prostate gland. *Biochem J* 104:1075–1081.

28. Ferro MA, Heinemann D, Smith PJB, Symes MO (1988) Effect of stilboestrol and testosterone on the incorporation of ^{75}selenomethionine by prostatic carcinoma cells. *Br J Urol* 62:166–172.

29. Robertson CN, Roberson KM, Padilla GM, O'Brien ET, Cook JM, Kim L-S, Fine RC (1996) Induction of apoptosis by diethylstilbestrol in hormone-insensitive prostate cancer cells. *J Natl Cancer Inst* 88:908–917.

30. Castle EP, Thrasher JB (2002) The role of soy phytoestrogens in prostate cancer. *Urol Clin North Am* 29:71–81.

31. Lau KM, LaSpina M, Long J, Ho SM (2000) Expression of estrogen receptor (ER)-α and ER-β in normal and malignant prostatic epithelial cells: Regulation by methylation and involvement in growth regulation. *Cancer Res* 60:3175–3182.

32. Latil A, Bièche I, Vidaud D, Lidereau R, Berthon P, Cussenot O, Vidaud M (2001) Evaluation of androgen, estrogen (ERα and ERβ), and progesterone

receptor expression in human prostate cancer by real-time quantitative reverse transcription-polymerase chain reaction assays. *Cancer Res* 61:1919–1926.

33. Signoretti S, Loda M (2001) Estrogen receptor β in prostate cancer: Brake pedal or accelerator? *Am J Pathol* 159:13–16.

34. Yeh S, Miyamoto H, Shima H, Chang C (1998) From estrogen to androgen receptor: A new pathway for sex hormones in prostate. *Proc Natl Acad Sci USA* 95:5527–5532.

35. Labrie F, Belanger A, Susan L, Labrie C, Simard J, Luu-The V, Diamond P, Gomez J-L, Candas B (1996) Histroy of LHRH agonist and combination therapy in prostate cancer. *Endocr-Rel Cancer* 3:243–278.

36. Dondi D, Limonta P, Moretti RM, Marelli MM, Garattini E, Motta M (1994) Antiproliferative effects of luteinizing hormone-releasing hormone (LHRH) agonists on human androgen-independent prostate cancer cell line DU 145: Evidence for an autocrine-inhibitory LHRH loop. *Cancer Res* 54:4091–4095.

37. Koppán M, Nagy A, Schally AV, Plonowski A, Halmos G, Arencibia JM, Groot K (1999) Targeted cytotoxic analog of luteinizing hormone-releasing hormone AN-207 inhibits the growth of PC-82 human prostate cancer in nude mice. *Prostate* 38:151–158.

38. Denis L (1998) European Organization for Research and Treatment of Cancer (EORTC) prostate cancer trials, 1976–1996. *Urology* 51(Suppl 5A): 50–57.

39. Seidenfeld J, Samson DJ, Hasselblad V, Aronson N, Albertsen PC, Bennett CL, Wilt TJ (2000) Single-therapy androgen suppression in men with advanced prostate cancer: A systematic review and meta-analysis. *Ann Intern Med* 132:566–577.

40. Tunn UW, Bargelloni U, Cosciani S, fiaccavento G, Guazzieri S, Pagano F (1998) Comparison of LH-RH analogue 1-month depot and 3-month depot by their hormone levels and pharmacokinetic profile in patients with advance prostate cancer. *Urol Int* 60(Suppl 1):9–16.

41. Stege R (2000) Potential side effects of endocrine treatment of long duration in prostate cancer. *Prostate Suppl* 10(Suppl):38–42.

42. Bubley GJ (2001) Is the flare phenomenon clinically significant? *Urology* 58(Suppl 2A):5–9.

43. Labrie F, Dupont A, Belanger A, Lachance R (1987) Flutamide eliminates the risk of disease flare in prostatic cancer patients treated with a luteinizing hormone-releasing hormone agonist. *J Urol* 138:804–806.

44. Cook T, Sheridan WP (2000) Development of GnRH antagonists for prostate cancer: New approaches to treatment. *Oncologist* 5:162–168.
45. Stricker HJ (2001) Luteinizing hormone-releasing hormone antagonists in prostate cancer. *Urology* 58(Suppl 2A):24–27.
46. McLeod D, Zinner N, Tomera K, Gleason D, Fotheringham N, Campion M, Garnick MB for the Abarelix Study Group (2001) A phase 3, multicenter, open-label, randomized study of abarelix versus leuprolide acetate in men with prostate cancer. *Urology* 58:756–761.
47. Tomera K, Gleason D, Gittelman M, Moseley W, Zinner N, Murdoch M, Menon M, Campion M, Garnick MB for the Abarelix Study Group (2001) The Gonadotropin-releasing hormone antagonist abarelix depot versus luteinizing hormone releasing hormone agonists leuprolide or goserelin: Initial results of endocrinological and biochemical efficacies in patients with prostate cancer. *J Urol* 165:1585–1589.
48. Trachtenberg J, Gittleman M, Steidle C, Barzell W, Friedel W, Pessis D, Fotheringham N, Campion M, Garnick MB and Abarelix Study Group (2002) A phase 3, multicenter, open-label, randomized study of abarelix versus leuprolide plus daily antiandrogen in men with prostate cancer. *J Urol* 167:1670–1674.
49. Labrie F, Dupont A, Giguere M, Borsanyi J-P, Lacouraere Y, Montette G, Emond J, Bergeron N (1998) Benefits of combination therapy with flutamide in patients relapsing after castration. *Br J Urol* 61:341–346.
50. Sandow J, von Rechenberg W, Engelbart K (1988) Pharmacological studies on androgen suppression in therapy of prostate carcinoma. *Am J Clin Oncol* 11(Suppl 1):S6–S10.
51. Prostate Cancer Trialists' Collaborative Group (2000) Maximum androgen blockade in advanced prostate cancer: An overview of the randomised trials. *Lancet* 355:1491–1498.
52. Boccardo F (2000) Hormone therapy of prostate cancer: Is there a role for antiandrogen monotherapy? *Crit Rev Oncol Hematol* 35:121–132.
53. Crawford ED, Eisenberger MA, McLeod DG, Spaulding JT, Benson R, Dorr A, Blumenstein BA, Davis MA, Goodman PJ. (1989) A controlled trial of leuprolide with and without flutamide in prostatic carcinoma. *N Engl J Med* 321:419–424.
54. Boccardo F, Pace M, Rubagotti A, Guarneri D, Decensi A, Oneto F, Martorana G, Giuliani L, Selvaggi F, Battaglia M, Ponti UD, Petracco S, Cortellini P, Ziveri M, Ferraris U, Bruttini GP, Epis R, Comeri G, Gallo G, and other participants in the Italian Prostatic Cancer Project (PONCAP)

Study Group (1993) Goserelin acetate with or without flutamide in the treatment of patients with locally advanced or metastatic prostate cancer. *Eur J Cancer* 29:1088–1093.

55. Denis LJ, Whelan P, de Moura JCL, Newling D, Bono A, De Pauw M, Sylvester R (1993) Goserelin acetate and flutamide versus bilateral orchiectomy: A phase III EORTC trial (30853). *Urology* 42:119–132.

56. Janknegt RA, Abbou CC, Bartoletti R, Bernstein-Hahn L, Bracken B, Brisset JM, Da Silva FC, Chisholm G, Crawford ED, Debruyne FMJ, Dijkman GD, Frick J, Goedhals L, Knönagel H, Venner PM (1993) Orchiectomy and nilutamide or placebo as treatment of metastatic prostatic cancer in a multinational double-blind randomized trial. *J Urol* 149:77–83.

57. Eisenberger MA, Blumenstein BA, Crawford ED, Miller G, McLeod DG, Loehrer PJ, Wilding G, Sears K, Culkin DJ, Thompson Jr IM, Lowe BA (1998) Bilateral orchiectomy with or without flutamide for metastatic prostate cancer. *N Engl J Med* 339:1036–1042.

58. Schmitt B, Wilt TJ, Schellhammer PF, De Masi V, Sartor O, Crawford ED, Bennett CL (2001) Combined androgen blockade with nonsteroidal antiandrogens for advanced prostate cancer: A systematic review. *Urology* 57:727–732.

59. Iversen P (2002) Antiandrogen monotherapy: Indications and results. *Urology* 60(Suppl 3A):64–71.

60. Delaere KPJ, Van Thillo EL (1991) Flutamide monotherapy as primary treatment in advanced prostatic carcinoma. *Semin Oncol* 18(Suppl 6):13–18.

61. Decensi AU, Boccardo F, Guarneri D, Positano N, Parletti MC, Costantini M, Martorano G, Giuliani L for the Italian Prostatic Cancer Project (1991) Monotherapy with nilutamide, a pure nonsteroidal antiandrogen, in untreated patients with metastatic carcinoma of the prostate. *J Urol* 146:377–381.

62. Dole EJ, Holdsworth MT (1997) Nilutamide: An antiandrogen for the treatment of prostate cancer. *Ann Pharmacother* 31:65–75.

63. Bales GT, Chodak GW (1996) A controlled trial of bicalutamide versus castration in patients with advanced prostate cancer. *Urology* 47(Suppl 1A): 38–43.

64. Tyrrell CJ, Kaisary AV, Iversen P, Anderson JB, Baert L, Tammela T, Chamberlain M, Webster A, Blackledge G (1998) A randomized comparison of 'Casodex'™ (bicalutamide) 150 mg monotherapy versus castration in the treatment of metastatic and locally advanced prostate cancer. *Eur Urol* 33:447–456.

65. Iversen P, Tyrrell CJ, Kaisary AV, Anderson JB, Van Poppel H, Tammela TLJ, Chamberlain M, Carroll K, Melezinek I (2000) Bicalutamide monotherapy

compared with castration in patients with nonmetastatic locally advanced prostate cancer: 6.3 years of followup. *J Urol* 164:1579–1582.

66. Chatelain C, Rousseau V, Cosaert J (1994) French multicentre trial comparing Casodex (ICI 176,334) monotherapy with castration plus nilutamide in metastatic prostate cancer: A preliminary report. *Eur Urol* 26(Suppl):10–14.

67. Boccardo F, Rubagotti A, Barichello M, Battaglia M, Carmignani G, Comeri G, Crucinni G, Dannino S, Delliponti U, Ditonno P, Ferraris V, Lilliu S, Montetiore F, Portoghese F, Spano G for the Italian Prostate Cancer Project (1999) Bicalutamide monotherapy versus flutamide plus goserelin in prostate cancer patients: Results of an Italian Prostate Cancer Project study. *J Clin Oncol* 17:2027–2038.

68. Katchen B, Buxbaum S (1975) Disposition of a new, nonsteroidal, antiandrogen, α,α,α-trifluoro-2-methy-4′-nitro-m-propionotoluidide (flutamide), in men following a single oral 200 mg dose. *J Clin Endocrinol Metab* 41:373–379.

69. McKillop D, Boyle GW, Cockshott ID, Jones DC, Phillips PJ, Yates RA (1993) Metabolism and enantioselective pharmacokinetics of Casodex in man. *Xenobiotica* 23:1241–1253.

70. See WA, Wirth MP, McLeod DG, Iversen P, Klimberg I, Gleason D, Chodak G, Montie J, Tyrrell C, Wallace DMA, Delaere KPJ, Vaage S, Tammela TLJ, Lukkarinen O, Persson BE, Carroll K, Kolvenbag GJCM (2002) Bicalutamide as immediate therapy either alone or as adjuvant to standard care of patients with localized or locally advanced prostate cancer: First analysis of the early prostate cancer program. *J Urol* 168:429–435.

71. Goldenberg SL, Bruchovsky N (1991) Use of cyproterone acetate in prostate cancer. *Urol Clin North Am* 18:111–122.

72. de Voogt HJ (1992) The position of cyproterone acetate (CPA), a steroidal anti-androgen, in the treatment of prostate cancer. *Prostate* 4(Suppl):91–95.

73. Gleave ME, Sato N, Goldenberg SL, Stothers L, Bruchovsky N, Sullivan LD (1997) Neoadjuvant androgen withdrawal therapy decreases local recurrence rates following tumor excision in the Shionogi tumor model. *J Urol* 157:1727–1730.

74. Aus G, Abrahamsson P-A, Ahlgren G, Hugosson J, Lundberg S, Schain M, Schelin S, Pedersen K (2002) Three-month neoadjuvant hormonal therapy before radical prostatectomy: A 7-year follow-up of a randomized controlled trial. *BJU Int* 90:561–566.

75. Hurtado-Coll A, Goldenberg SL, Klotz L, Gleave ME (2002) Preoperative neoadjuvant androgen withdrawal therapy in prostate cancer: The Canadian experience. *Urology* 60(Suppl 3A):45–51.

76. Soloway MS, Pareek K, Sharifi R, Wajsman I, McLeod D, Wood Jr DP, Puras-Baez A and the Lupron Depot Neoadjuvant Prostate Cancer Study Group (2002) Neoadjuvant androgen ablation before radical prostatectomy in $cT2bNxM_0$ prostate cancer: 5-year results. *J Urol* 167:112–116.

77. Klotz LH, Goldenberg SL, Jewett MAS, Fradet Y, Nam R, Barkin J, Chin J, Chatterjee S and the Canadian Uro-oncology Group (2003) Long-term followup of a randomized trial of 0 versus 3 months of neoadjuvant androgen ablation before radical prostatectomy. *J Urol* 170:791–794.

78. Gleave ME, Goldenberg L, Chin JL, Warner J, Saad F, Klotz LH, Jewett M, Kassabian V, Chetner M, Dupont C, Van Rensselaer S and the Canadian Uro-oncology Group (2001) Randomized comparative study of 3 versus 8-month neoadjuvant hormonal therapy before radical prostatectomy: Biochemical and pathological effects. *J Urol* 166:500–507.

79. DeKernion JB, Neuwirth H, Stein A, Dorey F, Stenzl A, Hannah J, Blyth B (1990) Prognosis of patients with stage D1 prostate carcinoma following radical prostatectomy with and without early endocrine therapy. *J Urol* 144:700–703.

80. Zincke H, Bergstralh E, Larson-Keller JJ, Farrow GM, Myers RP, Lieber MM, Barrett DM, Rife CC, Gonochoroff NJ (1992) Stage D1 prostate cancer treated by radical prostatectomy and adjuvant hormonal treatment: evidence for favorable survival in patients with DNA diploid tumors. *Cancer* 70(Suppl 1):311–323.

81. Zincke H, Lau W, Bergstralh E, Blute ML (2001) Role of early adjuvant hormonal therapy after radical prostatectomy for prostate cancer. *J Urol* 166:2208–2215.

82. Messing EM, Manola J, Sarosdy M, Wilding G, Crawford ED, Trump D (1999) Immediate hormonal therapy compared with observation after radical prostatectomy and pelvic lymphadenectomy in men with node-positive prostate cancer. *N Engl J Med* 341:1781–1788.

83. Walsh PC, DeWeese TL, Eisenberger MA (2001) A structures debate: Immediate versus deferred androgen suppression in prostate cancer: evidence for deferred treatment. *J Urol* 166:508–516.

84. Messing EM, Manola J, Yao J, Kiernan M, Crawford ED, Wilding G, di'SantAgnese PA (2004) Immediate *vs.* delayed hormonal therapy in patients with nodal positive prostate cancer who had undergone radical prostatectomy + pelvic lymphadenectomy: Results of central pathology review (Abstract). *J Urol* 171(Suppl 4):383.

85. Wirth M, Frohmüller H, Marx F, Bolten M, Theiß M (1997) Randomized multicenter trials on adjuvant flutamide therapy in locally advanced prostate

cancer after radical surgery — Interim analysis of treatment effect and prognostic factors (Abstract). *Br J Urol* 80:263.

86. Zietman AL, Nakfoor BM, Prince EA, Gerweck LE (1997) The effect of androgen deprivation and radiation therapy on an androgen-sensitive murine tumor: An *in vitro* and *in vivo* study. *Cancer J Sci Am* 3:31–36.

87. Joon DL, Hasegawa M, Sikes C, Khoo VS, Terry NH, Zagars GK, Meistrich ML, Pollack A (1997) Supraadditive apoptotic response of R3327-G rat prostate tumors to androgen ablation and radiation. *Int J Radiat Oncol Biol Phys* 38:1071–1077.

88. Pollack A, Salem N, Ashoori F, Hachem P, Sangha M, von Eschenbach AC, Meistrich ML (2001) Lack of prostate cancer radiosensitization by androgen deprivation. *Int J Radiat Oncol Biol Phys* 51:1002–1007.

89. Hara I, Miyake H, Yamada Y, Takechi Y, Hara S, Gotoh A, Fujisawa M, Okada H, Arakawa S, Soejima T, Sugimura K, Kamidono S (2002) Neoadjuvant androgen withdrawal prior to external radiotherapy for locally advanced adenocarcinoma of the prostate. *Int J Urol* 9:322–328.

90. Granfors T, Tomic R, Bergh A, Rydh M, Lofroth PO, Widmark A (1999) After radiation testosterone stimulation is unable to increase growth in the dunning R3327-PAP prostate tumor. *Urol Res* 27:357–361.

91. Kaminski JM, Hanlon A, Joon DL, Meistrich M, Pollack A (2002) The effect of sequencing of androgen ablation and radiation on prostate cancer growth (Abstract). *Int J Radiat Oncol Biol Phys* 54(Suppl):190–191.

92. Bolla M, Collette L, Blank L, Warde P, Dubois JB, Mirimanoff R-O, Storme G, Bernier I, Kuten A, Sternberg C, Mattelaer J, Torecilla JL, Pfeffer JR (2002) Long-term results with immediate androgen suppression and external irradiation in patients with locally advanced prostate cancer (an EORTC study): a phase III randomized trial. *Lancet* 360:103–108.

93. Pilepich MV, Caplan R, Byhardt RW, Lawton CA, Gallagher MJ, Mesic JB, Hanks GE, Coughlin CT, Porter A, Shipley WU, Grignon D (1997) Phase III trial of androgen suppression using goserelin in unfavorable-prognosis carcinoma of the prostate treated with definitive radiotherapy: Report of Radiation Therapy Oncology Group protocol 85-31. *J Clin Oncol* 15:1013–1021.

94. Pilepich MV, Winter K, Lawton C, Krisch RE, Wolkov H, Movsas B, Hug E, Asbell S, Grignon D (2003) Phase III trial of androgen suppression adjuvant to definitive radiotherapy. Long term results of RTOG study 85-31 (Abstract). *Am Soc Clin Oncol* 22:381A.

95. Shipley WU, Lu JD, Pilepich MV, Heydon K, Roach III M, Wolkov HB, Sause WT, Rubin P, Lawton CA, Machtay M (2002) Effect of a short course of neoadjuvant hormonal therapy on the response to subsequent androgen

suppression in prostate cancer patients with relapse after radiotherapy: A secondary analysis of the randomized protocol RTOG 86-10. *Int J Radiat Oncol Biol Phys* 54:1302–1310.

96. Horwitz EM, Winter K, Hanks GE, Lawton CA, Russell AH, Machtay M (2001) Subset analysis of RTOG 85-31 and 86-10 indicates an advantage for long-term *vs.* short-term adjuvant hormones for patients with locally advanced nonmetastatic prostate cancer treated with radiation therapy. *Int J Radiat Oncol Biol Phys* 49:947–956.

97. Hanks GE, Lu JD, Machtay M, Venkatesan VM, Pinover WH, Byhardt RW, Rosenthal SA (2000) RTOG protocol 92-02: A phase III trial of the use of long term total androgen suppression following neoadjuvant hormonal cytoreduction and radiotherapy in locally advanced carcinoma of the prostate (Abstract). *Int J Radiat Oncol Biol Phys* 48(Suppl):112.

98. Lee WR (2002) The role of androgen deprivation therapy combined with prostate brachytherapy. *Urology* 60(Suppl 3A):39–44.

99. Eisenberger MA, Simon R, O'Dwyer PJ, Wittes RE, Friedman MA (1985) A reevaluation of nonhormonal cytotoxic chemotherapy in the treatment of prostatic carcinoma. *J Clin Oncol* 3:827–841.

100. Gilligan T, Kantoff PW (2002) Chemotherapy for prostate cancer. *Urology* 60(Suppl 3A):94–100.

101. Pettaway CA, Pisters LL, Troncoso P, Slaton J, Finn L, Kamoi K, Logothetis CJ (1999) Neoadjuvant chemotherapy and hormonal therapy followed by radical prostatectomy: Feasibility and preliminary results. *J Clin Oncol* 18:1050–1057.

102. Kreis W, Budman DR, Calabro A (1997) Unique synergism or antagonism of combinations of chemotherapeutic and hormonal agents in human prostate cancer cell lines. *Br J Urol* 79:196–202.

103. Martikainen P, Isaacs J (1990) Role of calcium in the programmed death of rat prostatic glandular cells. *Prostate* 17:175–187.

104. Wang H-G, Pathan N, Ethell IM, Krajewski S, Yamaguchi Y, Shibazaki F, McKeon F, Babo T, Franke TF, Reed JC (1999) Ca^{2+}-induced apoptosis through calcineurin dephosphorylation of BAD. *Science* 284:339–343.

105. Hussain A, Dawson N, Amin P, Naslund M, Engstrom C, Chen T (2001) Docetaxel followed by hormone therapy after failure of definitive treatments for clinically localized/locally advanced prostate cancer: Preliminary results. *Semin Oncol* 28(Suppl 15):22–31.

106. Langeler EG, Connie JC, van Uffelen CJC, Blankenstein MA, van Steenbrugge GJ, Mulder E (1993) Effect of culture conditions on androgen sensitivity of the human prostatic cancer cell line LNCaP. *Prostate* 23:213–223.

107. Akakura K, Bruchovsky N, Goldernberg SL, Rennie PS, Buckley AR, Sullivan LD (1993) Effects of intermittent androgen suppression on andro-gen-dependent tumors. Apoptosis and serum prostate-specific antigen. *Cancer* 71:2782–2790.

108. Sato N, Gleave ME, Bruchovsky N, Rennie PS, Goldenberg SL, Lange PH, Sullivan LD (1996) Intermittent androgen suppression delays progression to androgen-independent regulation of prostate-specific antigen gene in the LNCaP prostate tumor model. *J Steroid Biochem Mol Biol* 58:139–146.

109. Klotz LH, Herr HW, Morse MJ, Whitmore Jr WF (1986) Intermittent endocrine therapy for advanced prostate cancer. *Cancer* 58:2546–2550.

110. Higano CS, Ellis W, Russel K, Lange PH (1996) Intermittent androgen sup-pression with leuprolide and flutamide for prostate cancer: A pilot study. *Urology* 48:800–804.

111. Crook JM, Szumacher E, Malone S, Huan S, Segal R (1999) Intermittent androgen suppression in the management of prostate cancer. *Urology* 53:530–534.

112. Egawa S, Takashima R, Matsumoto K, Mizoguchi H, Kuwano S, Baba S (2000) A pilot study of intermittent androgen ablation in advanced prostate cancer in Japanese men. *Jpn J Clin Oncol* 30:21–26.

113. Hurtado-Coll A, Goldenberg SL, Gleave ME, Klotz L (2002) Intermittent androgen suppression in prostate cancer: The Canadian experience. *Urology* 60(Suppl 3A):52–56.

114. Hall MC, Fritzsch RJ, Sagalowsky AI, Ahrens A, Petty B, Roehrborn CG (1999) Prospective determination of the hormonal response after cessation of lutenizing hormone-releasing hormone agonist treatment in patients with prostate cancer. *Urology* 53:898–903.

115. Oefelein MG (2003) Health related quality of life using serum testos-terone as the trigger to re-dose long acting depot luteinizing hormone-releasing hormone agonists in patients with prostate cancer. *J Urol* 169: 251–255.

116. Leibowitz RL, Tucker SJ (2001) Treatment of localized prostate cancer with intermittent triple androgen blockade: Preliminary results in 110 consecu-tive patients. *Oncologist* 6:177–182.

117. Boyle P, Gould AC, Roehrborn CG (1996) Prostate volume predicts outcome of treatment of benign prostatic hyperplasia with finasteride: meta-analysis of randomized clinical trials. *Urology* 48:398–405.

118. Ornstein DK, Smith DS, Andriole GL (1998) Biochemical response to tes-ticular androgen ablation among patients with prostate cancer for whom flu-tamide and/or finasteride therapy failed. *Urology* 52:1094–1097.

119. Kirby R, Robertson C, Turkes A, Griffiths K, Denis LJ, Boyle P, Altwein J, Schröder F (1999) Finasteride in association with either flutamide or goserelin as combination hormonal therapy in patients with stage M1 carcinoma of the prostate gland. International Prostate Health Council (IPHC) Trial Study Group. *Prostate* 40:105–114.

120. McNulty AM, Audia JE, Bemis KG, Goode RL, Rocco VP, Neubauer BL (2000) Kinetic analysis of LY320236: competitive inhibitor of type I and non-competitive inhibitor of type II human steroid 5α-reductase. *J Steroid Biochem Mol Biol* 72:13–21.

121. Miyamoto H, Messing EM (2004) Early versus late hormonal therapy for prostate cancer. *Curr Urol Rep* 5:188–196.

122. Miyamoto H, Messing EM, Chang C (2004) Androgen deprivation therapy for prostate cancer: Current status and future prospects. *Prostate*, in press.

123. Miyamoto H, Rahman MM, Chang C (2004) Molecular basis for the antiandrogen withdrawal syndrome. *J Cell Biochem* 91:3–12.

2

IMMUNOTHERAPIES FOR PROSTATE CANCER

Kelley M. Harsch, Jason E. Tasch and Warren D. W. Heston

The Cleveland Clinic Foundation, The Lerner Research Institute
Cleveland, Ohio 44195, USA

Introduction

Prostate cancer is the second leading cause of death in men, with approximately 220,000 new cases and an expected 28,000 deaths in the year 2003.[1] A decrease in prostate cancer related deaths has been attributed to early prostate-specific antigen (PSA) detection, more effective chemotherapy treatments, and immunotherapies. Although tumors can often evade an immune response by modulating their tumor antigens, reducing major histocompatibility complex-1 (MHC-I) expression or inhibiting cytotoxic T-cell activity, the use of immune modulation for prostate cancer is a relatively new concept because the prostate is not generally considered a site where immune processes typically occur. Since tumors arise when cancer cells evade the immune system, the prostate is an ideal target for immunotherapy.[2]

The four most common types of lesions associated with the prostate are acute/chronic prostatitis (bacterial/abacterial), proliferative inflammatory atrophy (PIA), benign prostatic hyperplasia (BPH), and prostate carcinoma.[3] The types of proliferative lesions that occur in the prostate are in different regions of the prostate. Most hyperplasias are prevalent in the transitional and periurethral zones, whereas carcinomas are found mostly in the peripheral zone.[4]

PIA, a newly recognized prostate lesion, is hypothesized to be a precursor to prostatic intraepithelial neoplasia (PIN) and to prostate cancer.

PIA lesions, which contain proliferating epithelial cells that fail to fully differentiate into columnar secretory cells, are typically present in the peripheral zone of the prostate, where prostate cancers arise, and are often directly juxtaposed to PIN and/or prostate cancers.[5–9] PIA may link inflammation with prostatic carcinogenesis.[6]

Inflammation

Virtually 100% of prostate specimens contain histological and immunological evidence of chronic inflammation.[10] Inflammation is a physiological response to a variety of stimuli such as infection, tissue injury, growth factors, or chemokines.[2,11] The distribution, location and histology of leukocytes determine the type of inflammation.[12] Persistent immune activation resulting in chronic inflammation often has pathological consequences. Acute/chronic inflammation is characterized by distinct cellular changes whereas precancerous lesions are associated with the change in the balance in the angiogenic and apoptotic cell cycle process.[11]

During the inflammation process, activated macrophages release various hydrolytic enzymes and reactive oxygen and nitrogen species that may contribute to tissue damage. Chemokines, plasma enzyme mediators (bradykinen, fibrinopeptidases), opsonins, leukotrienes, and prostaglandins are all mediators that have some role in the inflammatory process.[2] The normal prostate is populated by $\alpha\beta$ T-cells, B-cells and macrophages, with the T-cells being evenly distributed throughout the interstitium and between the epithelial cells.[13,14] There is some indication that the number of T-cells increases with age,[12] which correlates with the incidence of prostate inflammation during the aging process.

The proliferation and differentiation of prostate tissue are modulated by growth factors[15,16] as well as hormonal androgen therapy.[17,18] Evidence of hormonal impact on the prostate is seen in atrophy of the prostate following castration,[4] as well as treatment of BPH samples with a 5α-reductase inhibitor. When this inhibitor is given to patients, there is a regression of dihydrotestosterone (DHT) levels and a reduction in prostate volume.[19,20]

Recent data suggests that mutations in RNase L predispose men to an increased incidence of prostate cancer, which in some cases reflect more aggressive disease and/or decreased age of onset compared with non-RNase L linked cases. It is proposed that RNase L functions in counteracting prostate cancer by virtue of its ability to degrade RNA, thus initiating a cellular stress response that leads to apoptosis.[21] RNase L is a uniquely regulated endoribonuclease that requires 5'-triphosphorylated, 2',5'-linked oligoadenylates (2-5A) for its activity. The presence of both germline mutations in RNase L segregating with disease within HPC-affected families, and loss of heterozygosity (LOH) in tumor tissues suggest a novel role in the pathogenesis of prostate cancer. The association of mutations in RNase L with prostate cancer cases further suggests a relationship between innate immunity and tumor suppression.

Microbial activators may contribute to acute/chronic inflammatory processes, which could then lead to malignancy.[11] Differentiating between acute/chronic bacterial prostatitis and chronic abacterial prostatitis is done by quantification of bacterial cultures and microscopic examination of urine.[4] Depending on the severity and duration of the inflammation, acute bacterial prostatitis displays histological evidence of stromal leukocytic infiltration accompanied by increased elaboration of prostatic secretion or leukocytic infiltration within the glandular spaces.[4]

In contrast, bacterial/abacterial chronic prostatitis shows histological evidence of aggregation of numerous lymphocytes, plasma cells, macrophages, and neutrophils within the prostatic substance. Chemokines act as chemoattractants, which activate lymphocytes and other immune modulators into neighboring tissues via extravasation.[2] Since antibodies penetrate the prostate with poor efficiency, this type of inflammation is difficult to treat.[4] The normal aging process in the prostate results in aggregations of lymphocytes, which are prone to appear in the fibromuscular stroma of the gland. Frequently, this histology of the aging prostate is diagnosed as chronic prostatitis even though the macrophages and neutrophils are absent.[4]

Stromal-epithelial interactions are crucial for normal growth and homeostasis within the prostate.[22] These interactions are thought to influence the rate of development of BPH and prostate carcinoma.[22] BPH is characterized by diffuse infiltrates of activated T-lymphocytes in fibroblastic, fibromuscular, and stromal nodules.[14,23] Histological evidence of nodular hyperplasia or BPH is present in 20% of men 40 years of age, 70% by age 60, and 90% in men 70 years of age.[24] The usual BPH nodule weighs between 60–100 grams with some nodules weighing over 200 grams.[4] Studies indicate that BPH samples also display chronic mononuclear inflammation, which contain CD3[+] T-lymphocytes and express the T-cell receptor.[25] The epithelial cells associated with the inflammatory infiltrate were observed in the periglandular stroma[25] and were almost exclusively activated T-cells expressing CD45RO, and producing IL-2 and IFNγ.[3,24] Expression of IFN-γ, IL-2, and IL-4 mRNA in BPH suggests that the disease is associated with Th_1 and Th_2 response.[26]

The Immune System

The goal for cancer immunotherapy is to induce antibody and/or T-lymphocyte immune response targeted to the cancer cells. There are several branches of the immune system that can be targets for immunotherapy. They include antibody producing B-cells, CD8[+] cytotoxic T-cells, CD4[+] T-helper cells, natural killer (NK) cells, natural killer T (NKT)-cells, and monocytes. B-cells produce antibodies that kill antigen presenting cells via complement, antibody dependent cellular cytotoxicity (ADCC), or apoptosis.[27] Cell mediated response appears to play a major role in a tumor immune response. Many tumors induce a specific cytotoxic T-cell response that recognizes antigens presented by MHC-I, which can elicit a higher response.[2]

NKT-cells share several features with NK cells, such as CD161 and CD122 expression. These cells display intermediate levels of T-cell receptor (TCR) and are CD4[+] or CD4[-]/CD8[-]. NKT-cells produce IL-4, a pro-inflammatory cytokine, in response to engagement of the T-cell receptor.[28] In the presence of IL-18 and IL-12, NKT-cells will produce IFN-γ and kill target cells in a Fas ligand (FasL) dependent manner without engagement of the TCR.[29,30]

NK as well as NKT-cells recognize tumor cells through cell-cell contact and mediate killing with Fas/FasL or with the induction of cytokines or lytic enzymes.[27] NK cells recognize target cells based on expression of activating or inhibitory receptors. Since NK cells do not recognize target cells based on MHC expression, a decrease in MHC expression does not limit their activity. Also, some Fc receptors on NK cells can bind to antibody coated tumor cells leading to ADCC.[2]

Naïve T-cells require more than one signal for activation and subsequent proliferation into an effector cell. This activation is triggered by recognition of MHC-peptide complex and a co-stimulatory signal. Frequently, tumor cells give little or no co-stimulatory signals that can inhibit the activation of cytotoxic T-cells. The co-stimulatory signal occurs by interaction of B7 on antigen presenting cells and CD28 on the T-cells. CTLA-4 and CD28 are T-surface antigens, which bind to B7-1 or B7-2 ligands on antigen presenting cells to activate a T-cell response and control proliferation.[2] CD28 is expressed on resting and active cells while CTLA-4 is virtually undetectable on resting cells. Their ligands, B7-1 and B7-2, are two related forms of immunoglobulin superfamily members with similar extracellular domains but with different cytosolic domains. These ligands are constitutively expressed on dendritic cells and can be induced on macrophage and B-cells. Signaling through CD28 produces a positive co-stimulatory signal and increases CTLA-4 levels on the T-cells. Although CTLA-4 and CD28 are structurally similar, they act antagonistically. Surface levels of CTLA-4 are lower than CD28, but it competes favorably for B7 binding sites due to its high avidity.[2]

Targets of Immunotherapy

The complexity of the immune system presents many legitimate targets for the induction of an immune response. One aspect of the innate immune system present throughout the body, including the prostate epithelium and stroma, is the presence of toll-like receptors (TLR). TLRs are capable of recognizing foreign antigens and act as molecules with pattern recognition capabilities and may be soluble or cell-associated receptors. Pattern recognition receptors (PRR) are extracellular or present on cell membranes and target microbes or components in tissue fluids and blood. Typically, signals transduced through a TLR result in transcriptional activation, synthesis, and secretion of cytokines. This signaling process results in the activation of antigen presenting cells, all of which are involved in or promote inflammation.[2] For instance, TLR-5 mRNA is found in the prostate, testis, ovaries, and leukocytes. TLR-5 interacts with microbial lipoproteins leading to nuclear factor-kappa B (NF-κB) activation, cytokine secretion, and inflammation.[31,32] Other TLR activation induces secretion of cytokines, such as IFN-γ, MAPK pathways,[33] or acts as a target for CpG islands (found in bacterial DNA) or double stranded (ds)RNA.[11]

Cytokines

A second potential target for immunotherapy lies in the world of cytokines. Cytokines are low molecular weight regulatory proteins or glycoproteins that regulate the immune response, hematopoiesis, control of cellular proliferation and differentiation, and are involved in wound healing. Cytokines share many properties with hormones and growth factors in that they are secreted soluble factors that elicit biological effects. As cytokines are discovered, many can be grouped into families based on protein structural homology. Several examples of cytokine families are: interferons, tumor necrosis factors, and interleukins. These molecules are redundant and have overlapping functions. Once a cytokine encounters the appropriate receptor, it acts in an antigen non-specific manner and can induce a series of protein tyrosine phosphorylations. The two main cell types responsible for cytokine secretion are the T-helper cell and macrophage.[2]

Interferons are one of the major groups of cytokines that have been used for clinical cancer studies. IFN-α is produced by macrophages and increases MHC-I expression, activates NK cells, induces an anti-viral state, and inhibits cell division of normal or malignant transformed cells *in vitro*. IFN-β, produced by fibroblasts, increases MHC-I expression and activates NK cells. IFN-γ is produced by CD8$^+$ T-cells and NK cells and activates macrophages, increasing both MHC-I and MHC-II expression when foreign antigen is present. Data suggest that malignant tumors display a decrease in MHC-I expression and that the interferons may be responsible for restoring MHC-I expression, thereby increasing cytotoxic T-cell activity towards the tumor.[2] Daily injections of recombinant INF-α have been shown to induce partial or complete regression in hematological cancers (i.e. leukemia and lymphoma), as well as some solid tumors (i.e. breast and renal cancer).

Tumor necrosis factors TNF-α and TNF-β have been shown to display anti-tumor activity by direct killing of the tumor cells, reducing proliferation rate (while sparing the normal cells), and inhibiting angiogenesis by damaging vascular endothelial cells. Frequently, when treated with either factor, the tumor undergoes hemorrhagic necrosis and regression. Macrophages, mono-cytes, and other cell types including fibroblasts and T-cells secrete TNF-α. However, TNF-β is only produced by activated T-cells and B-cells and is a mediator of immune function and involved in wound healing. Both INF-γ and TNF-α are associated with chronic inflammation.[2] The complexity of cytokines and how they may potentially interact with each other has been one major obstacle of this type of therapy. Many cytokines have short half-lives and depending on the circumstances can act as either a pro-inflammatory or anti-inflammatory agent (i.e. IL-7, IL-9).[34,35] Systemic administration of a large amount of cytokines has led to serious consequences and has even been fatal, therefore these immunotherapies can be limiting.[2]

Growth Factors

Many tumors display high levels of growth factor receptors on their mem-branes making growth factor receptors a likely target for immunotherapy. Inappropriate expression of either a growth factor or its receptor can result in uncontrolled proliferation.[2] Vascular endothelial growth factor (VEGF) is a potent mitogen for cells and is one of the most well studied growth factors. VEGF mRNA expression is seen in breast cancer and is associated with poor prognosis of colon cancer and non-small cell lung carci-noma.[36,37] VEGF can be activated by *ras* oncogene causing inactivation of p53 and Von Hippel Landau (VHL), as well as cause activation of PKC.[38] VEGF is expressed in the epithelial and stromal areas of the human prostate, however, hyperplastic glands stain very poorly for the growth factor.[38,39] Several studies have shown that prostate cancer specimens dis-play 32% staining in the stroma and 56% staining in the epithelium.[40,41] In contrast, staining for VEGF in BPH displayed 73% staining of the stroma and 50% staining in the epithelium.[42,43] Of note is the use of the 5α-reductase inhibitor, Finasteride®, which has been shown to decrease expression of VEGF in prostatic tissue.[44]

Tumor Antigens

Tumor specific antigens may result from mutations that cause altered cellular proteins or may be normally expressed at certain stages of differentiation encoded by a variant form of the normal gene or may be exclusively expressed by the tumor.[2] Tumor associated glycoprotein-72 (TAG-72) is a mucin found on many adenocarcinomas including colorectal, pancreatic, gastric, ovarian, endometrial, and mammary, as well as some prostate cancers.[45,46]

Tumor antigens, while being specific for tumor tissue, can vary widely from tumor to tumor. The use of tissue specific antigens is usually undesirable, as normal tissue would also be targeted with the tumor. The case of prostate cancer is unique in that the prostate is not a vital organ and could be targeted without serious harm to the patient. This allows for the targeting of tissue specific antigens in the prostate. Several prostate specific antigens have been discovered and are targets of immunotherapy. These tissue specific antigens include PSA, prostate alkaline phosphatase (PAP) and prostate specific membrane antigen (PSMA). Although these self-proteins are not always immunogenic they do provide a basis for further development and testing.[27]

Monoclonal Antibody Therapy

Antigenic modulation in the treatment of many diverse cancers has been used for a number of years. In fact, the Food and Drug Administration has approved several monoclonal antibodies for treatment of various cancers and non-malignant diseases.[47] Ideally, by treating tumor cells with an antibody, one would hope for complete destruction of the tumor without recurrences. However, tumors seem to regenerate once the antibody treatment has ceased.[2] Passive administration of antibodies or active vaccination to induce antibodies can target cells that express antigenic proteins on their cell membranes.[27] Monoclonal antibodies are often conjugated to chemotherapeutic agents, biological toxins, radioactive compounds, or immunotoxins.[2,48,49] These immunoconjugates target the neoplastic cells expressing tumor specific or tumor-associated markers.[50] Problems with antibody specificity, delivery, and cost are often hurdles for therapy.[2,27] Unlike antibodies to Her2-*neu* for breast cancer or antibodies to CD20 for non-Hodgkin's lymphoma, there are limiting numbers of antibody targets for the treatment of prostate cancer.[27]

CC49, a murine IgG_1 antibody, recognizes TAG-72 and shows disease response when coupled to a radioisotope in ovarian cancer[45] and has been shown to be expressed in prostate cancer cells.[46] A clinical trial utilizing ^{131}I-CC49 failed to show any clinically relevant data.[51] However, when ^{131}I-CC49 was used in conjunction with INF-γ, up-regulation of TAG-72 and enhancement of the response was seen. The trial included 16 patients with androgen independent prostate cancer (AIPC), of which 12 patients had antibody localization to the tumor. None of the patients had a ≥50% decline in their PSA or a radiologic response, however several had moderate pain relief from bone metastases. Rapid production of anti-mouse antibodies and development of thrombocytopenia precluded further dosing.[52] In a subsequent clinical study, 14 patients were treated with IFN-α prior to the administration of ^{131}I-CC49.[53] Two patients had a minor radiographic response while 3 had a ≥50% reduction of their serum PSA levels. Therefore, IFN-α may be acting as an adjuvant yielding a greater response in comparison to just ^{131}I-CC49 therapy.

Since PSA is found in the serum, many researchers have used the antigen for a potential target for immunotherapy. *In vitro* data show that the generation of antibodies that recognize PSA and CD3 on T-cells would direct non-specific $CD3^+$ T-cells to PSA,[54] and in turn, this would re-direct preactivated peripheral mononuclear cells to lyse PSA expressing cells. Although demonstrated *in vivo*, a human trial is necessary. Since PSA is in the serum, directing antibodies to the prostate tissue would be difficult.[54]

PSMA is an ideal target for monoclonal antibody therapy since the target cell is always internalizing the protein and its internalization is augmented by monoclonal antibody contact[55] and is strongly expressed on nearly 100% of prostate tumors.[56,57] Prostacint® (7E11 from Cytogen) is an anti-PSMA antibody used to image the prostate. Prostacint® has been found to bind an intracellular epitope of PSMA and, therefore, likely binds areas of tumor necrosis. Second-generation anti-PSMA antibodies have been developed to target the extracellular domain of PSMA due to the fact that internal domain binding antibodies, such as 7E11 and PM2J0004.5 (Hybritech) do not bind viable cells.[58,59]

Most antibody therapies to PSMA have used J591, a mouse monoclonal antibody that is immunogenic. J591 has been genetically modified to eliminate the mouse antigens and is now fully "humanized," allowing

repeated dosing without generating anti-mouse antibodies. The unmodified antibody could focus the immune system on tumor sites to complement activation, however, dramatic responses to naked antibodies are
infrequent.[47,60] J591 binding to PSMA is rapidly internalized into the cell
and has been quite useful for imaging of known sites of metastasis.[47,60,61]

Antibodies to the extracellular domain of PSMA and coupled to toxins
or radioisotopes have been shown to have some effect in prostate cancer
cell lines and murine models.[50,62–64] In one study, J591, PEQ226.5, and
PM2P079.1 were conjugated with ricin A chain (RTA), a holotoxin containing an α subunit that inactivates protein synthesis and facilitates intracellular trafficking of RTA.[48,49] Since J591 and PEQ226.5 recognize the
same epitopes that are related to PSMA, a lower cytotoxic effect was
observed of the antibodies in cell monolayers in comparison to treatment
with RTA alone, while the specificity of PSMA expression of the tumors
was increased.[48,49]

A study performed by Dr. Bander and colleagues at the College of
Medicine of Cornell University enrolled 53 patients into a phase-I study
to assess disease staging, metastatic or recurrent disease. Twenty-nine
patients received ^{111}In/^{90}Y-DOTA-J591 while 24 patients received
[177]LU/DOTA-J591. The results indicated 98% of the patients had successful targeting of J591 to the bone and soft tissue with 87% having radiographic evidence of metastasis and 13% had zero visible lesions.
Remarkably, 16 of 18 patients with no evidence of metastasis showed positive J591 staining.[47] Other biotechnology companies have developed
external domain specific anti-PSMA antibodies using mice genetically
engineered to express human antibodies, resulting in the development of
monoclonal antibodies that are non-immunogenic. These anti-PSMA antibodies have demonstrated significant activity in clinical trials.[65]

Modulation of T-Cells

Modulation of the co-stimulatory signals required for T-cell activation
has been shown to be an effective therapy through blocking cytotoxic
T lymphocyte-associated antigen 4 (CTLA-4) with antibodies and
prolonging a T-cell response.[27] Anti-CTLA-4 blocks B7 binding to
CD28, preventing stimulation and decreasing expression of T-cells.[66,67]

Anti-CTLA-4 antibody treatment in animal models can induce tumor rejection in immunogenic tumors.[68] Coupled with an anti-tumor vaccination, it can induce rejection of minimally immunogenic tumors in the TRAMP animal model.[47] In a study of CTLA-4 blockade administered immediately after primary tumor resection, a reduction of metastatic relapse from 97.4% to 44% was observed. Consistent with this, lymph nodes obtained 2 weeks after treatment reveal marked destruction or complete elimination of C2 metastases in 60% of mice receiving adjunctive anti-CTLA-4 whereas 100% of control antibody-treated mice demonstrated progressive C2 lymph node replacement.[69]

Adjuvants are often used with various immunotherapies because they can increase B7 co-stimulation and activate macrophages. Activated macrophages can then cluster around tumors and are better T-helper activators. These increase both humoral and cell-mediated responses and correlate with tumor regression.[2] The Fc portion of human IgG has been fused to the B7 binding domain of CTLA-4 to produce a chimeric molecule, CTLA-Ig.[2] The human Fc portion gives the molecule a longer half-life and the B7 binding domain allows binding to CD28. A humanized antibody for CTLA-4, designated MDX-101 (Medarex, Inc.) has recently been tested in a Phase-I trial, which included 14 patients with AIPC. The study showed successful blocking of the co-stimulatory signaling with no T-cell activation occurring. The therapy was well tolerated and 2 patients had a $\geq$50% decline in PSA levels.[70]

Vaccines

Tumor vaccines cause induction of a cell-mediated response to antigens and are often composed of tumor-associated proteins mixed with a non-specific antigen.[2,27] Demonstrating that antigen specific T-cells are up-regulated by a particular vaccine strategy is important for immunologic therapies.[27] Antigen presentation is critical for any immunization technique and its enhancement can modulate tumor immunity. Anti-tumor vaccines that activate cytotoxic lymphocytes (CTLs) and human tumor infiltrating lymphocytes (HTLs) would be most desirable since HTLs induce CTLs. HTLs produce both IFN-γ and granulocyte macrophage colony stimulating factor (GM-CSF) and kill tumor cells. Therefore, vaccines that induce anti-tumor CTLs include MHC-II restricted epitopes, which would trigger a HTL response to tumor-associated antigens.[71] A method of activating these T-cells may be to use the antigen presenting dendritic cells to initiate the immune response.

Dendritic cells are the most potent antigen-presenting cells, capable of presenting antigen to $CD8^+$ (MHC-I restricted) and $CD4^+$ (MHC-II restricted) T-cells.[72] Dendritic cell-based vaccines use a patient's bone marrow derived antigen presenting cells that are able to sensitize naïve T-cells to new antigens. By combining dendritic cells with tumor antigens, the therapy supposes that the dendritic cells will then activate T-cells with tumor antigen.[27]

Mouse dendritic cells, pulsed with tumor fragments and incubated with GM-CSF, were re-infused into the mice to activate the T_H and CTL response to the tumor antigen.[73] Mouse tumor cells are immunogenic, therefore animals injected with killed tumor cells do not grow tumors when challenged with live tissue, a term designated protective immunity.[2] The same is true for humans. When tumor cells were transfected with GM-CSF and given back to the patient, they were able to secrete more GM-CSF and enhance the differentiation and activation of the host antigen presenting cells. As the dendritic cells surround the tumor cells, GM-CSF is secreted by the tumor and enhances presentation of antigen to the T_H and CTL cells.[2]

Dcnedron Corporation has developed Provenge®, a recombinant fusion protein with GM-CSF fused to prostate acid phosphatase (PAP), a prostate specific isozyme of acid phosphatase that is secreted by prostate cells.[27,74] This strategy uses autologous dendritic cells combined with human GM-CSF. Thirty-one patients with prostate cancer were enrolled in the clinical study and received three monthly infusions and one final boost at 24 months if the disease had not progressed. Results showed 38% of the patients had a T-cell response against native PAP while some had a decline in their PSA levels. T-cells collected after the treatment revealed the presence of IFN-γ, a reflection of successful activation.

The use of PAP as a vaccine has also been studied, since serum PAP levels increase with prostate cancer progression, from 33% up to 92%, making it a more important marker for advanced disease.[75] One study used a xenogenic homologue of PAP (mPAP), which was given to patients

with metastatic prostate cancer. The homologous mPAP possessed sufficient differences from self-antigen to render it immunogenic, but similar
enough that they would cross-react with human PAP. Seven out of
21 patients had stable disease following the vaccination beyond one year
while three patients had stable disease beyond three years. All of the
patients had T-cell immunity to mPAP and 11out of 21 had induced immunity to human PAP.[76,77]

A PAP peptide (termed PAP-5) capable of binding the HLA-A2 molecule was used to pulse an antigen presenting cell fraction containing dendritic cells isolated from a healthy HLA-A2 donor. The cells were
expanded and employed to elicit a CD8[+] CTL response. The peptide lysed
prostate tumors in an antigen specific manner. CTLs were evaluated for
peptide specific activity and potency in an *in vitro* chromium release
assay. The assay revealed that the CTLs generated after stimulation of
PAP-5 peptide loaded dendritic cells were able to endogenously process
the PAP-5 antigen.[74]

Human prostate cancer cells were removed at the time of surgery and
expanded in culture. They were transfected to secrete a high amount of
GM-CSF via *ex vivo* retroviral transduction with GM-CSF cDNA.[78] Eight
of 11 patients were then irradiated and given a subcutaneous injection of
their corresponding vaccine every 21 days (3–6 doses). Biopsies showed
the presence of macrophages, dendritic cells, T-cells, and eosinophils.
Delayed type hypersensitivity (DTH) *vs.* irradiated, unmodified, autologous tumor cells and recall antigen were tested pre/post treatment to
assess specific tumor cells and recall antigens to determine if a tumor specific response was achieved. Two of eight patients had a DTH response
prior to the vaccination while seven out of eight patients had a DTH
response post vaccination. Biopsies of the DTH sites showed that 80% of
the T-cells expressed CD45RO with the presence of Th_1 and Th_2 cells.[78]
Expression of CD45RO indicates that the T-cell has switched isoforms and
is now acting as an effector cell.[79]

A vaccine study targeting PSMA enrolled twenty-six patients with various stages of prostate cancer.[80] Patients were given either a cDNA plasmid encoding the extracellular domain of PSMA (with or without CD86),
an adenoviral vector expressing PSMA, or both in a prime-and-boost
strategy trial. Some of the patients received GM-CSF in addition to their

treatment. A DTH response to the PSMA expressing plasmid was seen in some of the patients including all 10 patients receiving the adenoviral vector. PSA decline was seen in some patients receiving vaccination only. Due to the various stages of disease and GM-CSF combination treatments, the results of this study are difficult to interpret.[27]

T-Bodies

A T-cell receptor that has been modified so the intra/extracellular part of the domain is the same but the most distal part of the receptor is replaced with a single chain antibody, is known as a T-body. The distal portion of the receptor being modified is the portion that would normally recognize the peptide antigen complex in the MHC cleft. A T-cell could then be activated to attach to a tumor using a specific antibody to a tumor specific antigen.[81] Sadelain *et al.* have created an artificial T-cell receptor (Pz-1) that is composed of an external PSMA-specific single chain antibody, linked to the CD8 hinge and transmembrane domain, followed by the cytoplasmic T-cell receptor signal transduction domain.[57] The receptor is capable of redirecting the specificity of the T-cell to target PSMA expressing cells, independent of MHC. *In vitro* data shows successful lysis of PSMA expressing prostate cancer cells lines and no effect on the non-PSMA expressing cells. These results indicate proliferation of modified T-cells in response to the presence of PSMA expression.[82]

Summary

More than 80% of prostate carcinoma tissue consists of tumor cells at advanced stages, with minor infiltration of inflammatory cells.[11] This indicates that the immune system is not involved. As a result, researchers have the opportunity to tap into a powerful natural defense system that can be augmented to involve prostate cancers. Immunotherapy can focus the immune system on a particular cancer with a wide range of alternatives that can be used singly or in concert to provide a tremendous benefit to the patient. By combining therapies involving biological response modifiers (i.e. cytokines and growth factors), conjugated monoclonal antibodies (including toxins and radiolabels), and cancer vaccines (tumor marker proteins with or without dendritic cell augmentation), the future of immunotherapeutic treatment of prostate cancer looks very promising.

References

1. Cancer Facts and Figures 2003 (2004) American Cancer Society Inc., Atlanta, GA, Ref Type: Report.
2. Goldsby RA, Kindt TJ, Osborne BAKJ (2003) *Immunology*, 5th ed. WH Freeman and Company, NY.
3. Meares EM, Jr (1991) Prostatitis. *Med Clin North Am* 75:405–424.
4. Cotran RS, Kumar VK, Collins TC (2004) *Robbins Pathologic Basis of Disease*. WB Saunders Company, Philadelphia.
5. De Marzo AM, DeWeese TL, Platz EA, Meeker AK, Nakayama M, Epstein JI, Isaacs WB, Nelson WG (2004) Pathological and molecular mechanisms of prostate carcinogenesis: Implications for diagnosis, detection, prevention, and treatment. *J Cell Biochem* 91:459–477.
6. De Marzo AM, Marchi VL, Epstein JI, Nelson WG (1999) Proliferative inflammatory atrophy of the prostate: Implications for prostatic carcinogenesis. *Am J Pathol* 155:1985–1992.
7. Putzi MJ, De Marzo AM (2000) Morphologic transitions between proliferative inflammatory atrophy and high-grade prostatic intraepithelial neoplasia. *Urology* 56:828–832.
8. Shah R, Mucci NR, Amin A, Macoska JA, Rubin MA (2001) Postatrophic hyperplasia of the prostate gland: Neoplastic precursor or innocent bystander? *Am J Pathol* 158:1767–1773.
9. Ruska KM, Sauvageot J, Epstein JI (1998) Histology and cellular kinetics of prostatic atrophy. *Am J Surg Pathol* 22:1073–1077.
10. Harmont TJ, Ratliff TL (1999) Prostate immunology. In: Kaisary AV, Murphy GP, Denis L, Griffiths K, eds. *Textbook of Prostate Cancer Pathology, Diagnosis and Treatment*. Martin Dunitz, London. 367 pp., illustrated (ISBN 1–85317–422–X).
11. Konig JE, Senge T, Allhoff EP, Konig W (2004) Analysis of the inflammatory network in benign prostate hyperplasia and prostate cancer. *Prostate* 58:121–129.
12. Steiner GE, Djavan B, Kramer G, Handisurya A, Newman ME, Lee C, Marberger M (2002) The picture of prostatic lymphokine network is becoming increasingly complex. *Rev Urol* 4:4171–4177.

13. Theyer G, Kramer G, Assmann I, Sherwood E, Preinfalk W, Marberger M, Zechner O, Steiner GE (1992) Phenotypic characterization of infiltrating leukocytes in benign prostatic hyperplasia. *Lab Invest* 66:96–107.

14. Steiner G, Gessl A, Kramer G, Schollhammer A, Forster O, Marberger M (1994) Phenotype and function of peripheral and prostatic lymphocytes in patients with benign prostatic hyperplasia. *J Urol* 151:480–484.

15. Gann PH, Klein KG, Chatterton RT, Ellman AE, Grayhack JT, Nadler RB, Lee C (1999) Growth factors in expressed prostatic fluid from men with prostate cancer, BPH, and clinically normal prostates. *Prostate* 40: 248–255.

16. Pisters LL, Troncoso P, Zhau HE, Li W, von Eschenbach AC, Chung LW (1995) c-met proto-oncogene expression in benign and malignant human prostate tissues. *J Urol* 154:293–298.

17. Bostwich DG (2000) Immunohistochemical changes in prostate cancer after androgen deprivation therapy. *Mol Urol* 4(3):101–106 (discussion 107).

18. Droller MJ (1997) Medical approaches in the management of prostatic disease. *Br J Urol* 79 (Suppl 2):42–52.

19. Walsh PC (1996) Treatment of benign prostatic hyperplasia. *N Engl J Med* 335:586–587.

20. Smith CJ, Gardner A (1987) *Current Concepts and Approaches to the Study of Prostate Cancer.* AR Liss, New York.

21. Silverman RH (2003) Implications for RNase L in prostate cancer biology. *Biochemistry* 42:1805–1812.

22. Robbins SG, Conaway JR, Ford BL, Roberto KA, Penn JS (1997) Detection of vascular endothelial growth factor (VEGF) protein in vascular and nonvascular cells of the normal and oxygen-injured rat retina. *Growth Factors* 14:229–241.

23. Bierhoff E, Vogel J, Benz M, Giefer T, Wernert N, Pfeifer U (1996) Stromal nodules in benign prostatic hyperplasia. *Eur Urol* 29:345–354.

24. Arrighi HM, Metter EJ, Guess HA, Fozzard JL (1991) Natural history of benign prostatic hyperplasia and risk of prostatectomy. The Baltimore Longitudinal Study of Aging. *Urology* 38:4–8.

25. Nadler RB, Humphrey PA, Smith DS, Catalona WJ, Ratliff TL (1995) Effect of inflammation and benign prostatic hyperplasia on elevated serum prostate specific antigen levels. *J Urol* 154:407–413.

26. Steiner GE, Stix U, Handisurya A, Willheim M, Haitel A, Reithmayr F, Paikl D, Ecker RC, Hrachowitz K, Kramer G, Lee C, Marberger M (2003) Cytokine expression pattern in benign prostatic hyperplasia infiltrating T cells and impact of lymphocytic infiltration on cytokine mRNA profile in prostatic tissue. *Lab Invest* 83:1131–1146.

27. Fong L, Small EJ (2003) Immunotherapy for prostate cancer. *Semin Oncol* 30:649–658.

28. Parkinson DR, Lotzova E (1990) Interleukin-2, killer cells and cancer therapy: an overview. *Nat Immun Cell Growth Regul* 9(4):237–241.

29. Leite-De-Moraes MC, Hameg A, Arnould A, Machavoine F, Koezuka Y, Schneider E, Herbelin A, Dy M (1999) A distinct IL-18-induced pathway to fully activate NK T lymphocytes independently from TCR engagement. *J Immunol* 163:5871–5876.

30. Leite-De-Moraes MC, Herbelin A, Gouarin C, Koezuka Y, Schneider E, Dy M (2000) Fas/Fas ligand interactions promote activation-induced cell death of NK T lymphocytes. *J Immunol* 165:4367–4371.

31. Rock FL, Hardiman G, Timans JC, Kastelein RA, Bazan JF (1998) A family of human receptors structurally related to Drosophila Toll. *Proc Natl Acad Sci USA* 95:588–593.

32. Chaudhary PM, Ferguson C, Nguyen V, Nguyen O, Massa HF, Eby M, Jasmin A, Trask BJ, Hood L, Nelson PS (1998) Cloning and characterization of two Toll/Interleukin-1 receptor-like genes TIL3 and TIL4: Evidence for a multi-gene receptor family in humans. *Blood* 91:4020–4027.

33. Papatsoris AG, Papavassiliou AG (2001) Molecular 'palpation' of BPH: A tale of MAPK signalling? *Trends Mol Med* 7:288–292.

34. Feghali CA, Wright TM (1997) Cytokines in acute and chronic inflammation. *Front Biosci* 2:d12–d26.

35. Fisman EZ, Motro M, Tenenbaum A (2003) Cardiovascular diabetology in the core of a novel interleukins classification: The bad, the good and the aloof. *Cardiovasc Diabetol* 2:11.

36. Leung DW, Cachianes G, Kuang WJ, Goeddel DV, Ferrara N (1989) Vascular endothelial growth factor is a secreted angiogenic mitogen. *Science* 246: 1306–1309.

37. Fontanini G, Faviana P, Lucchi M, Boldrini L, Mussi A, Camacci T, Mariani MA, Angeletti CA, Basolo F, Pingitore R (2002) A high vascular count and overexpression of vascular endothelial growth factor are associated with unfavorable prognosis in operated small cell lung carcinoma. *Br J Cancer* 86:558–563.

38. Walsh K, Sriprasad S, Hopster D, Codd J, Mulvin D (2002) Distribution of vascular endothelial growth factor (VEGF) in prostate disease. *Prostate Cancer Prostatic Dis* 5:119–122.

39. Ferrer FA, Miller LJ, Andrawis RI, Kurtzman SH, Albertsen PC, Laudone VP, Kreutzer DL (1997) Vascular endothelial growth factor (VEGF) expression in human prostate cancer: *in situ* and *in vitro* expression of VEGF by human prostate cancer cells. *J Urol* 157:2329–2333.

40. Berkman RA, Merrill MJ, Reinhold WC, Monacci WT, Saxena A, Clark WC, Robertson JT, Ali IU, Oldfield EH (1993) Expression of the vascular permeability factor/vascular endothelial growth factor gene in central nervous system neoplasms. *J Clin Invest* 91:153–159.

41. Warren RS, Yuan H, Matli MR, Gillett NA, Ferrara N (1995) Regulation by vascular endothelial growth factor of human colon cancer tumorigenesis in a mouse model of experimental liver metastasis. *J Clin Invest* 95:1789–1797.

42. Brown LF, Berse B, Jackman RW, Tognazzi K, Manseau EJ, Dvorak HF, Senger DR (1993) Increased expression of vascular permeability factor (vascular endothelial growth factor) and its receptors in kidney and bladder carcinomas. *Am J Pathol* 143:1255–1262.

43. Suzuki K, Hayashi N, Miyamoto Y, Yamamoto M, Ohkawa K, Ito Y, Sasaki Y, Yamaguchi Y, Nakase H, Noda K, Enomoto N, Arai K, Yamada Y, Yoshihara H, Tujimura T, Kawano K, Yoshikawa K, Kamada T (1996) Expression of vascular permeability factor/vascular endothelial growth factor in human hepatocellular carcinoma. *Cancer Res* 56:3004–3009.

44. Steinberg DM, Sauvageot J, Piantadosi S, Epstein JI (1997) Correlation of prostate needle biopsy and radical prostatectomy Gleason grade in academic and community settings. *Am J Surg Pathol* 21:566–576.

45. Alvarez RD, Partridge EE, Khazaeli MB, Plott G, Austin M, Kilgore L, Russell CD, Liu T, Grizzle WE, Schlom J, LoBuglio AF, Meredith RF (1997) Intraperitoneal radioimmunotherapy of ovarian cancer with 177Lu-CC49: A phase I/II study. *Gynecol Oncol* 65:94–101.

46. Myers RB, Meredith RF, Schlom J, LoBuglio AF, Bueschen AJ, Wheeler RH, Stockard CR, Grizzle WE (1994) Tumor associated glycoprotein-72 is highly expressed in prostatic adenocarcinomas. *J Urol* 152:243–246.

47. Bander NH, Trabulsi EJ, Kostakoglu L, Yao D, Vallabhajosula S, Smith-Jones P, Joyce MA, Milowsky M, Nanus DM, Goldsmith SJ (2003) Targeting metastatic prostate cancer with radiolabeled monoclonal antibody J591 to the extracellular domain of prostate specific membrane antigen. *J Urol* 170:1717–1721.

48. Thrush GR, Lark LR, Clinchy BC, Vitetta ES (1996) Immunotoxins: An update. *Annu Rev Immunol* 14:49–71.

49. Kreitman RJ (2001) Quantification of immunotoxin number for complete therapeutic response. *Methods Mol Biol* 166:111–123.

50. Fracasso G, Bellisola G, Cingarlini S, Castelletti D, Prayer-Galetti T, Pagano F, Tridente G, Colombatti M (2002) Anti-tumor effects of toxins targeted to the prostate specific membrane antigen. *Prostate* 53:9–23.

51. Meredith RF, Bueschen AJ, Khazaeli MB, Plott WE, Grizzle WE, Wheeler RH, Schlom J, Russell CD, Liu T, LoBuglio AF (1994) Treatment of metastatic prostate carcinoma with radiolabeled antibody CC49. *J Nucl Med* 35:1017–1022.

52. Slovin SF, Scher HI, Divgi CR, Reuter V, Sgouros G, Moore M, Weingard K, Pettengall R, Imbriaco M, El Shirbiny A, Finn R, Bronstein J, Brett C, Milenic D, Dnistrian A, Shapiro L, Schlom J, Larson SM (1998) Interferon-gamma and monoclonal antibody 131I-labeled CC49: Outcomes in patients with androgen-independent prostate cancer. *Clin Cancer Res* 4:643–651.

53. Meredith RF, Khazaeli MB, Macey DJ, Grizzle WE, Mayo M, Schlom J, Russell CD, LoBuglio AF (1999) Phase II study of interferon-enhanced 131I-labeled high affinity CC49 monoclonal antibody therapy in patients with metastatic prostate cancer. *Clin Cancer Res* 5:3254s–3258s.

54. Katzenwadel A, Schleer H, Gierschner D, Wetterauer U, Elsasser-Beile U (2000) Construction and *in vivo* evaluation of an anti-PSA x anti-CD3 bispecific antibody for the immunotherapy of prostate cancer. *Anticancer Res* 20:1551–1555.

55. Liu H, Rajasekaran AK, Moy P, Xia Y, Kim S, Navarro V, Rahmati R, Bander NH (1998) Constitutive and antibody-induced internalization of prostate-specific membrane antigen. *Cancer Res* 58:4055–4060.

56. Ghosh A, Heston WD (2003) Effect of carbohydrate moieties on the folate hydrolysis activity of the prostate specific membrane antigen. *Prostate* 57: 140–151.

57. Tasch J, Gong M, Sadelain M, Heston WD (2001) A unique folate hydrolase, prostate-specific membrane antigen (PSMA): A target for immunotherapy? *Crit Rev Immunol* 21:249–261.

58. Danshe M, Gardner JM, Donovan GP, Schulke N, Hopf C, Cohen M (2003) Fully human anti-PSMA antibodies for prostate cancer therapy. *Proc Am Assoc Cancer Res* 44:1483 (Ref Type: Abstract).

59. Chang SS, Reuter VE, Heston WD, Bander NH, Grauer LS, Gaudin PB (1999) Five different anti-prostate-specific membrane antigen (PSMA) antibodies confirm PSMA expression in tumor-associated neovasculature. *Cancer Res* 59:3192–3198.

60. Bander NH, Nanus DM, Milowsky MI, Kostakoglu L, Vallabahajosula S, Goldsmith SJ (2003) Targeted systemic therapy of prostate cancer with a monoclonal antibody to prostate-specific membrane antigen. *Semin Oncol* 30:667–676.

61. Chang SS, Bander NH, Heston WD (2004) Biology of PSMA as a diagnostic and therapeutic target. In: Klein EA, ed. *Management of Prostate Cancer,* 2nd ed. Humana Press, Totowa NJ.
62. Vallabhajosula S, Smith-Jones PM, Navarro V, Goldsmith SJ, Bander NH (2004) Radioimmunotherapy of prostate cancer in human xenografts using monoclonal antibodies specific to prostate specific membrane antigen (PSMA): Studies in nude mice. *Prostate* 58:145–155.
63. Nanus DM, Milowsky MI, Kostakoglu L, Smith-Jones PM, Vallabahajosula S, Goldsmith SJ, Bander NH (2003) Clinical use of monoclonal antibody HuJ591 therapy: Targeting prostate specific membrane antigen. *J Urol* 170:S84–S88.
64. Smith-Jones PM, Vallabhajosula S, Navarro V, Bastidas D, Goldsmith SJ, Bander NH (2003) Radiolabeled monoclonal antibodies specific to the extracellular domain of prostate-specific membrane antigen: Preclinical studies in nude mice bearing LNCaP human prostate tumor. *J Nucl Med* 44:610–617.
65. Smith S (2001) Technology evaluation: C242-DM1, ImmunoGen Inc. *Curr Opin Mol Ther* 3:198–203.
66. Egen JG, Kuhns MS, Allison JP (2002) CTLA-4: New insights into its biological function and use in tumor immunotherapy. *Nat Immunol* 3:611–618.
67. Chambers CA, Kuhns MS, Egen JG, Allison JP (2001) CTLA-4-mediated inhibition in regulation of T cell responses: Mechanisms and manipulation in tumor immunotherapy. *Annu Rev Immunol* 19:565–594.
68. Hurwitz AA, Foster BA, Kwon ED, Truong T, Choi EM, Greenberg NM, Burg MB, Allison JP (2000) Combination immunotherapy of primary prostate cancer in a transgenic mouse model using CTLA-4 blockade. *Cancer Res* 60:2444–2448.
69. Kwon ED, Foster BA, Hurwitz AA, Madias C, Allison JP, Greenberg NM, Burg MB (1999) Elimination of residual metastatic prostate cancer after surgery and adjunctive cytotoxic T lymphocyte-associated antigen 4 (CTLA-4) blockade immunotherapy. *Proc Natl Acad Sci USA* 96:15074–15079.
70. Davis TA, Korman A, Keler T (2002) MDX-010 (human anti-CTLA4): A phase I trial in hormone refractory prostate carcinoma (HRPC). *Proc Am Soc Clin Oncol* 21:74 (Ref Type: Abstract).
71. Kobayashi H, Omiya R, Sodey B, Yanai M, Oikawa K, Sato K, Kimura S, Senju S, Nishimura Y, Tateno M, Celis E (2003) Identification of naturally processed helper T-cell epitopes from prostate-specific membrane antigen using peptide-based *in vitro* stimulation. *Clin Cancer Res* 9:5386–5393.
72. Guery JC, Adorini L (1995) Dendritic cells are the most efficient in presenting endogenous naturally processed self-epitopes to class II-restricted T cells. *J Immunol* 154:536–544.

73. Dranoff G, Jaffee E, Lazenby A, Golumbek P, Levitsky H, Brose K, Jackson V, Hamada H, Pardoll D, Mulligan RC (1993) Vaccination with irradiated tumor cells engineered to secrete murine granulocyte-macrophage colony-stimulating factor stimulates potent, specific, and long-lasting antitumor immunity. *Proc Natl Acad Sci USA* 90:3539–3543.

74. Peshwa MV, Shi JD, Ruegg C, Laus R, van Schooten WC (1998) Induction of prostate tumor-specific CD8+ cytotoxic T-lymphocytes *in vitro* using antigen-presenting cells pulsed with prostatic acid phosphatase peptide. *Prostate* 36:129–138.

75. Jacobs EL, Haskell CM (1991) Clinical use of tumor markers in oncology. *Curr Probl Cancer* 15:299–360.

76. Fong L, Brockstedt D, Benike C, Breen JK, Strang G, Ruegg CL, Engleman EG (2001) Dendritic cell-based xenoantigen vaccination for prostate cancer immunotherapy. *J Immunol* 167:7150–7156.

77. Fong L, Benike C, Brockstedt D, *et al.* (1999) Immunization with dendritic cells pulsed with xenogenic prostatic acid phosphatase administered via different routes induces cellular immune response in prostate cancer patients. *Proc Am Assoc Cancer Res* 40:85 (Ref Type: Abstract).

78. Simmons SJ, Tjoa BA, Rogers M, Elgamal A, Kenny GM, Ragde H, Troychak MJ, Boynton AL, Murphy GP (1999) GM-CSF as a systemic adjuvant in a phase II prostate cancer vaccine trial. *Prostate* 39:291–297.

79. Suarez A, Mozo L, Gutierrez C (2002) Generation of CD4(+)CD45RA(+) effector T cells by stimulation in the presence of cyclic adenosine 5′-monophosphate-elevating agents. *J Immunol* 169:1159–1167.

80. Mincheff M, Tchakarov S, Zoubak S, Loukinov D, Botev C, Altankova I, Georgiev G, Petrov S, Meryman HT (2000) Naked DNA and adenoviral immunizations for immunotherapy of prostate cancer: A phase I/II clinical trial. *Eur Urol* 38:208–217.

81. Kramer G, Steiner GE, Handisurya A, Stix U, Haitel A, Knerer B, Gessl A, Lee C, Marberger M (2002) Increased expression of lymphocyte-derived cytokines in benign hyperplastic prostate tissue, identification of the producing cell types, and effect of differentially expressed cytokines on stromal cell proliferation. *Prostate* 52:43–58.

82. Gong MC, Latouche JB, Krause A, Heston WD, Bander NH, Sadelain M (1999) Cancer patient T cells genetically targeted to prostate-specific membrane antigen specifically lyse prostate cancer cells and release cytokines in response to prostate-specific membrane antigen. *Neoplasia* 1:123–127.

3

RADIATION THERAPY AND HORMONAL THERAPY FOR PROSTATE CANCER

Ralph A. Brasacchio

Department of Radiation Oncology and JP Wilmot Cancer Center
University of Rochester Medical Center
Rochester, New York, USA

Introduction

Prostate cancer is the most common cancer among American men (33% of the estimated 699,560 new cancer cases in males in 2004) and is second only to lung cancer in male cancer-related deaths (10% of the estimated 290,890 cancer deaths in males in 2004).[1] Because the incidence of prostate cancer increases more rapidly with age, and the average age of the American male is increasing, the number of patients with prostate cancer is expected to steadily increase over the next decade. Therefore, prostate cancer has become a major health concern.

Several treatment options exist for prostate cancer depending on the stage of disease and other prognostic factors. These include orchiectomy, prostatectomy, radiation therapy (RT) [external beam (EBRT) and brachytherapy], hormonal therapy, and chemotherapy. Clinicians frequently combine these options in treating the disease in order to optimize results.

This review will focus on the use of RT in the treatment of localized prostate cancer and the role and mechanisms of hormonal therapy in combination with RT.

Conventional and Conformal Radiation Therapy

Localized Prostate Cancer

External beam radiation therapy (EBRT), conventional and more recently three-dimensional conformal radiation therapy (3D-CRT) with dose escalation, including intensity modulated radiation therapy (IMRT), has proven to be a highly effective treatment for men with localized prostate cancer. Treatment results from several series for patients with favorable prognostic factors of prostate-specific antigen (PSA) $\leq$ 10 ng/ml, Gleason score $<$ 7 (i.e. well-moderately differentiated), and T_1–T_{2a} (i.e. locally-confined, low volume) disease, have been excellent. In a large series from MD Anderson Cancer Center, patients with favorable risk factors experienced a freedom from biochemical failure rate of 88% at 5 years and 84% at 10 years.[2] Similar results have been seen in a number of other series across multiple institutions.[3–5]

Despite these reports showing the clinical benefit of RT in early-stage, low-risk prostate cancer, patients with intermediate risk prognostic factors and with high risk/locally advanced disease [i.e. clinical stage T_{2B}, extensive unilateral disease, or Gleason score 7 (i.e. moderately–poorly differentiated), PSA 10–20 ng/ml; and clinical stage $\geq T_{2C}$, bilateral often bulky disease, Gleason score ≥ 8 (i.e. poorly differentiated) and PSA ≥ 20 ng/ml] have a 25%–50% and a greater than 50% risk of bio-chemical recurrence in 5 years.[6] Ten-year survival rates of only 40% have been observed with standard RT alone for patients with locally advanced disease.[7,8] The rates of survival free of biochemical failure at 5 years were 69% for intermediate risk patients and 47% for high risk patients in a multi-institutional review.[3]

These relatively poor results of RT in patients with intermediate and high risk disease have led to trials investigating radiation dose-escalation using conformal RT methods, such as 3D-CRT and IMRT, and external beam combined with hormonal therapy, which is the main subject of this review.

In one trial of dose escalation performed at Fox Chase Cancer Center, an improvement in PSA-relapse free survival (RFS) was observed among the subgroup of patients with PSA $>$ 10 when the RT dose was increased from 68 Gy to 79 Gy.[9] The 5-year biochemical disease-free survival (DFS) was significantly improved for patients with pre-treatment PSA > 10 who received greater than 76 Gy. Patients with an initial PSA of 10.0–19.9 had a 5-year biochemical DFS of 29%, 57%, and 73% if they received <71.5 Gy, 71.5–75.6 Gy, and ≥75.6 Gy respectively (p = 0.02). Patients with an initial PSA > 20 had a 5-year biochemical DFS rate of 8%, 28% and 30% if they received <71.5 Gy, 71.5–75.6 Gy and ≥75.6 Gy, respectively (p = 0.02).[10]

Similar dose-response results have been observed at Memorial Sloan Kettering Cancer Center, indicating improvement in biochemical DFS for patients with intermediate and high-risk disease who received a dose of ≥75.6 Gy (p ≤ 0.05).[11] The study from Memorial Sloan Kettering showed that clinical response was dose dependent, with 90% of the patients receiving 75.6 Gy or 81.0 Gy achieving a PSA nadir < 1.0 ng/ml compared with 76% and 56% for those treated with 70.2 Gy and 64.8 Gy (p < 0.001). Five-year actuarial PSA-RFS for patients with favorable prognostic indicators (stage T_{1-2}, PSA < 10.0, Gleason score < 6/10) was 85% compared with 65% for those with intermediate prognosis and 35% for the group with unfavorable prognosis (≥2 indicators with high risk features) (p < 0.001).[11] Positive biopsy rates also were significantly less in those receiving the higher doses.

In a large series of patients, analyzed at the University of Michigan,[12] 3D-CRT with dose escalation reduced the risk of biochemical failure among intermediate risk patients. Hormonal therapy was not associated with reduced rate of failure in patients with intermediate risk features, although for patients with high-risk features, adjuvant and neoadjuvant hormonal therapy significantly increased failure-free survival in radiation treated patients (p < 0.05), as is also reported in the randomized trial discussed below.

A French study accrued 164 patients to a dose escalation trial. The patients had clinical T_{1b}–T_3 disease and were prescribed doses ranging from 66 Gy to 80 Gy, with group 1 patients receiving a standard dose of 66–70 Gy, and group 2 patients receiving a dose of 74–80 Gy. Although mean follow-up was short for both groups (32 months for group 1, n = 46; 17.5 months for group 2, n = 118) the probability of achieving nadir PSA ≤ 1 ng/ml was significantly higher for group 2 patients.[13]

The results of a randomized study from MD Anderson Cancer Center comparing 70 Gy *vs.* 78 Gy showed an improvement in 5-year freedom from PSA failure, most significant in patients with pre-treatment PSA > 10 ng/ml.[2,14] The 5-year freedom from failure (FFF) rate was 75% for the patients in the high risk arm *vs.* 48% for those in the control group (p = 0.011). Updated results at 60 months showed an improvement in crude biochemical failure rate for the experimental group (21% *vs.* 32%, p = 0.03).[15] Kaplan-Meier analysis[16] showed that although FFF rates were improved in the experimental group the differences narrowed, with longer follow-up, to 6% at 6 years. Improvements in FFF were most significant for patients with intermediate to high risk disease (6-year FFF rate of 43% *vs.* 62% for the control and experimental arms, respectively). There also appeared to be a reduction in freedom from distant metastasis at 6 years for patients with pre-treatment PSA > 10 ng/ml (88% for the 70 Gy arm *vs.* 98% for the 78 Gy arm [p = 0.056]). There was no overall survival difference seen at 6 years.

Therefore, both radiation dose escalation and randomized series show a more pronounced effect of dose escalation in patients with intermediate risk prostate cancer. Patients with more favorable disease may not benefit from higher doses because conventional doses are adequate to eradicate these tumors. Patients with high risk disease may have a local control benefit from high dose RT; however, due to the high likelihood of occult metastases, long term biochemical no evidence of disease (NED) and DFS may not be affected. For this high-risk group of patients, adjuvant hormonal therapy and possibly chemotherapy may be necessary in addition to dose escalation. It is also not clear that dose escalation is without potential toxicity with longer follow-up[15] and particularly when higher doses are used, although studies in general report an improvement in late sequelae of 3D-CRT and IMRT dose escalation.[17–19]

Radiation Therapy With or Without Androgen Ablation Therapy

As discussed in the previous section, several retrospective and prospective dose escalation trials have suggested that the use of higher radiation doses, particularly in intermediate risk groups (clinical stage T_{2B} or Gleason score 7, PSA 10–20 ng/ml) of prostate cancer patients, may lead to improvements in biochemical control and DFS. However, the optimum radiation dose has yet to be determined, and in especially high-risk patients, RT dose escalation alone may not be adequate. In addition, the more long-term results of dose-escalation have yet to be assessed. Therefore, investigators have attempted to improve the outcome for patients with localized but locally-advanced prostate cancer by the addition of hormonal therapy to EBRT. Green *et al.*[20] was one of the early workers in this area. In 1975, he reported a study including 80 patients treated with RT for prostate cancer, 35 of whom also received estrogen during the radiation and for the subsequent 3 months. The majority of the patients had locally advanced but non-metastatic disease. The author noted that the most favorable tumor response was seen in those who received estrogen along with radiation compared with those who received radiation or estrogens alone.

This same investigator later reported on a group of 35 patients with pelvic or pelvic and para-aortic lymph node metastasis. These patients were treated with 3 mg of diethylstilbesterol (DES) for 8 weeks prior to and continuing during RT, then discontinued after 6 months in the majority of patients. The study suggested a benefit of DES regarding cytoreduction and the role of estrogen therapy in allowing RT to improve control of disease.[21] Green *et al.* also reported on 36 patients with bulky prostate cancer of whom 25 received 3 mg DES before RT and were compared with a similar group of 11 patients treated with RT alone. With a median follow-up of 4 years, the group reported a local control rate of 72% for the combined group compared to 53% local control for the RT alone group.[22]

Other nonrandomized studies have investigated the role of hormonal therapy (estrogens) with RT. van der Werf-Messing *et al.*[23] retrospectively analyzed patients with T_3–$T_4N_XM_0$ prostate cancer, 26 of whom received orchiectomy and hormones (1 mg DES) alone, 30 were treated with external RT alone, and 30 received hormones and external RT. Patients in the RT alone group had a significantly greater overall survival at 4 years than the other groups. There were 10 cardiovascular deaths in the groups treated with hormones that likely accounted for the decreased survival. The combined therapy group also had a greater percentage of patients with poorly-differentiated tumors.

The first randomized series comparing hormonal therapy plus radiation to radiation alone was initiated by Del Regato in 1967.[24] This was a multi-institutional trial including patients with locally-advanced (stage T_3/T_4) prostate cancer. DES was started at the end of RT and continued indefinitely, most patients continuing for several years and many permanently. The long-term results of the trial encompassed patients treated at MD Anderson. Seventy-eight patients were randomized to RT plus DES at 2 mg or 5 mg daily, or RT alone. There was an improvement in disease freedom, although a survival difference due to adjuvant DES was not observed, despite a median follow-up of 14.5 years.[25] This may have been related to small patient numbers since large numbers of patients must be studied because of the large number of intercurrent deaths in the elderly prostate cancer population; and to the association of DES with increased cardiac mortality, which may have counterbalanced any potential survival benefit from the hormonal therapy.

Pilepich *et al.* have reported a Radiation Therapy Oncology Group (RTOG) Phase II trial investigating potential benefit of hormonal cytoreduction in locally advanced prostate cancer. This trial compared the efficacy and toxicity of megastrol versus DES as cytoreductive agents before and during RT. Patients had locally-advanced adenocarcinoma of the prostate, stage B_2 and C with or without pelvic lymph node involvement, and were stratified by stage, grade and nodal status. They were randomized to receive either 40 mg megastrol 3 times daily (tid) or 1 mg DES orally, tid. The drugs were started 2 months before RT, continued during RT, and then discontinued. This study accrued 203 patients, of which 197 were evaluable. With a median follow-up of 32 months, only 6.5% of all evaluable patients manifested evidence of local failure. There was no significant difference between DES and megastrol regarding tumor clearance, although the DES appeared to be more effective in suppressing testosterone. This came with an increased rate of toxicity, especially gynecomastia and fluid retention. Patients with medical conditions predisposing them to thromboembolic phenomenon were excluded from this trial because of the risk of DES contributing to cardiovascular events.[26]

These preliminary investigations evaluating the role of neoadjuvant and/or adjuvant androgen deprivation therapy plus RT in the treatment of locally advanced prostate cancer have led to a number of randomized trials.

RTOG 85-31 randomized 977 patients with clinical stage T_3 disease (57%), post-prostatectomy patients with seminal vesicle or extracapsular disease (15%), and T_1/T_2 patients with node positive disease (28%), to either indefinite androgen deprivation *vs.* no androgen deprivation therapy with goserelin (LHRH analog therapy) following EBRT and goserelin continued indefinitely. Improved outcome was observed for those treated with the combination with regard to local, biochemical, and distant control (p < 0.0001). At median follow-up of 5.6 years there was numerical, although not statistically significant (p = 0.52), improvement in overall survival at 5 and 8 years for all patients. In a subgroup of patients with centrally reviewed biopsy (Gleason score 8–10), and who did not undergo prostatectomy, there was a significant improvement in the estimated 8-year overall and cause-specific survival (p = 0.036 and 0.019, respectively) with immediate hormonal therapy. However, results of subset analysis should be reviewed with caution and require confirmation in an appropriately randomized and stratified study.[27,28]

The EORTC studied 415 men with T_1–T_4 prostate cancer, the majority of whom had T_3–T_4 disease without evidence of lymph node involvement. Men with clinically localized disease had a Gleason score of 8–10. Patients were randomized to immediate hormonal therapy with LHRH agonist goserelin monthly starting on the first day of radiotherapy and continuing for 3 years, also receiving an antiandrogen for 1 week before and for 2–4 weeks after the first LHRH agonist injection in order to ameliorate possible LHRH agonist flare reaction. Those in the control arm received the same hormonal therapy at clinical progression. The initial analysis was reported in 1997, and showed overall survival at 5 years for the RT plus adjuvant hormonal therapy of 79% *vs.* 62% for the RT alone group. PSA-determined DFS at 5 years was significantly improved with the addition of hormonal manipulation, 85% *vs.* 48%. Local control was 97% for the combined group *vs.* 77% for the RT alone group. An update with median follow-up of 66 months continued to show a statistically significant survival benefit (78% *vs.* 62%; p = 0.0002) and clinical DFS benefit (74% *vs.* 40%; p = 0.0001) for the patients treated with combined therapy *vs.* RT alone respectively.[29,30]

The RTOG has conducted a number of randomized trials addressing the potential benefit of cytoreduction given neoadjuvantly to RT. In the RTOG 86-10 trial, patients with locally advanced prostate cancer, i.e. bulky T_2–T_4 disease with palpable tumor >25 cc, with or without pelvic lymph node involvement, were randomized to receive goserelin 3.6 mg subcutaneously every 4 weeks and the antiandrogen flutamide, 250 mg tid, for 2 months before and 2 months during RT (arm I) or RT alone (arm II). Of the 456 patients determined to be eligible at median follow-up of 4.5 years (471 patients accrued), arm I showed a significant improvement in local progression compared with arm II, 46% vs. 75% (p < 0.001) and progression-free survival 36% vs. 15% (p < 0.001). There was a trend toward improvement in distant metastasis-free survival (p = 0.09) but not improvement in overall survival.[31] Their data indicated that the combined treatment results in an additive effect over RT alone in freedom from relapse or rising PSA.

In an update of this trial[32] with median follow-up of 6.7 years and 8.6 years for surviving patients, there was a statistical benefit for neoadjuvant hormonal therapy plus RT in local failure, NED survival, biochemical NED survival with PSA < 4 ng/ml, biochemical survival with PSA < 1.5 ng/ml, and cause-specific failure. Patients who seemed to benefit the most from cytoreduction therapy were patients with Gleason score 2–6, who also had an improvement in overall survival. The survival improvement was not seen in the higher Gleason score groups who only showed an improvement in biochemical NED survival.

Subset analysis of RTOG 85-71 and 86-10 supported that the use of long-term hormonal therapy for locally-advanced but non-metastatic prostate cancer, was beneficial for patients with Gleason score 7 and 8–10. These patients showed an improvement in both cause-specific and overall survival with long-term hormonal therapy.[33]

In order to attempt to answer the question of long vs. short-term hormonal therapy with RT, RTOG protocol 92-02 randomized 1554 men with clinical stage T_2–T_4 disease and PSA < 150 ng/ml, to goserelin given for 2 years after neoadjuvant total androgen blockade (goserelin and - flutamide for 2 months before and 2 months during radiotherapy) and radiotherapy, or to neoadjuvant total androgen blockade and radiation followed by no further therapy. At a median follow-up of 4.8 years, the group receiving long term hormonal therapy showed a statistically significant improvement in estimated 5-year DFS, 46% vs. 28% (p < 0.001); clinical local progression, 6% vs. 12% (p = 0.001); distant metastasis, 12% vs. 17% (p = 0.0035); and biochemical failure 28% vs. 56% (p = 0.001). The 5-year survival rate for both groups was comparable at this early endpoint. Patients in the study were stratified according to pretreatment Gleason score. In the subset of patients with Gleason score 8–10, there was an improvement in estimated 5-year overall survival (80% *vs.* 69%; p = 0.02) and disease-specific survival (90% *vs.* 75%; p = 0.0007) favoring the long term arm.[34]

RTOG 94-13 was a 4-arm randomized trial which accrued 1327 patients with clinical stage T_{2C}–T_4 disease with pretreatment PSA < 100 ng/ml and estimated >15% risk of lymph node involvement based on the equation: % + LN = 2/3PSA + ([GS − 6] × 10).[35] The randomization was to neoadjuvant hormonal manipulation with LHRH agonist plus antiandrogen for 2 months before and during RT or the same hormonal manipulation for 4 months after RT. Patients were also randomized between whole-pelvis RT plus prostate boost versus radiation to the prostate only. With a median follow-up of nearly 5 years, patients receiving neoadjuvant hormonal therapy and RT had a 4-year progression-free survival of 53% *vs.* 48% for the adjuvant hormonal arm (p = 0.33). Patients treated with whole-pelvis RT plus a boost had a 4-year progression-free survival rate of 56% *vs.* 46% for the prostate only RT (p = 0.014). In the whole pelvis RT plus neoadjuvant hormonal manipulation arm, the progression-free survival rate was 61% at 4.5 years *vs.* 45% for the prostate only plus neoadjuvant hormonal manipulation, 49% for the whole-pelvis plus - adjuvant hormonal therapy arm, and 47% for the prostate only without adjuvant hormonal therapy (p = 0.005). Overall survival was not statistically significant for any of the arms (p = 0.15), being 88% for the whole-pelvis plus neoadjuvant hormonal therapy *vs.* 81–83% for each of the remaining three arms.[36]

Two additional randomized studies have been reported: Laverdiere accrued 120 patients to a 3-arm trial of RT alone, *vs.* RT plus 3 months of neoadjuvant hormonal manipulation with LHRH-agonist, *vs.* RT plus neoadjuvant LHRH-agonist and an additional 6 months of adjuvant LHRH-agonist. Patients were eligible if they had clinically measurable disease by digital-rectal exam and no distant metastasis. At 12 and 24 months there was a statistically significant decrease in the positive biopsy rate in favor of the radiation plus hormonal therapy arms and an increase in biochemical control at 12 months in the hormonal and radiation arms, although this was not apparent at 24 months.[37]

Finally, Granfors *et al.* randomized men to hormonal therapy and radiation versus RT alone, with hormonal therapy deferred until clinical disease progression. All patients underwent pelvic lymph node staging prior to randomization and both node-positive and node-negative patients were included. The patient population in this study was small since the study was closed early due to a significant difference in the two arms. The hormonal therapy was orchiectomy performed approximately one month before radiotherapy. Pelvic radiation fields were given. At a median follow-up of 9.3 years, immediate orchiectomy was associated with an increase in median survival of more than 3 years. Overall survival was 62% in the immediate therapy group *vs.* 39% in the deferred therapy group ($p = 0.02$). When the results were analyzed by node status at study entry, the survival difference favoring immediate therapy was only seen in the node positive patients ($p = 0.007$), which may reflect the lower number of events in node negative, i.e. more favorable patients.[38]

In summary, the available data from trials comparing RT plus androgen ablation to RT alone have shown significant differences based on endpoints such as biochemical failure and biopsy positivity. Two studies have demonstrated an improved overall survival for immediate hormonal therapy.[29,30,38] Two have shown no significant difference in survival between immediate and deferred therapy[8,25,28] and it is too early to draw definitive conclusions from the RTOG 92-02 and RTOG 94-13 studies. A difference in the studies, which may partially explain these differences in survival, may be that the hormonal therapy was commenced before the patients underwent the first RT treatment, whereas in those studies in which no survival benefit was seen, the hormonal therapy was commenced at the end of the course of RT. Patients with clinical T_3 tumor with favorable Gleason score (≤ 6) seem to benefit from short course neoadjuvant total androgen blockade with LHRH agonist and antiandrogen (flutamide) for 4 months (2 months before RT and during RT). Patients with any T stage with Gleason score 8–10 seem to benefit from LHRH treatment (≥ 2 years). Based on a metanalysis of RTOG protocols, patients with T_3 Gleason score 7 tumors also appear to benefit from long term hormonal manipulation. This may more likely reflect the control of micrometastatic disease.[39] Finally, a study recently completed by the RTOG (RTOG 99-10) is investigating, in a randomized fashion, 2 months *vs.* 7 months total androgen blockade prior to definitive RT in intermediate risk prostate cancer patients.

It appears therefore, that there are benefits to the combination of hormonal therapy and RT for patients with adenocarcinoma of the prostate, likely as a result of its potential for cytoreduction, as well as for control of metastatic disease.

Hormone Therapy and Brachytherapy

No randomized trial has been completed analyzing the role of hormone suppression in patients treated with brachytherapy, i.e. the placement of radioactive seeds within the prostate. A retrospective matched-pair analysis failed to identify an improvement in survival for low risk patients treated with hormone therapy and brachytherapy *vs.* brachytherapy alone. Stratification by Gleason score and pretreatment PSA also failed to reveal a subpopulation that benefited from hormonal therapy.[40]

In a series from Seattle, the addition of hormone suppression did not significantly increase freedom from PSA failure in patients treated with the combination of EBRT and brachytherapy.[41] However, Stone and Stock[42] reported improved freedom from biochemical failure at 4 years for intermediate-risk patients treated with 6 months of hormonal therapy and brachytherapy compared to brachytherapy alone. High risk patients appeared to have a similar benefit in another report.[43] However, at this time the primary benefit of short-term use of hormonal therapy with brachytherapy is limited to reduction of prostate volume. It is possible that intermediate-risk patients may benefit from hormonal therapy in association with brachytherapy, although the majority of studies have short follow-up and therefore the effect of hormonal therapy is difficult to interpret, as it may be masking PSA failure in the combination arm.

Potential Mechanisms of Androgen Ablation and Radiation Therapy

Androgen dependence of the prostate was described more than 100 years ago when the effect of castration on prostate hypertrophy was demonstrated.[44] Higgins and Hodges in 1941 showed the androgen dependence of prostate adenocarcinoma through orchiectomy and measuring the levels of acid phosphatase in patients with metastatic disease.[45] This work ultimately led to that of Walsh, who summarized the mechanism of action of androgens on prostate growth.[46] Histologic changes resulting from androgen deprivation in malignant prostate cancer cells include glandular shrinkage, cytoplasmic vacuolization, nuclear pyknosis, and degeneration of the tumor cells.[47]

The mechanism by which malignant and non-malignant tissues balance cell numbers are being better elucidated. Various factors are capable of tilting the balance in one direction or another. Active prostate cell cycling, for example, may be promoted by androgens through stimulation of growth factors and through bcl-2-mediated gene products. Programmed cell death (apoptosis) may conversely be triggered by androgen deprivation, influencing expression of cathepsin-D by abnormal p53 gene expression and by radiation. The role of apoptosis is supported by the presence of pyknosis and nuclear fragments.[48]

The mechanism of radiation cell kill in prostate cancer remains uncertain. DNA double-strand breaks are responsible, as well as induction of apoptosis. A number of investigators have shown radiation-induced apoptosis in a variety of cell systems.[49,50] Pollack *et al.* demonstrated apoptosis following radiation of prostate adenocarcinoma in the Dunning R3327 rat model.[51]

The rationale for androgen ablation (AA) plus RT may be divided by the treatment strategies of neoadjuvant *vs.* adjuvant AA. Neoadjuvant AA decreases clonogen numbers, leaving fewer cells for radiation to eradicate. The addition of RT leads to an additive cell kill, which is more likely to be curative to patients who otherwise might have failed single modality treatment. Neoadjuvant AA plus RT may also enhance cell death by a supra-additive effect, i.e. cells "weakened" (but not eradicated) by the hormonal therapy become more susceptible to cell killing by RT. This latter mechanism may also be that by which adjuvant AA, i.e. hormonal therapy started during or immediately after RT has its beneficial effect. This may occur via apoptosis, with radiation and hormonal therapies shunting more cells down the apoptotic pathway than either therapy alone. Additive cell killing may also be a mechanism for the effect of adjuvant AA.

Work by Joon *et al.* using the Dunning R3327 rat model showed that radiation alone or castration alone induced apoptotic indices of about 2% or less, primarily through propagation of the cell cycle, but when AA preceded RT, approximately 10% apoptotic indices were noted, representing a 5-fold increase. In a protracted course of fractionated RT this may total a significant degree of additional cell kill. The maximum effect was sequence and timing dependent, since apoptosis was significantly enhanced when AA was given 3 days before 7 Gy radiation and no supra-additive effect was achieved when AA was initiated at the same time as radiation or when radiation was given 3–4 weeks after AA.[52] These data suggest that neoadjuvant AA may be preferable to adjuvant AA although fractionation studies are needed to investigate the impact of fractionation on cell killing. It should also be noted, somewhat paradoxically, that it has been reported that some patients with abnormal p53 expression may fare more poorly if androgen deprivation is part of their therapy, than if it is not.[53]

The Shionogi tumor system has been an important model for prostate cancer as it is androgen-sensitive and progresses in an androgen-independent manner following androgen deprivation. In a series of studies, the radiation dose required to control 50% of the tumors (TCD_{50}) was reduced 50% by both neoadjuvant and adjuvant androgen deprivation; however, the effect of androgen deprivation was greatest when it preceded radiation and if radiation was deferred until maximal tumor regression. If the period of neoadjuvant deprivation is extended too far, however, the advantage is largely lost. The degree of response to neoadjuvant androgen deprivation can also be used in the system as a predictor of response to subsequent radiation, since some tumors which showed a slow response to androgen deprivation had a significantly higher TCD_{50}, then those that had a rapid response to androgen deprivation. Androgen deprivation given after RT also reduces TCD_{50}, but to a lesser degree than neoadjuvant therapy. It is possible that the neoadjuvant approach leads to a synergistic effect with RT, while the adjuvant approach reflects the effect of independent cell killing.[54,55]

Other mechanisms may also be involved in the favorable results of hormonal therapy and RT, including volume reduction leading to improved oxygenation of tumor, which through the production of free oxygen radicals, leads to increased radiation sensitivity.

Future Directions

The use of hormonal therapy in the treatment of prostate cancer has moved from castration, to the use of estrogen and similar compounds, and now to the use of LHRH agonists. The use of GnRH antagonists, which inhibit LH production and cause suppression of testosterone and dihydrotestosterone, is also being investigated.[56-58] GnRH antagonists do not stimulate LH and testosterone production, which may cause a temporary worsening of cancer or symptoms, as is the case when LHRH agonists are initiated. The optimal combinations of hormonal therapy, whether LHRH alone, or with antiandrogen, or the use of other new agents to be used in conjunction with RT, have yet to be fully defined. In addition, the optimal timing and duration of hormonal therapy and which group of patients stand to benefit the most, taking into account potential for disease control, side effects, and possible survival benefit, still need to be elucidated. The integration of chemotherapy and other therapies, e.g. gene therapy[59] and AA, with RT in the treatment of prostate cancer also represents important challenges to improving the results of treatment. It is hoped that such improvements will lead to a positive impact on the lives of the many patients with this disease.

References

1. Jemal A, Tiwari RC, Murray T, Ghafoor A, Samuels A, Ward E, Fewer EJ, Thun MJ (2004) Cancer Statistics, 2004. *CA Cancer J Clin* 54:8–29.
2. Pollack A, Zagars GK (1997) External beam radiotherapy dose response of prostate cancer. *Int J Radiat Oncol Biol Phys* 39:1011–1018.
3. Shipley WU, Thames HD, Sandler HM, Hanks GE, Zietman AL, Perez CA, Kuban DA, Hancock SL, Smith CD (1999) Radiation therapy for clinically localized prostate cancer: A multi-institutional pooled analysis. *JAMA* 281: 1598–1604.
4. Keyser D, Kupelian PA, Zippe CD, Levin HS, Klein EA (1997) Stage T1-2 prostate cancer with pretreatment prostate-specific antigen level < or = 10 ng/ml: Radiation therapy or surgery? *Int J Radiat Oncol Biol Phys* 38:723–729.
5. Brachman DG, Thomas T, Hilbe J, Beyer DC (2000) Failure-free survival following brachytherapy alone or external beam irradiation alone for T1-2

prostate tumors in 2222 patients: Results from a single practice. *Int J Radiat Oncol Biol Phys* 48:111–117.

6. D'Amico AV, Whittington R, Malkowicz SB, Schultz D, Blank K, Broderick GA, Tomaszewski JE, Renshaw AA, Kaplan I, Beard CJ, Wein A (1998) Biochemical outcome after radical prostatectomy, external beam radiation therapy, or interstitial radiation therapy for clinically localized prostate cancer. *JAMA* 280:969–974.

7. del Regato JA, Trailins AH, Pittman DD (1993) Twenty years follow-up of patients with inoperable cancer of the prostate (stage C) treated by radiotherapy: Report of a national cooperative study. *Int J Radiat Oncol Biol Phys* 26:197–201.

8. Zagars GK, von Eschenbach AC, Ayala AG (1993) Prognostic factors in prostate cancer. Analysis of 874 patients treated with radiation therapy. *Cancer* 72:1709–1725.

9. Hanks GE, Lee WR, Hanlon AL, Hunt M, Kaplan E, Epstein BE, Movsas B, Schultheiss TE (1996) Conformal technique dose escalation for prostate cancer: Biochemical evidence of improved cancer control with higher doses in patients with pretreatment prostate-specific antigen > or = 10 ng/ml. *Int J Radiat Oncol Biol Phys* 35:861–868.

10. Hanks GE, Hanlon AL, Pinover WH, Horwitz EM, Price RA, Schultheiss T (2000) Dose selection for prostate cancer patients based on dose comparison and dose response studies. *Int J Radiat Oncol Biol Phys* 46:823–832.

11. Zelefsky MJ, Leibel SA, Gaudin PB, Kutcher GJ, Fleshner NE, Venkatramen ES, Reuter VE, Fair WR, Ling CC, Fuks Z (1998) Dose escalation with three-dimensional conformal radiation therapy affects the outcome in prostate cancer. *Int J Radiat Oncol Biol Phys* 41:491–500.

12. Symon Z, Griffith KA, McLaughlin PW, Sullivan M, Sandler HM (2003) Dose escalation for localized prostate cancer: Substantial benefit observed with 3D conformal therapy. *Int J Radiat Oncol Biol Phys* 57:384–390.

13. Bey P, Carrie C, Beckendorf V, Ginestet C, Aletti P, Madelis G, Luporsi E, Pommier P, Cowen D, Gonzague-Casablanca L, Simonian-Sauve M, Maingon P, Naudy S, Lagrange JL, Marcie S (2000) Dose escalation with 3D-CRT in prostate cancer: French study of dose escalation with conformal 3D radiotherapy in prostate cancer—preliminary results. *Int J Radiat Oncol Biol Phys* 48:513–517.

14. Pollack A, Zagars GK, Smith LG, Lee JJ/von Eschenbach AC, Antolak JA, Starkschall G, Rosen I (2000) Preliminary results of a randomized radiotherapy dose-escalation study comparing 70 Gy with 78 Gy for prostate cancer. *J Clin Oncol* 18:3904–3911.

15. Pollack A, Zagars GK, Starkschall G, Antolak JA, Lee JJ, Huang E, von Eschenbach AC, Kuban DA, Rosen I (2002) Prostate cancer radiation dose response: Results of the M. D. Anderson phase III randomized trial. *Int J Radiat Oncol Biol Phys* 53:1097–1105.

16. Kaplan EL, Meier P (1958) Nonparametric estimation from incomplete observations. *J Am Stat Assoc* 53:457–481.

17. Michalski JM, Winter K, Purdy JA, Wilder R, Perez CA, Roach M, Parliament M, Pollack A, Markoe A, Harms WB, Sandler H, Cox JD (2002) Trade-off to low-grade toxicity with conformal radiation therapy for prostate cancer on Radiation Therapy Oncology Group 9406. *Semin Radiat Oncol* 12:75–80.

18. Perez CA, Michalski JM, Purdy JA, Wasserman TH, Williams K, Lockett MA (2000) Three-dimensional conformal therapy or standard irradiation in localized carcinoma of prostate: Preliminary results of a nonrandomized comparison. *Int J Radiat Oncol Biol Phys* 47:629–637.

19. Zelefsky MJ, Cowen D, Fuks Z, Shike M, Burman C, Jackson A, Venkatramen ES, Leibel SA (1999) Long term tolerance of high dose three-dimensional conformal radiotherapy in patients with localized prostate carcinoma. *Cancer* 85:2460–2468.

20. Green N, Melbye RW, Lipsett J, Kurohara SS, George FW 3rd, Cosgrove M, Morrow J (1975) Prostate carcinoma: Measures to improve therapeutic response and prevent complications. *Urology* 6:287–290.

21. Green N, Bodner H, Broth E, Garrett G, Goldberg H, Goldstein A, Polse S, Skaist L, Treible D, Wallack H (1981) Response of lymph node metastasis to sequential estrogen and radiation therapy in prostate carcinoma. *Urology* 18:137–142.

22. Green N, Bodner H, Broth E, Chiang C, Garrett J, Goldstein A, Goldberg H, Gualtieri V, Gray R, Jaffe J, Kaplan R, Polse S, Ross S, Skaist L, Treible D, Valz A, Wallack H (1984) Improved control of bulky prostate carcinoma with sequential estrogen and radiation therapy. *Int J Radiat Oncol Biol Phys* 10:971–976.

23. van der Werf-Messing B, Sourek-Zikova V, Blonk DI (1976) Localized advanced carcinoma of the prostate: Radiation therapy versus hormonal therapy. *Int J Radiat Oncol Biol Phys* 1:1043–1048.

24. del Regato JA (1979) Long-term curative results of radiotherapy of patients with inoperable prostatic carcinoma. Erskine Memorial Lecture 1978. *Radiology* 131:291–297.

25. Zagars GK, Johnson DE, von Eschenbach AC, Hussey DH (1988) Adjuvant estrogen following radiation therapy for stage C adenocarcinoma of the

prostate: Long-term results of a prospective randomized study. *Int J Radiat Oncol Biol Phys* 14:1085–1091.

26. Pilepich MV, Krall JM, John MJ, Rubin P, Porter AT, Marcial VA, Martz KL (1989) Hormonal cytoreduction in locally advanced carcinoma of the prostate treated with definitive radiotherapy: Preliminary results of RTOG 83-07. *Int J Radiat Oncol Biol Phys* 16:813–817.

27. Pilepich MV, Caplan R, Byhardt RW, Lawton CA, Gallagher MJ, Mesic JB, Hanks GE, Coughlin CT, Porter A, Shipley WU, Grignon D (1997) Phase III trial of androgen suppression using goserelin in unfavorable-prognosis carcinoma of the prostate treated with definitive radiotherapy: Report of Radiation Therapy Oncology Group Protocol 85-31. *J Clin Oncol* 15:1013–1021.

28. Lawton CA, Winter K, Murray K, Machtay M, Mesic JB, Hanks GE, Coughlin CT, Pilepich MV (2001) Updated results of the phase III Radiation Therapy Oncology Group (RTOG) trial 85-31 evaluating the potential bene-fit of androgen suppression following standard radiation therapy for unfa-vorable prognosis carcinoma of the prostate. *Int J Radiat Oncol Biol Phys* 49:937–946.

29. Bolla M, Collette L, Blank L, Warde P, Dubois JB, Mirimanoff RO, Storme G, Bernier J, Kuten A, Sternberg C, Mattelaer J, Lopez Torecilla J, Pfeffer JR, Lino Cutajar C, Zurlo A, Pierart M (2002) Long-term results with immediate androgen suppression and external irradiation in patients with locally advanced prostate cancer (an EORTC study): A phase III randomized trial. *Lancet* 360:103–106.

30. Bolla M, Gonzalez D, Warde P, Dubois JB, Mirimanoff RO, Storme G, Bernier J, Kuten A, Sternberg C, Gil T, Collette L, Pierart M (1997) Improved survival in patients with locally advanced prostate cancer treated with radio-therapy and goserelin. *N Engl J Med* 337:295–300.

31. Pilepich MV, Krall JM, al-Sarraf M, John MJ, Doggett R, Sause WT, Lawton CA, Abrams RA, Rotman M, Rubin P, Shipley WU, Grignon D, Caplan R, Cox JD (1995) Androgen deprivation with radiation therapy com-pared with radiation therapy alone for locally advanced prostatic carcinoma: A randomized comparative trial of the Radiation Therapy Oncology Group. *Urology* 45:616–623.

32. Pilepich MV, Winter K, John MJ, Mesic JB, Sause W, Rubin P, Lawton C, Machtay M, Grignon D (2001) Phase III radiation therapy oncology group (RTOG) trial 86-10 of androgen deprivation adjuvant to definitive radiother-apy in locally advanced carcinoma of the prostate. *Int J Radiat Oncol Biol Phys* 50:1243–1252.

33. Horwitz EM, Winter K, Hanks GE, Lawton CA, Russell AH, Machtay M (2001) Subset analysis of RTOG 85-31 and 86-10 indicates an advantage for long-term vs. short-term adjuvant hormones for patients with locally advanced nonmetastatic prostate cancer treated with radiation therapy. *Int J Radiat Oncol Biol Phys* 49:947–956.

34. Hanks GE, Pajak TF, Porter A, Grignon D, Brereton H, Venkatesan V, Horwitz EM, Lawton C, Rosenthal SA, Sandler HM, Shipley WU (2003) Radiation Therapy Oncology Group. Phase III trial of long-term adjuvant androgen deprivation after neoadjuvant hormonal cytoreduction and radiotherapy in locally advanced carcinoma of the prostate: The Radiation Therapy Oncology Group Protocol 92-02. *J Clin Oncol* 21:3972–3978.

35. Roach M 3rd, Marquez C, Yuo HS, Narayan P, Coleman L, Nseyo UO, Navvab Z, Carroll PR (1994) Predicting the risk of lymph node involvement using the pre-treatment prostate specific antigen and Gleason score in men with clinically localized prostate cancer. *Int J Radiat Oncol Biol Phys* 28:33–37.

36. Roach M 3rd, Lu JD, Lawton C, Hsu IC, Machtay M, Seider MJ, Rotman M, Jones C, Asbell SO, Valicenti RK, Han S, Thomas CR, Jr., Shipley WS (2001) A phase III trial comparing whole-pelvic (WP) to prostate only (PO) radiotherapy and neoadjuvant to adjuvant total androgen suppression (TAS): Preliminary analysis of RTOG 94-13. *Int J Radiat Oncol Biol Phys* 51:3.

37. Laverdiere J, Gomez JL, Cusan L, Suburu ER, Diamond P, Lemay M, Candas B, Fortin A, Labrie F (1997) Beneficial effect of combination hormonal therapy administered prior and following external beam radiation therapy in localized prostate cancer. *Int J Radiat Oncol Biol Phys* 37:247–252.

38. Granfors T, Modig H, Damber JE, Tomic R (1998) Combined orchiectomy and external radiotherapy versus radiotherapy alone for nonmetastatic prostate cancer with or without pelvic lymph node involvement: A prospective randomized study. *J Urol* 159:2030–2034.

39. Roach M 3rd, Lu J, Pilepich MV, Asbell SO, Mohuidden M, Terry R, Grignon D, Lawton C, Shipley W, Cox J (2000) Predicting long-term survival, and the need for hormonal therapy: A meta-analysis of RTOG prostate cancer trials. *Int J Radiat Oncol Biol Phys* 47:617–627.

40. Potters L, Torre T, Ashley R, Leibel S (2000) Examining the role of neoadjuvant androgen deprivation in patients undergoing prostate brachytherapy. *J Clin Oncol* 18:1187–1192.

41. Sylvester JE, Blasko JC, Grimm PD, Meier R, Malmgren JA (2003) Ten-year biochemical relapse-free survival after external beam radiation and

brachytherapy for localized prostate cancer: The Seattle experience. *Int J Radiat Oncol Biol Phys* 57:944–952.

42. Stone NN, Stock RG (1999) Prostate brachytherapy: Treatment strategies. *J Urol* 162:421–426.

43. Lee LN, Stock RG, Stone NN (2002) Role of hormonal therapy in the management of intermediate- to high-risk prostate cancer treated with permanent radioactive seed implantation. *Int J Radiat Oncol Biol Phys* 52:444–452.

44. White JW (1893) The present position of the surgery of the hypertrophied prostate. *Ann Surg* 18:152–188.

45. Higgins C, Hodges C (1941) The effects of castration, of estrogen and of androgen injection of serum phosphatase in metastatic carcinoma of the prostate: Studies of prostate cancer. *Cancer Res* 1:293–297.

46. Walsh PC (1975) Physiologic basis for hormonal therapy in carcinoma of the prostate. *Urol Clin North Am* 2:125–140.

47. Hellstrom M, Haggman M, Brandstedt S, de la Torre M, Pedersen K, Jarlsfeldt I, Wijkstrom H, Busch C (1993) Histopathological changes in androgen-deprived localized prostatic cancer. A study in total prostatectomy specimens. *Eur Urol* 24:461–465.

48. Gleave M, Hsieh JT, Gao CA, von Eschenbach AC, Chung LW (1991) Acceleration of human prostate cancer growth *in vivo* by factors produced by prostate and bone fibroblasts. *Cancer Res* 51:3753–3761.

49. Fuks Z, Haimowitz-Friedman A, Kolesnick RN (1995) The role of the sphingomyelin pathway and protein kinase C in radiation-induced cell kill. In: Devita VT, Hellman S, Rosenberg SA, eds. *Important Advances in Oncology.* JB Lippincott, Philadelphia, pp. 15–31.

50. Meyn RE, Stephens LC, Ang KK, Hunter NR, Brock WA, Milas L, Peters LJ (1993) Heterogeneity in the development of apoptosis in irradiated murine tumours of different histologies. *Int J Radiat Oncol Biol Phys* 64:583–591.

51. Joon DL, Hasegawa M, Wu CS, Sikes C, Khoo VS, Zagars GK, Terry NHA, Meistrich ML, Pollack A (1996) Supra-additive apoptotic response in predominantly quiescent prostate tumors when treated with androgen ablation and radiotherapy. *Int J Radiat Oncol Biol Phys* 36:191 (Abstract).

52. Joon DL, Hasegawa M, Sikes C, Khoo VS, Terry NHA, Zagars GK, Meistrich ML, Pollack A (1997) Supraadditive apoptotic response of R3327-G rat prostate tumors to androgen ablation and radiation. *Int J Radiat Oncol Biol Phys* 38:1071–1077.

53. Grignon DJ, Caplan R, Sarkar FH, Lawton CA, Hammond EH, Pilepich MV, Forman JD, Mesic J, Fu KK, Abrams RA, Pajak TF, Shipley WU, Cox JD

(1997) p53 status and prognosis of locally advanced prostatic adenocarcinoma: A study based on RTOG 86-10. *J Natl Cancer Inst* 89:158–165.

54. Zietman AL, Nakfoor BM, Prince EA, Gerweck LE (1997) The effect of androgen deprivation and radiation therapy on an androgen-sensitive murine tumor: An *in vitro* and *in vivo* study. *Cancer J Sc Am* 3:31–36.

55. Zietman AL, Prince EA, Nakfoor BM, Park JJ (1997) Androgen deprivation and radiation therapy: Sequencing studies using the Shionogi *in vivo* tumor system. *Int J Radiat Oncol Biol Phys* 38:1067–1070.

56. Campion M, Kuca B, Garnick MB (1999) The magnitude of Lupron® (L) or Zoladex® (Z) testosterone (T) and Luteinizing Hormone (LH) surge is dependent on formulation: Comparative results of L and Z vs abarelix-Depot (A-D), a GnRH antagonist devoid of androgen surge. *Proc Am Soc Clin Oncol* 18:320a (Abstract).

57. Garnick MB, Gittelman M, Steidle C, *et al.* (1998) Abarelix (PPI-149), a novel and potent GnRH antagonist, induces a rapid and profound prostate gland volume reduction (PGVR) and androgen suppression before brachytherapy (BT) or radiation therapy (XRT). *J Urol* 159:222a (Abstract).

58. Garnick MB, Tomera K, Campion M *et al.* (1999) Abarelix-depot (A-D A sustained-release (SR) formulation of a potent GnRH pure antagonist in patients (pts) with prostate cancer (PrCA): Phase II clinical results and endocrine comparison with superagonist Lupron® (L) and Zoladex® (Z). *Proc Am Soc Clin Oncol* 18:321a (Abstract).

59. Teh BS, Aguilar-Cordova E, Kernen K, Chou CC, Shalev M, Vlachaki MT, Miles B, Kadmon D, Mai WY, Caillouet J, Davis M, Ayala G, Wheeler T, Brady J, Carpenter LS, Lu HH, Chiu JK, Woo SY, Thompson T, Butler EB (2001) Phase I/II trial evaluating combined radiotherapy and *in situ* gene therapy with or without hormonal therapy in the treatment of prostate cancer — a preliminary report. *Int J Radiat Oncol Biol Phys* 51:605–613.

4

GENE THERAPY FOR PROSTATE CANCER

Juan Antonio Jiménez, Chinghai Kao, Sang-Jin Lee,
Chaeyong Jung and Thomas A. Gardner

*Urology Research Laboratory, Departments of Urology, Microbiology
and Immunology, Walther Oncology Center
Indiana University Medical Center
Indianapolis, Indiana, USA*

Introduction

In 2003, it was estimated that prostate cancer would account for the most new cancer diagnoses, aside from skin cancer, at 220,900 men in the United States and was the second most common cause of cancer deaths at 28,900 men. A steady decline in the annual age-adjusted prostate cancer death rates over the past five years as recorded in the SEER Cancer Statistics Review would suggest improvements in early detection and treatment of locally confined prostate cancer.[1] While this may be true, at the present time, treatment options prolong life; however, most patients will eventually experience local recurrence or develop advanced disease. Androgen ablation therapy slows the dissemination of the disease but once the cancer changes its androgen status, tumors become refractory to hormonal treatment. A greater understanding of the molecular events underlying cancer and the subsequent development of metastatic disease allows gene therapy approaches targeted against these molecular events to be developed. Our laboratory has focused its energy on the development and application of tissue-specific promoters such as *osteocalcin* (*OC*) and *prostate-specific enhancer sequence* (*PSES*) as well as the development of molecular therapy for androgen-independent primary and metastatic prostate cancer.[2–6]

Gene Therapy Strategy

The ultimate goals of research in this area are to develop treatment modalities that increase survival, enhance quality of life, and cure men afflicted with prostate cancer. In order to do so, four factors must be considered when developing strategies. These include the selection of the disease to be targeted, the genetic material to transfer, the method of delivery, and the route of administration. The safety and efficacy of the trial underlie each of these factors.

The discussion begins with the selection of the disease and patient to target. The progression of prostate cancer from benign dysplasia to malignancy to metastatic disease is well known and results from the accumulation of multiple genetic defects. Several stages of prostate cancer are susceptible to treatment with gene therapy. Currently, most of the stages in the progression from localized prostate cancer to metastatic disease have been targeted; however, many more can be targeted as vector development and understanding of the molecular events continue. Lack of conventional therapies for locally advanced, locally recurrent, or metastatic prostate cancer makes these patients excellent candidates to target. Of course, as with most therapies, the ability to treat men with low volume disease should enhance the success of the therapy. This is a critical point for the therapeutic approaches discussed below.

With further research into the genetic determinants of prostate cancer progression, a protective approach could be used to decrease the morbidity and mortality associated with conditions such as benign prostatic hyperplasia (BPH) and prostatic intraepithelial neoplasia (PIN). Current studies have demonstrated a prophylactic effect against the development of prostate cancer with conventional therapies for BPH.[7] As prostate-specific targeting and tumor killing efficacy continue to increase, the laboratory vision of a molecular prostatectomy may soon translate into a clinical reality. Because the prostate is a non-essential organ post-fertility and the side effects from chemotherapy, radiation, and surgical intervention are so great, molecular ablation has vast appeal.

The genetic material for transfer is determined by the objective of the therapy. For example, gene therapy for prostate cancer can provide corrective therapy for genetic alterations that give the cancer a survival advantage such as those affecting tumor suppressors or growth-promoting oncogenes; however, because multiple mutations occur in the pathogenesis and progression of cancer, correction of one genetic insult may not be sufficient to change the cancer cell phenotype. Nevertheless, *in vivo* correction of single gene defects has been successful in several preclinical studies.[8–11] Targets for corrective therapy include the proto-oncogenes *p53, p21, p16*, and *retinoblastoma (Rb)*, and certain cell adhesion molecules (CAMs), as well as oncogenes *ras, myc*, and *bcl-2*. A second objective of molecular therapy for prostate cancer is to deliver genes that are capable of destroying tumor cells either directly or indirectly. Such cytoreductive therapies include the direct killing of prostate cancer cells by replication-competent oncolytic viruses and the indirect killing of cancer cells through the delivery of suicide genes such as pro-drug enzyme and apoptosis-inducing genes. The final objective of gene therapy for prostate cancer is to enhance the body's antitumor immune response. Current approaches involve *ex vivo* gene therapy of autologous tumor cells and subsequent vaccination with the irradiated cells now expressing cytokines such as interleukin-2 (IL-2) and granulocyte-macrophage colony-stimulating factor (GM-CSF), *ex vivo* gene transfer of genes encoding tumor antigens and subsequent vaccination leading to enhanced induction of T-cell immunity, *in vivo* intratumoral gene transfer of cytokine genes, and delivery of naked tumor DNA or RNA and the subsequent uptake and expression by antigen presenting cells such as dendrites.[12] Table 1 summarizes these objectives as they appear in clinical trials registered with the Office of Biologic Activities (OBA).

The currently available methods of delivery of genetic information are listed in Table 2. The ideal method of delivery would transfer the genetic material efficiently and specifically to the targeted organ, not be harmful to the patient, and be inexpensive to produce and administer. Each vector has advantages and disadvantages as couriers of genetic information. Adenovirus, perhaps the most commonly administered vector, clearly has its advantages and disadvantages. For example, adenovirus can deliver large amounts of genetic information with high efficiency regardless of the cell cycle status; however, it is highly immunogenic. To further compound this issue, it is believed that up to 75% of the population have humoral immunity to several serotypes of adenovirus due to prior infection.

J. A. Jiménez et al.

Table 1. Current Approaches for Prostate Cancer Gene Therapy

Strategy	Vector(s)	DNA Transferred
Corrective	Retrovirus	p53
	Adenovirus	p16
		c-myc
Cytoreductive	Adenovirus	TK
(suicide)		CD
		TK/CD
		NIS
		OC promoter
(oncolytic)		PB/PSA promoter
		PB/PSE promoter
Immunotherapy	Retrovirus	GM-CSF
	Vaccinia/fowl	MUC-1/IL-2
		PSA
	Liposome	PSA
		hTERT
		PSMA
		IL-2
	RNA	Tumor RNA
	AAV	GM-CSF
	Adenovirus	IL-12
		Inf-α

Efforts have been made to create less immunogenic forms of the virus as well as gutless forms of the virus that are incapable of replicating in immunocompromised patients. Such replication-deficient adenoviruses are achieved by deleting the early genes responsible for the control of viral replication.[13]

Finally, the route of administration is determined by a combination of the previous three factors. At the present time, most prostate cancer gene therapy trials involve the intratumoral injection of the vector which is quite suitable given the ability to visualize the prostate using ultrasound and its convenient transrectal access. Ultimately, the desired route of administration is systemic intravenous transfusion of the vector. Limiting factors include vector half-life, hematologic inactivation of the vector, and

Table 2. Comparison of Vector Systems in Gene Therapy

Attribute	Retrovirus/ Lentivirus	Adenovirus (Ad)/'gutless'	Adeno-associated Virus (AAV)	Vaccinia/ Fowlpox Virus	Non-viral (Liposome)
In vivo gene transfer rate	**Low**/High	High	High	High	Low
Size limit of DNA transfer	8 kb	10/35 kb	**<5 kb**	>30 kb	? Limit
Cell cycling dependent	**Yes**/No	No	No	No	No
Genome integrating	**Yes**	No	**Yes**	No	No
DNA expression stability	Stable	Transient/ stable	Stable	Transient	Transient
Immunoreactive	No	Yes/No	No	Yes	No
Use in previous clinical trial	Yes/**No**	Yes/**No**	Yes	Yes	Yes

This table lists the important attributes of the currently used gene therapy vectors for prostate cancer. The bold items are felt to be the particular vector.

infection of non-target organs. As prostate-specific promoter systems become more effective, gene therapy may become the silver-bullet that seeks and destroys cancer cells in the prostate and distant metastatic sites.

Tissue-Specific Promoters

Recently, much effort has been made to develop tissue-specific delivery systems that eliminate the threat of harm to the patient. Several studies have demonstrated the importance of tissue-specific vectors, revealing systemic toxicity with the administration of high doses of nonspecific vectors.[14,15] Essentially, viral vectors can transfer their therapeutic genes to any cell in the body, provided that it expresses the correct receptors for the virus. Through the use of prostate-specific promoters and enhancers, the expression of a therapeutic gene can be limited to cells that contain the appropriate activators and transcription factors. One limitation to this technology is low level leaky activation of prostate-specific promoters in non-prostatic tissues; however, the development of chimeric promoters promises greater prostate-specificity.

Osteocalcin Promoter

OC is a highly conserved bone gamma-carboxyglutamic acid protein (BGP) that has been shown to be transcriptionally regulated by 1,25-dihydroxyvitamin D_3.[16] This noncollagenous bone protein constitutes 1–2% of the total protein in bone, and its expression is limited to differentiated osteoblasts and osteotropic tumors.[17] Figure 1 depicts expression of *OC* RNA and protein in primary and metastatic prostate cancers. The osteoblastic nature of osseous prostate cancer metastases is well characterized,[18] and the mechanism is believed to be via its osteomimetic properties, specifically its ability to express bone-related proteins such as OC.[19] The human *OC* promoter contains numerous regulatory elements including a vitamin D-responsive element (VDRE), making it inducible by vitamin D_3 administration,[20,21] a glucocorticoid response element (GRE), an AP-1 binding site,[22] and an AML-1 binding site which has been shown to be responsible for 75% of *OC* expression.[23] The *OC* promoter retains its tissue specificity in a recombinant *OC* promoter-driven thymidine kinase (TK)-expressing adenoviral vector (Ad-OC-TK). Following infection with Ad-OC-TK, only cells of osteoblastic lineage expressed TK; furthermore, Ko *et al.* demonstrated that the addition of acyclovir (ACV) resulted in osteoblast-specific cell toxicity.[24] A similar strategy has been developed for the intralesional injection of Ad-OC-TK to osseous prostate cancer metastases followed by administration of valcyclovir (VAL). In phase I clinical trials, this therapy induced apoptosis in every lesion treated without serious adverse effects to the patients.[3,6]

Prostate-Specific Enhancer Sequence

Prostate-specific proteins such as prostate-specific antigen (PSA) and prostate-specific membrane antigen (PSMA) are released into the bloodstream when the prostatic basement membrane is compromised, such as

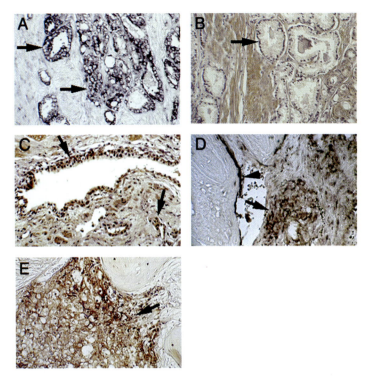

Fig. 1. Expression of OC RNA and protein in primary and metastatic prostate cancers. Nine primary tumors and ten osseous metastases stained positive for OC protein. RNA *in situ* hybridization was to characterize the expression of OC in prostate cancer cells. OC RNA transcripts were detected in the majority of primary (**A**) and metastatic (**D**) prostate cancers. OC protein was detected by immunohistochemical staining with OC4-30 anti-OC antibody (Takara Shuzo Co., LTD, Shiga, Japan). In three primary tumors, OC-positive staining was homogeneous (**C**); however, the other six had more OC-negative glands than positive glands (**B**). On the other hand, all ten osseous metastases stained OC-positive (**E**). Arrows indicate prostate cancer. The arrowhead indicates an osteoblast.

occurs in prostate cancer, and therefore is used as a sensitive marker for diagnosis and progression of prostate cancer.[25] PSA expression is androgen receptor (AR)-dependent, and its transcript levels are significantly reduced in the absence of androgen.[26] AR regulates *PSA* expression by binding to an androgen-responsive enhancer core (AREc) in the upstream 5′ flanking region of the *PSA* gene.[27,28] This promoter confers high tissue specificity and has been used in several gene therapy studies;[29–31] however, its utility in men undergoing androgen ablation therapy is limited. On the other hand, PSMA expression is upregulated under androgen-depleted conditions.[32] Its expression is elevated higher in prostate cancer than in benign hyperplasia or normal prostate.[33] In addition, serum PSMA levels are highest in patients with metastatic disease, suggesting enhanced PSMA expression as prostate cancer progresses.[34] Recently, the PSMA enhancer (PSME) was discovered within the third intron of the PSMA gene, *FOLH1*[35] and has been used for prostate-specific gene delivery under low androgen levels.[36] Our laboratory hypothesized that AREc and PSME could function synergistically and developed a novel chimeric promoter, prostate-specific enhancer sequence (PSES), with high transcriptional activity and strong prostate specificity.

Through deletion and linker scan mutagenesis, PSES was developed by locating the minimal sequences, AREc3 and PSME(del2) in AREc and PSME, respectively and placing AREc3 upstream from PSME(del2). AREc3 contains six GATA transcription factor binding sites and three AR binding sites leading to high enhancer activity once surrounding silencer regions are deleted. PSME(del2) contains eight AP-1 and three AP-3[37] binding sites acting as positive regulators in the absence of androgen and a downstream deletion of an *Alu* repeat that functions as a transcriptional silencer. As depicted in Fig. 2, PSES drives luciferase activity five-fold higher than universal promoter RSV and slightly higher than CMV promoter, and luciferase expression was detected in several PSA- and PSMA-positive prostate cancer cell lines, but not in PSA- and PSMA-negative prostate cells or non-prostate cell lines. PSES retains its prostate-specific nature in recombinant adenoviral vectors as well. Figure 3 shows the results after injection of *BALB/c* nude mice with Ad-CMV-luc and Ad-PSES-luc.[4] Due to its small size, high level of tissue specificity, and strong promoter activity in the presence or absence of androgen, PSES is an ideal promoter for use in prostate cancer gene therapy.

Human Telomerase Promoter

Telomeres are tandem repeat structures found at the termini of chromosomes that maintain chromosomal integrity by preventing DNA rearrangements, degradation, and end-to-end fusions. In most normal

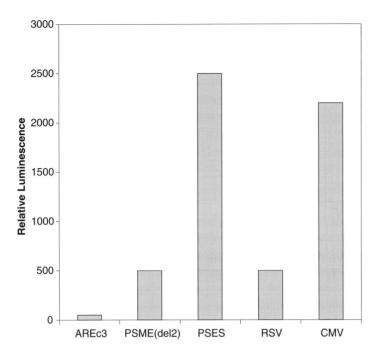

Fig. 2. Comparison of strength of promoter activities. 0.5 μg of pGL3/TATA containing AREc3, PSME(del2), PSES, RSV, or CMV promoters along with pRL-SV40 (*Renilla* luciferase) were transfected. Cells were grown in the absence of androgen. PSES demonstrates strong promoter activity at 5-fold the activity of RSV and slightly higher than that of CMV promoter. Furthermore, the activity of PSES is greater than the activity of AREc3 and PSME(del2) combined, suggesting a synergistic effect.

somatic cells, the telomeric cap is shortened with each cycle of DNA replication and cell division. When telomeres shorten to a critical length, cells progress toward irreversible arrest of growth and cellular senescence.[38] In contrast, tumor cells have evolved a means to prevent telomere shortening through the activation of the catalytic component of human telomerase reverse transcriptase (hTERT).[39] The *hTERT* promoter region has been cloned and characterized, and has high GC content. Unlike most promoters, it does not contain TATA or CAAT boxes.[40] Importantly, the *hTERT* promoter is active in most cancer cells including prostate cancer[41] and inactive in normal cells, thereby providing a unique tool to target cancer cells. Promising results have been reported using the *hTERT* promoter

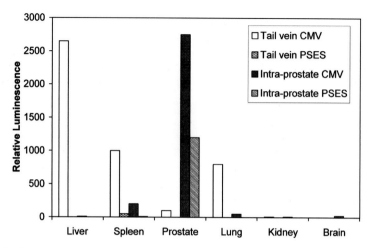

Fig. 3. *In vivo* PSES prostate-specificity comparison. Recombinant adenoviruses Ad-CMV-luc and Ad-PSES-luc were injected into male athymic mice, 7×10^{10} virus particles by tail vein injection or 1.4×10^{10} virus particles by intra-prostate injection. Mice were sacrificed and organs were harvested for luciferase activity 2 days post-injection. Following systemic injection, negligible levels of PSES-driven luciferase activity were detected in organs expected to take up adenovirus, mainly liver, spleen, and lung. To overcome the low infectivity of the prostate, intraprostatic injections were performed, revealing high PSES activity in the prostate.

to deliver TRAIL, an inducer of apoptosis[42] and to control the replication of an oncolytic adenovirus.[43] Our laboratory is investigating the use of the *hTERT* promoter in conjunction with a prostate-specific promoter to control adenoviral replication in a prostate cancer-specific manner.

Past Approaches

Over the past ten years, three categories of gene therapy approaches for prostate cancer have emerged, corrective gene therapy, cytoreductive gene therapy, and immunotherapy. Each molecular therapy has a strong foundation of preclinical data allowing for the approval of several clinical studies. Currently, 56 gene transfer protocols registered with the OBA are targeted against prostate cancer. This accounts for 15% of all cancer protocols listed to date.[44] Table 3 highlights the details of the prostate cancer

Table 3. Prostate Cancer Gene Therapy Trials (OBA Protocol List, 17 December 2003)[44]

Principal Investigator	Institution	Vector	Genetic Material	Year Reviewed
1. Simons, JW	Johns Hopkins, MD	Retrovirus	GM-CSF	1994
2. Steiner, MS	Vanderbilt Univ., TN	Retrovirus	c-myc	1995
3. Chen, AP	Nat. Naval Med, MD	Vaccinia/ fowlpox	PSA	1995
4. Paulson, DF	Duke Univ., NC	Liposome	IL-2	1995
5. Scardino, PT	MSKCC, NY	Adenovirus	HSV-TK	1996
6. Eder, JP	Dana-Farber, MD	Vaccinia/ fowlpox	PSA	1996
7. Sanda, MG	Univ. of Michigan, MI	Vaccinia/ fowlpox	PSA	1997
8. Belldegrun, AS	UCLA, CA	Liposome	IL-2	1997
9. Hall, SJ	Mt. Sinai, NY	Adenovirus	HSV-TK	1997
10. Belldegrun, AS	UCLA, CA	Adenovirus	p53	1997
11. Simons, JW	Johns Hopkins, MD	Retrovirus	GM-CSF	1997
12. Logothetis, CJ	MD Anderson, TX	Adenovirus	p53	1997
13. Kadmon, D	Baylor College, TX	Adenovirus	HSV-TK	1998
14. Simons, JW	Johns Hopkins, MD	Adenovirus	PSA	1998
15. Figlin, RA	UCLA, CA	Vaccinia/ fowlpox	MUC-1/IL-2	1998
16. Gardner, TA	Univ. of Virginia, VA	Adenovirus	OC-HSV-TK	1998
17. Eder, JP	Dana-Farber, MD	Vaccinia/ fowlpox	PSA	1999
18. Small, EJ	UCSF, CA	Retrovirus	GM-CSF	1999
19. Kaufman, HL	Albert Einstein, NY	Vaccinia/ fowlpox	PSA	1999
20. Vieweg, J	Duke Univ., NC	RNA	PSA	1999
21. Belldegrun, AS	UCLA, CA	Liposome	IL-2	1999
22. Small, EJ	UCSF, CA	Retrovirus	GM-SCF	1999

Table 3 (*Continued*)

Principal Investigator	Institution	Vector	Genetic Material	Year Reviewed
23. Kim, JH	Henry Ford Hosp., MI	Adenovirus	CD/TK	1999
24. Aguilar-Cordova, E	Harvard Univ., MA	Adenovirus	TK	1999
25. Gingrich, JR	Univ. of Tenn., TN	Adenovirus	p16	1999
26. Terris, MK	Stanford Univ., CA	Adenovirus	PSA	1999
27. Wilding, G	Univ. Of Wisc., WI	Adenovirus	PSA	1999
28. Belldegrun, AS	UCLA, CA	Liposome	IL-2	1999
29. Dahut, WL	NIH/NCI	Vaccinia/ fowlpox	PSA	1999
30. Arlen, PM	NIH/NCI	Vaccinia/ fowlpox	PSA	2000
31. Vieweg, J	Duke Univ., NC	RNA	Tumor RNA	2000
32. Pollack, A	Univ. of Texas, TX	Adenovirus	p53	2000
33. Gardner, TA	Indiana Univ., IN	Adenovirus	OC promoter	2000
34. Freytag, SO	Henry Ford Hosp., MI	Adenovirus	CD/TK	2000
35. Lubaroff, DM	Univ. of Iowa, IA	Adenovirus	PSA	2001
36. Miles, BJ	Baylor College, TX	Adenovirus	IL-12	2001
37. DeWeese, TL	Johns Hopkins, MD	Adenovirus	PB/PSE promoter	2001
38. Small, EJ	UCSF, CA	Adenovirus	PB/PSE promoter	2001
39. Dula, E	West Coast Clin. Res.	AAV	GM-CSF	2001
40. Freytag, SO	Henry Ford Hosp., MI	Adenovirus	CD/TK	2001
41. Scher, H	MSKCC, NY	Liposome	PSMA	2001
42. Corman, J	VA Puget Sound, VA	AAV	GM-CSF	2001
43. Pantuck, AJ	UCLA, LA	Vaccinia/ fowlpox	MUC-1/IL-2	2001
44. Vieweg, J	Duke, NC	RNA	hTERT	2001
45. Corman, J	VA Puget Sound, VA	Adenovirus	PSE promoter	2001
46. Vieweg, J	Duke, NC	RNA	PSA	2001
47. Dinney, CP	MD Anderson, TX	Adenovirus	Inf-α	2002
48. Dahut, W	NIH/NCI	Vaccinia/ fowlpox	PSA	2002

Table 3 (*Continued*)

Principal Investigator	Institution	Vector	Genetic Material	Year Reviewed
49. Morris, J	Mayo Clinic, MN	Adenovirus	NIS	2002
50. Kaufman, HL	Columbia, NY	Vaccinia/ fowlpox	PSA	2002
51. Zanetti, M	Univ. of Calif., CA	Liposome	hTERT	2002
52. Malkowicz, SB	Univ. of Penn., PA	Liposome	PSA	2002
53. Arlen, PM	NIH/NCI	Vaccinia/ fowlpox	PSA	2002
54. Corman, J	Virginia Mason, WI	Adenovirus	PSA	2003
55. Freytag, S	Henry Ford Hosp., MI	Adenovirus	HSV-TK	2003
56. Kantoff, P	Dana-Farber, MD	Vaccinia/ fowlpox	PSA	2003

trials registered with the OBA. Prostate cancer will remain a focus for laboratories due to the limited availability of treatments for advanced disease and the large population that is affected.

Corrective Gene Therapy

This approach repairs inherited or acquired genetic defects affecting the regulation of the cell growth cycle. A single prostate cancer cell may harbor several such mutations, giving it a survival advantage. The replacement of a damaged gene with the wild-type is often sufficient to suppress the growth of the cancer or lead to apoptosis, as evidenced in the pre-clinical and clinical trials outlined below.

p53

Tumor suppressor p53 is referred to as the molecular gatekeeper, protecting the integrity of the genome.[45] When cellular DNA damage occurs, wild type p53 is activated and stimulates the expression of *GADD45* (growth arrest and DNA damage) and the cyclin-dependent kinase (CDK) inhibitor, *p21*. p21 inhibits the CDK-cyclin D complex required to phosphorylate Rb, thereby halting the cell at the G_1/S checkpoint to allow for DNA repair. If GADD45-mediated DNA repair is unsuccessful, p53 activates *bax* which mediates apoptosis.[46] p53 mutations occur in approximately one third of early prostate cancers,[47] and this increases in patients with advanced and metastatic disease.[48] Replacement of wild-type p53 with recombinant adenoviral vectors (Ad-p53) has resulted in growth inhibition and induction of apoptosis in prostate cancer both *in vitro*[9,49] and *in vivo*.[50] In addition, intratumoral administration of Ad-p53 has been shown to slow the progression of prostate cancer to metastatic disease.[51] Perhaps the most powerful use of p53 replacement is in combination with conventional therapies. Ad-p53 has been shown to sensitize prostate cancer cells *in vitro* and *in vivo* to chemotherapeutic agents[52] and *in vitro* to radiation therapy.[53] Clinical trials are ongoing to determine the safety of such therapies.[54,55]

p16

Similar to p53, tumor suppressor *p16* is a negative regulator of the cell growth cycle, preventing the phosphorylation of Rb by sequestering CDK4 of the CDK-cyclin D complex. Hypophosphorylated Rb arrests the cell at G_1, and loss of normal *p16* function is common in prostate cancer.[46] Small homozygous deletions have been identified as the major mechanism of inactivation of *p16*, which occurs in 40% of primary prostate cancers and 71% of advanced androgen-independent prostate cancers.[56–58] Replacement of *p16* using adenoviral vectors suppressed cell growth and induced senescence in several prostate cancer cell lines including LNCaP (androgen-dependent) and C4-2, DU-145, PPC-1 and PC-3 (androgen-independent).[10,59,60] Furthermore, intratumoral injection of Ad-CMV-p16 inhibited the growth of PC-3 tumor xenografts in experimental animal models and prolonged the animals' survival.[60] Currently, one clinical trial utilizing *p16* is in progress.

c-myc

The oncogene *c-myc* plays an important role in the progression of the cell cycle. As a transcription factor, it regulates the expression of CDC25 phosphatases that control CDK activity.[61] c-myc amplification is a common mutation in prostate cancer and its levels correlate with increasing tumor grade.[62] The approach developed to suppress the overexpression of oncogenes delivers antisense RNA complimentary to the sense strand for that gene. This approach not only inhibits cancer cell growth, but also induces apoptosis through the down-regulation of *bcl-2* resulting from *c-myc* suppression. Steiner *et al.* developed a replication-incompetent retroviral vector to deliver antisense *c-myc* transcripts intratumorily in DU-145 nude mice xenografts. Reduction in tumor size and even complete tumor obliteration were observed.[11] One *c-myc* clinical trial is in progress.

Cytoreductive Gene Therapy

This approach to the molecular therapy of prostate cancer results in the direct or indirect killing of prostate cancer cells by replication-competent oncolytic viruses such as Ad-OC-E1a, pro-drug enzyme genes such as thymidine kinase, and apoptosis-inducing genes such as TRAIL. Perhaps one of the most successful approaches to the molecular therapy of prostate cancer, several clinical trials are ongoing to explore cytoreductive treatments.

Oncolytic Virus Therapy

Previous studies have shown that a replication-competent adenovirus injected intra-organ is sufficient to kill prostate cancer cells.[63] Although this therapy alone might be effective, adenovirus is taken up by the liver and lungs. This has the potential to cause hepatic and respiratory distress in immune-compromised cancer patients.[64] Controlling the replication of adenovirus solely to prostate cancer cells increases the safety of this tumor-eliminating therapy. The replication of adenovirus can be controlled by placing the early gene, *E1a*, a transcriptional activator of adenoviral late genes, under the control of a tissue-specific promoter. Without the expression of the essential late genes, the virus cannot reassemble and propagate in the host cell.[65] Recently, Henderson *et al.* demonstrated the ability to conditionally drive the replication of adenovirus by a prostate-specific enhancer (PSE) resulting in regression of *in vivo* androgen-independent LNCaP tumors.[66]

Our laboratory has developed a conditional replication-competent adenoviral vector (Ad-OC-E1a) using the mouse *OC* promoter to restrict the expression of *E1a* to prostate epithelia and its supporting bone stroma in osseous metastases of prostate cancer. This virus appears to be more effective than the PSE-controlled virus at killing a broader spectrum of prostate cancer cells including LNCaP, C4-2, and ARCaP (PSA-positive), as well as PC-3 and DU-145 (PSA-negative). Intratumoral injection of Ad-OC-E1a was effective at obliterating subcutaneous androgen-independent PC-3 tumors in athymic mice. In addition, intraosseous C4-2 prostate cancer xenografts responded very well to the systemic administration of Ad-OC-E1a. One hundred percent of the treated mice responded with a drop in the serum PSA below detectable levels. At the conclusion of the study, 40% of the treated mice were cured of prostate cancer as no PSA rebound or prostate cancer cells in the skeleton were detected.[5] Figure 4 shows the X-ray of a mouse with a C4-2 bone tumor before and after treatment with Ad-OC-E1a.

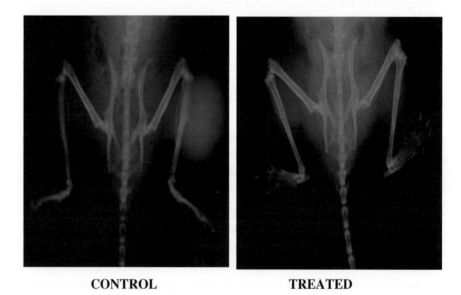

CONTROL   **TREATED**

Fig. 4. Therapeutic effect of Ad-OC-E1a on prostate bone tumors. C4-2 prostate cancer cells were injected into the bone marrow space of the right tibia in SCID mice. The left panel shows the X-ray of an untreated mouse with a large mass and deformed tibia. The right panel shows the X-ray of a mouse following intravenous administration of Ad-OC-E1a.

It has been shown that controlling the expression of the early gene *E1b*, in addition to *E1a*, results in better viral replication control.[67] For this reason, we developed a second replication-competent adenoviral vector, Ad-hOC-E1, containing a single bidirectional human *OC* promoter to control the expression of both *E1a* and *E1b*. Under the control of this VDRE-containing promoter, viral replication is induced 10-fold higher than wild-type viral replication and cytotoxicity is enhanced with the administration of vitamin D.[68] Although still controversial,[69] some preclinical studies indicate that vitamin D has an antiproliferative effect on androgen independent prostate cancer.[70,71] In our preclinical studies, administration of vitamin D_3 in nude mice with subcutaneous DU-145 xenografts demonstrated a therapeutic effect; however, the systemic administration of Ad-hOC-E1 in combination with vitamin D showed marked repression of the tumors, indicating the potential for clinical use.[68] The previously outlined preclinical findings have translated into a phase I clinical trial of *OC*-driven oncolytic adenoviral intratumoral therapy for androgen-independent prostate cancer.

Pro-drug Enzyme Gene Therapy

The efficacy of this approach depends on the conversion of a non-toxic pro-drug to an active cytotoxic drug by the enzymatic product of a delivered gene not normally expressed in human cells. Following systemic administration of the pro-drug, high concentrations of the lethal metabolite are only found locally at the tumor site, avoiding systemic toxicity. Fortunately, the toxic effect is not limited to the cells that produced the cytotoxic drug, but extends to neighboring cells via the bystander effect. This bystander effect is mediated by intercellular gap junctions and phagocytosis of debris from dying cells. By these means, the cytotoxic effect is amplified, compensating for low gene transfer efficiencies. The most widely applied pro-drug gene therapy in prostate cancer utilizes thymidine kinase from the herpes simplex virus (HSV-TK) and any one of several anti-herpetic agents such as ganciclovir (GCV), acyclovir (ACV), or valacyclovir (VAL). These nucleoside analogues are phosphorylated specifically by HSV-TK. The phosphorylated forms of the drugs are incorporated into cellular DNA during DNA replication resulting in chain termination and ultimately cell death.

The TK/pro-drug system is widely favored because it is a safe approach for cancer gene therapy for a number of reasons. First, apoptosis is induced in the transduced cell only when it divides, allowing the gene therapist to target cancer cells that divide more rapidly than noncancerous cells. Second, the toxic effect only occurs when the pro-drug is administered allowing the cessation of treatment in the event of adverse effects. Third, several anti-herpetic nucleoside analogue drugs are clinically available, simplifying the approval process for the use of the pro-drug in clinical trials. Finally, the bystander effect greatly increases the killing efficiency of the therapy.

Previously, Eastham *et al.* demonstrated the sensitivity of human prostate cancer cells PC-3 and DU-145 to GCV cytotoxicity following the *in vitro* transduction of the cells with *HSV-TK* using a recombinant replication-deficient adenoviral vector. Similar results were obtained *in vivo* in subcutaneous xenografts of murine and human cancer models following the intralesional injection of Ad-RSV-TK and Ad-CMV-TK.[72–74] Placing *TK* under the control of universal promoters such as RSV or CMV allows for the potential of *TK* activation in any cell without discrimination between normal and cancer cells. Therefore, intratumoral injection of the vector is required to prevent systemic dissemination of the virus. Scardino *et al.* developed the initial TK clinical trial in which a replication-deficient adenoviral vector was injected intralesionally to deliver *HSV-TK*, preceding the administration of GCV, in men with locally recurrent prostate cancer one or more years after definitive external beam radiotherapy. This trial realized the potential of this therapy by demonstrating the tumoricidal activity of this TK/GCV therapy as evidenced by sustained decreases in serum PSA and improved biopsies. As a result of adenoviral leakage from the injection site through the bloodstream and tracking to the liver, several of the patients experienced a self-limiting toxicity and one patient experienced moderate but reversible hepatic dysfunction and thrombocytopenia.[15] To circumvent toxicity to the patient, Chung *et al.* developed a replication-deficient adenovirus to deliver *HSV-TK* driven by the *PSA* promoter.[29]

Our laboratory developed a clinical protocol to test the hypothesis that the *OC* promoter can regulate *HSV-TK* expression specifically within a prostate cancer cell and the supportive stroma of a metastasis. We performed a phase I clinical trial enrolling 11 patients with locally recurrent or metastatic prostate cancer. Two post-surgical local recurrences and nine metastatic lesions (five osseous and 4 lymph node) were injected with replication-defective Ad-OC-TK vector followed by the administration of oral valacyclovir.[3] All patients tolerated this therapy with no severe adverse effects. Of the eleven men, local cancer cell death was observed in seven patients; however, the treated lesions of all eleven men showed histological changes as a result of the treatment. One patient demonstrated regression and stabilization of the treated lesion for 317 days post-treatment without alternative treatments, as demonstrated in Fig. 5.[6] This trial opened the door to the development of future adenoviral vectors for the systemic treatment of osseous and visceral prostate cancer metastases.

Suicide Gene Therapy

Tumor necrosis factor-related apoptosis-inducing ligand (TRAIL), also known as Apo-2 ligand, is a member of the tumor necrosis factor (TNF)

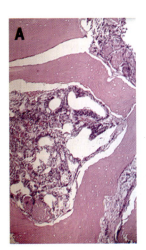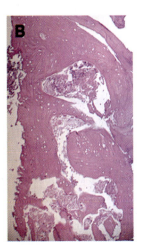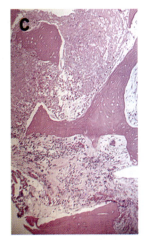

Fig. 5. Histomorphologic study of prostate cancer bone metastases treated with Ad-OC-TK. Tissue biopsies were collected from one patient and H&E-stained before (**A**), during (day 8) (**B**), and after (day 30) (**C**) treatment with Ad-OC-TK and VAL. Malignant prostate cancer cells surround healthy bone tissue before treatment (A). During treatment, cancer cells are replaced and fibrosis occurs (B). By day 30, malignant cells disappear and are replaced completely by fibrosis and inflammatory cells (C).

family and has been shown to preferentially kill tumor cells. Originally discovered because of its similarity to Fas-ligand, TRAIL is a 32 kDa type II transmembrane protein, whose C-terminal extracellular domain (amino acids 114–281) is homologous with other members of the TNF family.[75,76] TRAIL induces apoptosis by binding to the death domain-containing receptors DR4 and DR5; however, the death signal is not transduced via the adaptor molecule FADD. Instead, the death protease FLICE2 is believed to be engaged, cleaving the initiating caspase 8 and beginning the caspase cascade.[77]

The selectivity of TRAIL for cancer cells over normal cells makes it a prime candidate for anticancer therapy. TRAIL expression has been detected in several normal human tissues which suggests that TRAIL is not toxic to those cells *in vivo*.[78] In essence, these cells are protected from the apoptotic effects of TRAIL by an antagonistic decoy receptor, TRID, which lacks an intracellular domain and is found on the surface membrane of TRAIL-resistant cells.[77] Many prostate cancer cell lines including ALVA-31, DU-145, and PC-3 are extremely sensitive to TRAIL and undergo apoptosis when exposed; however, other cell lines such as LNCaP are highly resistant.[79] This resistance has been shown to be reversed by simultaneous administration of the chemotherapeutic agents doxorubicin, cisplatin, or etoposide[80] or by infection of those cells with adenovirus.[81] For this reason, TRAIL is a promising suicide gene to consider for prostate cancer gene therapy; however, recent studies suggest that cultured human hepatocytes may be sensitive to TRAIL.[82] Recombinant forms of TRAIL with reduced hepatotoxicity are being investigated[83] in addition to mono-clonal antibodies that antagonize the TRAIL receptor in hepatocytes.[84]

Immunotherapy

Prostate cancer, like most cancers, has developed mechanisms to evade the host immune system. Such mechanisms include the down-regulation of class I major histocompatibility complex (MHC) molecules on the tumor cell surface[85] as well as the down-regulation of the co-stimulatory B7 molecules.[86] These means of evasion result in decreased presentation of tumor antigens to cytotoxic T lymphocytes (CTLs). The goal of immunotherapy is to enhance the host immune response to prostate cancer cells. Although several clinical trials have been initiated, only limited results have been published.

GM-CSF

After demonstrating that immunostimulatory molecules could transform cancer cells to activate a tumor-directed immune response,[87] Simons *et al.* developed the first gene therapy clinical trial protocol for prostate cancer. In this study, eight men with metastatic prostate cancer discovered during radical prostatectomy were administered autologous, *ex vivo GM-CSF* transduced, irradiated cancer vaccines. Unfortunately, due to the large number of *ex vivo* manipulations, the vaccination rate decreased, from the original enrollment number of eleven men to eight. Side effects were limited to pruritis, erythema, and swelling at the site of vaccination. Delayed-type hypersensitivity (DTH) reactions to untransduced autologous prostate cancer cells were positive in seven of the eight men, demonstrating the ability to mount a T cell response. Furthermore, new antibodies against prostate cancer polypeptides were discovered in the sera of three of the eight men, suggesting a B cell response to vaccination.[88] A subsequent clinical trial demonstrated no therapeutic value of systemic administration of recombinant GM-CSF, thereby suggesting the importance of local secretion of GM-CSF by the cancer vaccines.[89] Multiple clinical trials are in progress that employ a simple vaccine composed of irradiated prostate cancer cell line allografts expressing *GM-CSF*, which allows for multiple dosing.

IL-2

More recently, *in vivo* immunotherapy approaches have been used. Belldegrun *et al.* developed a gene therapy protocol in which 24 men with locally advanced prostate cancer were administered a DNA-liposome complex encoding the *IL-2* gene intraprostatically. This therapy was well tolerated, with side effects including mild hematuria, transient rectal bleeding, and perineal discomfort. Immunohistochemical analysis of the tumor site demonstrated T cell infiltration. Decreased serum PSA levels were observed in 16 of the 24 men on day 1 and 14 of the 24 by day 8.[90] Similar clinical trials are still in progress.

Future Directions

Among clinical trials that have been launched to demonstrate the safety and efficacy of adenoviral-based gene therapy on prostate cancer in the past few years, the most exciting results have come from the study of tumor/tissue-restricted replicative adenovirus (TRRA). This strategy allows the viral vector to propagate from a limited number of infected cells to the whole tumor mass, overcoming the problem of inadequate *in vivo* infectivity or biodistribution of the vector; however, TRRA-based therapy is not without its limitations. One of the major limitations of this therapy is the induction of the host immune system, targeted to eliminate the adenovirus from the body.

It will become critical to temporarily suppress the host's immune system or enhance the killing activity of the virus so that it can eliminate tumors within a shorter period of time, allowing it to escape from host immune attack. Among immune regulators, TGF-β and Fas-ligand are likely the best candidates for incorporation into TRRA for cancer gene therapy. There are five members reported in the TGF-β family; three of them (TGF-β1, TGF-β2, and TGF-β3) are expressed in mammals. These three isoforms share a high degree of sequence homology in the mature domain, and have similar actions on cells in tissue culture. Suppression of the immune response includes the inhibition of T and B cell proliferation, the down-regulation of natural killer cell activity and CTL response, and the regulation of macrophage activation.[91] TGF-β is a mediator of immune suppression that allows tumors to escape from immune surveillance, and its use has been explored to suppress the inflammatory and alloreactive immune responses in liver transplantation.[92] Besides TGF-β, Fas-ligand is another immune modulator that has been explored for use in kidney transplant patients to suppress alloreactive lymphocytes.[93] Fas-ligand, also known as CD95 or APO-1, is a membrane-bound protein of the TNF family, and it is expressed in several cell types including tumors, T cells, and B cells. Cells expressing the Fas receptor undergo apoptosis when they encounter Fas-ligand.[94] Besides their immune modulation function, TGF-β and Fas-ligand are also strong growth inhibitors and induce apoptosis in a variety of cancers, including prostate cancer.[95] Therefore, incorporating TGF-β or Fas-ligand into a TRRA will potentially enhance the tumoricidal activity of the vector and blanket the tumor site from the immune system, allowing the TRRA to complete its mission.

Once the TRRA is armed with immune suppressors, the need for tight regulation of viral replication increases. In addition to controlling *E1a* and *E1b* with prostate-specific promoters, *E4* should be considered. The *E4* transcription unit encodes regulatory genes that are critical for viral replication, involving the shut-down of host gene expression and the facilitation of late viral gene expression.[96] Mutant adenoviral vectors lacking the *E4* region are severely replication defective and can only propagate in *E4*-expressing cells.[97] Placing *E4* under the control of a prostate-specific promoter should provide additional safety. TK should also be considered for incorporation into a TRRA. In addition to enhancing the tumor-killing activity of a TRRA, TK will allow a gene therapist to monitor adenoviral replication *in vivo* via positron emission tomography (PET) imaging.[98]

Finally, because all tissue-specific promoters have basal activity levels in non-target tissues, the potential exists for accumulation of adenovirus in the liver, resulting in undesirable toxic effects caused by significant expression of therapeutic genes in the liver. Modification of the adenoviral fiber knob can increase viral tropism toward cancers and away from the liver and other vital organs.[99,100] This is also beneficial because it is well known that expression of the coxsackievirus-adenovirus receptor (CAR) is frequently down-regulated in cancers. Our laboratory is currently investigating an Ad-5/35 hybrid adenovirus for use in prostate cancer gene therapy whose infectivity is CAR-independent and lacks liver tropism.

Conclusion

The safety and efficacy of gene therapy for prostate cancer has been demonstrated through various preclinical and clinical trials. In recent years, interest in this field has expanded and will continue to do so. It is conceivable that, in the near future, a safe gene therapy modality will be developed to replace hormone ablation therapy which causes unpleasant side effects, decreases the quality of life of the patient, and only temporarily controls the disease. Due to its convenient administration through ultrasound-guided transrectal injection, it is also conceivable that gene therapy applied in an outpatient clinic may someday replace radical prostatectomy and radiation therapy to treat early prostate cancer. Factors that limit the disseminated use of gene therapy as a standard of care include time, funding, and fear from the general public; however, these should diminish as the number of successful clinical trials increase.

References

1. Jemal A, Murray T, Samuels A, Ghafoor A, Ward E, Thun MJ (2003) Cancer Statistics, 2003. *CA Cancer J Clin* 53:5–26.
2. Gardner TA, Ko SC, Kao C, Shirakawa T, Cheon J, Gotoh A, Wu T, Sikes RA, Zhau HE, Cui Q, Balian G, Chung LWK (1998) Exploiting stromal-epithelial interaction for model development and new strategies of gene therapy for prostate cancer and osteosarcoma metastases. *Gene Therapy Mol Bio* 2:41–58.
3. Koeneman KS, Kao C, Ko SC, Yang L, Wada Y, Kallmes DF, Gillenwater JY, Zhau HE, Chung LW, Gardner TA (2000) Osteocalcin-directed gene therapy for prostate-cancer bone metastasis. *World J Urol* 18:102.
4. Lee SJ, Kim HS, Yu R, *et al.* (2002) Novel prostate-specific promoter derived from PSA and PSMA enhancers. *Mol Ther* 6:415–421.
5. Matsubara S, Wada Y, Gardner TA, *et al.* (2001) A conditional replication-competent adenoviral vector, Ad-OC-E1a, to cotarget prostate cancer and bone stroma in an experimental model of androgen-independent prostate cancer bone metastasis. *Cancer Res* 61:6012–6019.
6. Kubo H, Gardner TA, Wada Y, *et al.* (2003) Phase I dose escalation clinical trial of adenovirus vector carrying osteocalcin promoter-driven herpes simplex virus thymidine kinase in localized and metastatic hormone-refractory prostate cancer. *Hum Gene Ther* 14:227–241.
7. Thompson IM, Goodman PJ, Tangen CM, *et al.* (2003) The influence of finasteride on the development of prostate cancer. *N Engl J Med* 349: 215–224.
8. Bookstein R, Shew JY, Chen PL, Scully P, Lee WH (1990) Suppression of tumorigenicity of human prostate carcinoma cells by replacing a mutated RB gene. *Science* 247:712–715.
9. Eastham JA, Hall SJ, Sehgal I, *et al.* (1995) *In vivo* gene therapy with p53 or p21 adenovirus for prostate cancer. *Cancer Res* 55:5151–5155.
10. Allay JA, Steiner MS, Zhang Y, Reed CP, Cockroft J, Lu Y (2000) Adenovirus p16 gene therapy for prostate cancer. *World J Urol* 18:111–120.
11. Steiner MS, Anthony CT, Lu Y, Holt JT (1998) Antisense c-myc retroviral vector suppresses established human prostate cancer. *Hum Gene Ther* 9:747–755.

12. Wei C, Willis RA, Tilton BR, *et al.* (1997) Tissue-specific expression of the human prostate-specific antigen gene in transgenic mice: Implications for tolerance and immunotherapy. *Proc Natl Acad Sci USA* 94:6369–6374.

13. Hay RT (1985) The origin of adenovirus DNA replication: Minimal DNA sequence requirement *in vivo*. *EMBO J* 4:421–426.

14. Brand K, Arnold W, Bartels T, *et al.* (1997) Liver-associated toxicity of the HSV-tk/GCV approach and adenoviral vectors. *Cancer Gene Ther* 4:9–16.

15. Herman JR, Adler HL, Aguilar-Cordova E, *et al.* (1999) *In situ* gene therapy for adenocarcinoma of the prostate: A phase I clinical trial. *Hum Gene Ther* 10:1239–1249.

16. Pan LC, Price PA (1984) The effect of transcriptional inhibitors on the bone gamma-carboxyglutamic acid protein response to 1,25-dihydroxyvitamin D3 in osteosarcoma cells. *J Biol Chem* 259:5844–5847.

17. Jung C, Ou YC, Yeung F, Frierson HF, Jr, Kao C (2001) Osteocalcin is incompletely spliced in non-osseous tissues. *Gene* 271:143–150.

18. Wu TT, Sikes RA, Cui Q, *et al.* (1998) Establishing human prostate cancer cell xenografts in bone: Induction of osteoblastic reaction by prostate-specific antigen-producing tumors in athymic and SCID/bg mice using LNCaP and lineage-derived metastatic sublines. *Int J Cancer* 77:8878–8894.

19. Koeneman KS, Yeung F, Chung LW (1999) Osteomimetic properties of prostate cancer cells: A hypothesis supporting the predilection of prostate cancer metastasis and growth in the bone environment. *Prostate* 39:246–261.

20. Bortell R, Owen TA, Bidwell JP, *et al.* (1992) Vitamin D-responsive protein-DNA interactions at multiple promoter regulatory elements that contribute to the level of rat osteocalcin gene expression. *Proc Natl Acad Sci USA* 89:6119–6123.

21. Lian JB, Stein GS, Stein JL, van Wijnen AJ (1999) Regulated expression of the bone-specific osteocalcin gene by vitamins and hormones. *Vitam Horm* 55:443–509.

22. Banerjee C, Stein JL, Van Wijnen AJ, Frenkel B, Lian JB, Stein GS (1996) Transforming growth factor-beta 1 responsiveness of the rat osteocalcin gene is mediated by an activator protein-1 binding site. *Endocrinology* 137: 1991–2000.

23. Banerjee C, Hiebert SW, Stein JL, Lian JB, Stein GS (1996) An AML-1 consensus sequence binds an osteoblast-specific complex and transcriptionally activates the osteocalcin gene. *Proc Natl Acad Sci USA* 93:4968–4973.

24. Ko SC, Cheon J, Kao C, *et al.* (1996) Osteocalcin promoter-based toxic gene therapy for the treatment of osteosarcoma in experimental models. *Cancer Res* 56:4614–4619.

25. Stamey TA, Yang N, Hay AR, McNeal JE, Freiha FS, Redwine E (1987) Prostate-specific antigen as a serum marker for adenocarcinoma of the prostate. *N Engl J Med* 317:909–916.

26. Cleutjens KB, van der Korput HA, van Eekelen CC, van Rooij HC, Faber PW, Trapman J (1997) An androgen response element in a far upstream enhancer region is essential for high, androgen-regulated activity of the prostate-specific antigen promoter. *Mol Endocrinol* 11:148–161.

27. Schuur ER, Henderson GA, Kmetec LA, Miller JD, Lamparski HG, Henderson DR (1996) Prostate-specific antigen expression is regulated by an upstream enhancer. *J Biol Chem* 271:7043–7051.

28. Pang S, Dannull J, Kaboo R, *et al.* (1997) Identification of a positive regulatory element responsible for tissue-specific expression of prostate-specific antigen. *Cancer Res* 57:495–499.

29. Gotoh A, Ko SC, Shirakawa T, *et al.* (1998) Development of prostate-specific antigen promoter-based gene therapy for androgen-independent human prostate cancer. *J Urol* 160:220–229.

30. Wu L, Matherly J, Smallwood A, *et al.* (2001) Chimeric PSA enhancers exhibit augmented activity in prostate cancer gene therapy vectors. *Gene Ther* 8:1416–1426.

31. Lu Y, Carraher J, Zhang Y, *et al.* (1999) Delivery of adenoviral vectors to the prostate for gene therapy. *Cancer Gene Ther* 6:64–72.

32. Wright GL, Jr, Grob BM, Haley C, *et al.* (1996) Upregulation of prostate-specific membrane antigen after androgen-deprivation therapy. *Urology* 48:326–334.

33. Xiao Z, Adam BL, Cazares LH, *et al.* (2001) Quantitation of serum prostate-specific membrane antigen by a novel protein biochip immunoassay discriminates benign from malignant prostate disease. *Cancer Res* 61:6029–6033.

34. Sweat SD, Pacelli A, Murphy GP, Bostwick DG (1998) Prostate-specific membrane antigen expression is greatest in prostate adenocarcinoma and lymph node metastases. *Urology* 52:637–640.

35. Watt F, Martorana A, Brookes DE, *et al.* (2001) A tissue-specific enhancer of the prostate-specific membrane antigen gene, FOLH1. *Genomics* 73:2432–2454.

36. Uchida A, O'Keefe DS, Bacich DJ, Molloy PL, Heston WD (2001) *In vivo* suicide gene therapy model using a newly discovered prostate-specific membrane antigen promoter/enhancer: A potential alternative approach to androgen deprivation therapy. *Urology* 58:13213–13219.

37. Lee SJ, Lee K, Yang X, *et al.* (2003) NFATc1 with AP-3 site binding specificity mediates gene expression of prostate-specific-membrane-antigen. *J Mol Biol* 330:749–760.

38. Chiu CP, Harley CB (1997) Replicative senescence and cell immortality: The role of telomeres and telomerase. *Proc Soc Exp Biol Med* 214:99–106.
39. Kim NW, Piatyszek MA, Prowse KR, *et al.* (1994) Specific association of human telomerase activity with immortal cells and cancer. *Science* 266: 2011–2015.
40. Horikawa I, Cable PL, Afshari C, Barrett JC (1999) Cloning and characterization of the promoter region of human telomerase reverse transcriptase gene. *Cancer Res* 59:826–830.
41. Sommerfeld HJ, Meeker AK, Piatyszek MA, Bova GS, Shay JW, Coffey DS (1996) Telomerase activity: A prevalent marker of malignant human prostate tissue. *Cancer Res* 56:218–222.
42. Lin T, Huang X, Gu J, *et al.* (2002) Long-term tumor-free survival from treatment with the GFP-TRAIL fusion gene expressed from the hTERT promoter in breast cancer cells. *Oncogene* 21:8020–8028.
43. Lanson NA, Jr, Friedlander PL, Schwarzenberger P, Kolls JK, Wang G (2003) Replication of an adenoviral vector controlled by the human telomerase reverse transcriptase promoter causes tumor-selective tumor lysis. *Cancer Res* 63:7936–7941.
44. 2003 Office of Biotechnology Activities' Recombinant DNA and Gene Transfer Web Page, http://www4.od.nih.gov/oba/rdna.htm
45. Levine AJ (1997) p53, the cellular gatekeeper for growth and division. *Cell* 88:323–331.
46. Sherr CJ (1996) Cancer cell cycles. *Science* 274:1672–1677.
47. Downing SR, Russell PJ, Jackson P (2003) Alterations of p53 are common in early stage prostate cancer. *Can J Urol* 10:1924–1933.
48. Eastham JA, Stapleton AM, Gousse AE, *et al.* (1995) Association of p53 mutations with metastatic prostate cancer. *Clin Cancer Res* 1: 1111–1118.
49. Yang C, Cirielli C, Capogrossi MC, Passaniti A (1995) Adenovirus-mediated wild-type p53 expression induces apoptosis and suppresses tumorigenesis of prostatic tumor cells. *Cancer Res* 55:4210–4213.
50. Ko SC, Gotoh A, Thalmann GN, *et al.* (1996) Molecular therapy with recombinant p53 adenovirus in an androgen-independent, metastatic human prostate cancer model. *Hum Gene Ther* 7:1683–1691.
51. Eastham JA, Grafton W, Martin CM, Williams BJ (2000) Suppression of primary tumor growth and the progression to metastasis with p53 adenovirus in human prostate cancer. *J Urol* 164:814–819.
52. Gurnani M, Lipari P, Dell J, Shi B, Nielsen LL (1999) Adenovirus-mediated p53 gene therapy has greater efficacy when combined with chemotherapy

against human head and neck, ovarian, prostate, and breast cancer. *Cancer Chemother Pharmacol* 44:143–151.

53. Colletier PJ, Ashoori F, Cowen D, *et al.* (2000) Adenoviral-mediated p53 transgene expression sensitizes both wild-type and null p53 prostate cancer cells *in vitro* to radiation. *Int J Radiat Oncol Biol Phys* 48:1507–1512.

54. Pantuck AJ, Zisman A, Belldegrun AS (2000) Gene therapy for prostate cancer at the University of California, Los Angeles: Preliminary results and future directions. *World J Urol* 18:143–147.

55. Sweeney P, Pisters LL (2000) Ad5CMVp53 gene therapy for locally advanced prostate cancer — where do we stand? *World J Urol* 18:121–124.

56. Jarrard DF, Bova GS, Ewing CM, *et al.* (1997) Deletional, mutational, and methylation analyses of CDKN2 (p16/MTS1) in primary and metastatic prostate cancer. *Genes Chromosomes Cancer* 19:90–96.

57. Liggett WH Jr, Sidransky D (1998) Role of the p16 tumor suppressor gene in cancer. *J Clin Oncol* 16:1197–1206.

58. Isaacs WB (1995) Molecular genetics of prostate cancer. *Cancer Surv* 25:357–379.

59. Steiner MS, Zhang Y, Farooq F, Lerner J, Wang Y, Lu Y (2000) Adenoviral vector containing wild-type p16 suppresses prostate cancer growth and prolongs survival by inducing cell senescence. *Cancer Gene Ther* 7:360–372.

60. Gotoh A, Kao C, Ko SC, Hamada K, Liu TJ, Chung LW (1997) Cytotoxic effects of recombinant adenovirus p53 and cell cycle regulator genes (p21 WAF1/CIP1 and p16CDKN4) in human prostate cancers. *J Urol* 158: 636–641.

61. Galaktionov K, Chen X, Beach D (1996) Cdc25 cell-cycle phosphatase as a target of c-myc. *Nature* 382:511–517.

62. Jenkins RB, Qian J, Lieber MM, Bostwick DG (1997) Detection of c-myc oncogene amplification and chromosomal anomalies in metastatic prostatic carcinoma by fluorescence *in situ* hybridization. *Cancer Res* 57:524–531.

63. Deng J, Xia W, Hung MC (1998) Adenovirus 5 E1A-mediated tumor suppression associated with E1A-mediated apoptosis *in vivo*. *Oncogene* 17:2167–2175.

64. van der Eb MM, Cramer SJ, Vergouwe Y, *et al.* (1998) Severe hepatic dysfunction after adenovirus-mediated transfer of the herpes simplex virus thymidine kinase gene and ganciclovir administration. *Gene Ther* 5:451–458.

65. Robbins PD, Tahara H, Ghivizzani SC (1998) Viral vectors for gene therapy. *Trends Biotechnol* 16:35–40.

66. Rodriguez R, Schuur ER, Lim HY, Henderson GA, Simons JW, Henderson DR (1997) Prostate attenuated replication competent adenovirus (ARCA)

CN706: A selective cytotoxic for prostate-specific antigen-positive prostate cancer cells. *Cancer Res* 57:2559–2563.

67. Yu DC, Sakamoto GT, Henderson DR (1999) Identification of the transcriptional regulatory sequences of human kallikrein 2 and their use in the construction of calydon virus 764, an attenuated replication competent adenovirus for prostate cancer therapy. *Cancer Res* 59:1498–1504.

68. Hsieh CL, Yang L, Miao L, *et al.* (2002) A novel targeting modality to enhance adenoviral replication by vitamin D(3) in androgen-independent human prostate cancer cells and tumors. *Cancer Res* 62:3084–3092.

69. Konety BR, Johnson CS, Trump DL, Getzenberg RH (1999) Vitamin D in the prevention and treatment of prostate cancer. *Semin Urol Oncol* 17:77–84.

70. Getzenberg RH, Light BW, Lapco PE, *et al.* (1997) Vitamin D inhibition of prostate adenocarcinoma growth and metastasis in the Dunning rat prostate model system. *Urology* 50:999–1006.

71. Zhao XY, Feldman D (2001) The role of vitamin D in prostate cancer. *Steroids* 66:293–300.

72. Eastham JA, Chen SH, Sehgal I, *et al.* (1996) Prostate cancer gene therapy: Herpes simplex virus thymidine kinase gene transduction followed by ganciclovir in mouse and human prostate cancer models. *Hum Gene Ther* 7: 515–523.

73. Hall SJ, Mutchnik SE, Chen SH, Woo SL, Thompson TC (1997) Adenovirus-mediated herpes simplex virus thymidine kinase gene and ganciclovir therapy leads to systemic activity against spontaneous and induced metastasis in an orthotopic mouse model of prostate cancer. *Int J Cancer* 70:183–187.

74. Cheon J, Kim HK, Moon DG, Yoon DK, Cho JH, Koh SK (2000) Adenovirus-mediated suicide-gene therapy using the herpes simplex virus thymidine kinase gene in cell and animal models of human prostate cancer: Changes in tumour cell proliferative activity. *BJU Int* 85:759–766.

75. Wiley SR, Schooley K, Smolak PJ, *et al.* (1995) Identification and characterization of a new member of the TNF family that induces apoptosis. *Immunity* 3:673–682.

76. Pitti RM, Marsters SA, Ruppert S, Donahue CJ, Moore A, Ashkenazi A (1996) Induction of apoptosis by Apo-2 ligand, a new member of the tumor necrosis factor cytokine family. *J Biol Chem* 271:12687–12690.

77. Pan G, Ni J, Wei YF, Yu G, Gentz R, Dixit VM (1997) An antagonist decoy receptor and a death domain-containing receptor for TRAIL. *Science* 277:815–818.

78. Pan G, O'Rourke K, Chinnaiyan AM, *et al.* (1997) The receptor for the cytotoxic ligand TRAIL. *Science* 276:111–113.

79. Nesterov A, Lu X, Johnson M, Miller GJ, Ivashchenko Y, Kraft AS (2001) Elevated AKT activity protects the prostate cancer cell line LNCaP from TRAIL-induced apoptosis. *J Biol Chem* 276:10767–10774.

80. Munshi A, McDonnell TJ, Meyn RE (2002) Chemotherapeutic agents enhance TRAIL-induced apoptosis in prostate cancer cells. *Cancer Chemother Pharmacol* 50:46–52.

81. Voelkel-Johnson C, King DL, Norris JS (2002) Resistance of prostate cancer cells to soluble TNF-related apoptosis-inducing ligand (TRAIL/Apo2L) can be overcome by doxorubicin or adenoviral delivery of full-length TRAIL. *Cancer Gene Ther* 9:164–172.

82. Jo M, Kim TH, Seol DW, *et al.* (2000) Apoptosis induced in normal human hepatocytes by tumor necrosis factor-related apoptosis-inducing ligand. *Nat Med* 6:564–567.

83. Lawrence D, Shahrokh Z, Marsters S, *et al.* (2001) Differential hepatocyte toxicity of recombinant Apo2L/TRAIL versions. *Nat Med* 7:383–385.

84. Mori E, Thomas M, Motoki K, *et al.* (2003) Human normal hepatocytes are susceptible to apoptosis signal mediated by both TRAIL-R1 and TRAIL-R2. *Cell Death Differ* 11:203–207.

85. Bander NH, Yao D, Liu H, *et al.* (1997) MHC class I and II expression in prostate carcinoma and modulation by interferon-alpha and -gamma. *Prostate* 33:233–239.

86. Kwon ED, Hurwitz AA, Foster BA, *et al.* (1997) Manipulation of T cell co-stimulatory and inhibitory signals for immunotherapy of prostate cancer. *Proc Natl Acad Sci USA* 94:8099–8103.

87. Sanda MG, Ayyagari SR, Jaffee EM, *et al.* (1994) Demonstration of a rational strategy for human prostate cancer gene therapy. *J Urol* 151:622–628.

88. Simons JW, Mikhak B, Chang JF, *et al.* (1999) Induction of immunity to prostate cancer antigens: Results of a clinical trial of vaccination with irradiated autologous prostate tumor cells engineered to secrete granulocyte-macrophage colony-stimulating factor using *ex vivo* gene transfer. *Cancer Res* 59:5160–5168.

89. Simmons SJ, Tjoa BA, Rogers M, *et al.* (1999) GM-CSF as a systemic adjuvant in a phase II prostate cancer vaccine trial. *Prostate* 39:291–297.

90. Belldegrun A, Tso CL, Zisman A, *et al.* (2001) Interleukin 2 gene therapy for prostate cancer: Phase I clinical trial and basic biology. *Hum Gene Ther* 12:883–892.

91. Huang X, Lee C (2003) From TGF-beta to cancer therapy. *Curr Drug Targets* 4:243–250.

92. Narumoto K, Saibara T, Maeda T, *et al.* (2000) Transforming growth factor-beta 1 derived from biliary epithelial cells may attenuate alloantigen-specific immune responses. *Transpl Int* 13:21–27.

93. Ke B, Coito AJ, Kato H, *et al.* (2000) Fas ligand gene transfer prolongs rat renal allograft survival and down-regulates anti-apoptotic Bag-1 in parallel with enhanced Th2-type cytokine expression. *Transplantation* 69: 1690–1694.

94. Winoto A (1997) Cell death in the regulation of immune responses. *Curr Opin Immunol* 9:365–370.

95. Norris JS, Hyer ML, Voelkel-Johnson C, Lowe SL, Rubinchik S, Dong JY (2001) The use of Fas Ligand, TRAIL and Bax in gene therapy of prostate cancer. *Curr Gene Ther* 1:123–136.

96. Tauber B, Dobner T (2001) Molecular regulation and biological function of adenovirus early genes: The E4 ORFs. *Gene* 278:1–23.

97. Krougliak V, Graham FL (1995) Development of cell lines capable of complementing E1, E4, and protein IX defective adenovirus type 5 mutants. *Hum Gene Ther* 6:1575–1586.

98. Pantuck AJ, Berger F, Zisman A, *et al.* (2002) CL1-SR39: A noninvasive molecular imaging model of prostate cancer suicide gene therapy using positron emission tomography. *J Urol* 168:1193–1198.

99. Campbell M, Qu S, Wells S, Sugandha H, Jensen RA (2003) An adenoviral vector containing an arg-gly-asp (RGD) motif in the fiber knob enhances protein product levels from transgenes refractory to expression. *Cancer Gene Ther* 10:559–570.

100. Vigne E, Dedieu JF, Brie A, *et al.* (2003) Genetic manipulations of adenovirus type 5 fiber resulting in liver tropism attenuation. *Gene Ther* 10: 153–162.

5

CHEMOTHERAPY FOR PROSTATE CANCER

Samuel K. Kulp, Kuen-Feng Chen
and Ching-Shih Chen

Division of Medicinal Chemistry and Pharmacognosy
College of Pharmacy, The Ohio State University
Columbus, OH, USA

Introduction

For several decades, androgen deprivation has been the mainstay of therapy for metastatic prostate cancer. The high response rates to this approach, which near 90% by PSA criteria,[1] underscore the activity of this treatment modality in prostate cancer patients. However, satisfaction with the efficacy of androgen deprivation therapy is tempered by the transience of its effects on disease progression. The median time to progression has been reported to range from 9 to 30 months.[1,2] Although secondary hormonal maneuvers will further benefit a subset of these patients, they are characterized by even shorter durations of response (<6 months).[3,4] Continued progression in the face of castrate levels of androgen and the lack of responsiveness to hormonal therapies defines the emergence of hormone-refractory prostate cancer (HRPC) for which the prognosis is bleak. The treatment of hormone-refractory tumors constitutes a significant challenge in the management of patients with prostate cancer.

Although HRPC has historically been considered a chemorefractory disease, chemotherapy has an established role in the management of patients with HRPC. Evidence obtained over the last decade has shown some chemotherapeutic regimens to be unquestionably active in these patients.[5] Indeed, guidelines set forth by the National Comprehensive

Cancer Network (NCCN) currently identify six chemotherapeutic regimens as options for the management of HRPC.[6] These options, however, are solely palliative. The oft-cited caveat that applies to these active chemotherapeutic regimens is that none have been shown definitively to extend the survival of HRPC patients beyond the typically reported median of 12–16 months.[3,7] Certainly, palliation and improvement or maintenance of quality of life are important and valuable clinical goals in the management of HRPC patients, but the short duration of response and the lack of clear survival benefit of current chemotherapeutic options emphasize the need for new agents and strategies for the treatment of HRPC.

Opportunities for the development of therapies that achieve, not only palliation, but also prolonged survival, emerge from the elucidation of the cellular and genetic abnormalities that underlie prostate carcinogenesis, malignant progression, prostate cancer cell survival, and resistance to therapy. Such findings from the "bench" have revealed promising targets that can guide the rational development of novel therapeutic agents that make sense in the context of prostate cancer biology.

This chapter is broadly organized into two parts. The first is a brief overview of the current combinatorial chemotherapeutic regimens identified by the NCCN as options for treatment of HRPC. Thorough reviews of the clinical findings of trials utilizing these regimens, as well as their component agents as monotherapy have been presented elsewhere.[3,8–11] The second section discusses investigational agents designed to target specific molecules within pathways involved in cancer cell survival with a specific focus on signaling through phosphoinositide-3-kinase (PI3K)/Akt.

Present Chemotherapies for HRPC

The NCCN recommends combination chemotherapies as a treatment option in the management of patients with HRPC.[6] It is understood that these regimens are solely palliative and yield no definitive survival benefit. Nonetheless, their inclusion in these guidelines illustrates the diminished pessimism associated with chemotherapy for HRPC. These regimens include ketoconazole/doxorubicin, mitoxantrone/prednisone, and various estramustine-based combinations that include etoposide, vinblastine, paclitaxel and docetaxel. Among these combinations are two major chemotherapeutic approaches that represent the most frequently used regimens in the management of HRPC: mitoxantrone/prednisone and estramustine/antimicrotubule agents.[3,12]

Mitoxantrone-Based Regimens

Mitoxantrone is a semisynthetic anthracenedione. Two large, randomized trials of corticosteroids alone *vs.* in combination with mitoxantrone demonstrated that the combination regimens (mitoxantrone plus prednisone or hydrocortisone) achieved greater palliation and better quality of life in symptomatic HRPC patients. Despite these important clinical benefits, overall survival was not affected.[3,12] Nonetheless, the improved palliation and improvements in quality of life led to the FDA approval of this combination for patients with HRPC.

Estramustine Phosphate/Antimicrotubule Agent Combinations

Estramustine phosphate (EMP) is a conjugate of 17β-estradiol and nitrogen mustard. As such, it possesses both estrogenic and alkylating activities; however, its cytotoxic effects on cancer cells are apparently unrelated to its alkylating actions. EMP induces cell death through its binding to microtubule-associated proteins resulting in microtubule disassembly.[13,14] In combination with cytotoxic antimicrotubule agents, such as the vinca alkaloids and taxanes, antitumor effects were potentiated preclinically and translated to clinical trials in which enhanced palliation and antitumor activity were documented.[3,15] No significant effects on overall survival, however, were observed. However, tantalizing findings from Phase II trials of combinations containing EMP and paclitaxel or docetaxel reveal median overall survival durations as high as 20 months.[3] These promising results have yet to be confirmed in larger, randomized clinical trials.

Future Therapies for HRPC

Despite the valuable palliative role of current chemotherapeutic regimens for HRPC patients, improvement in the survival rates of these patients will require novel approaches. Efforts to develop new, more selective, and potentially less toxic, molecularly targeted agents have benefited from recent experimental advances identifying genetic and cellular aberrations implicated in prostate cancer cell survival and progression against which these agents can be directed. Signal transduction pathways and networks are frequently altered in cancer cells and represent promising targets for novel therapeutic interventions. The recent clinical successes of trastuzumab (Herceptin, Genentech) and imatinib mesylate (STI571; Gleevec; Novartis) in patients with defined abnormalities in HER2 and bcr-abl or c-kit, respectively,[16–18] has spurred enthusiasm for the discovery and development of novel therapeutic agents targeting aberrant signaling molecules in cancer cells. The PI3K/Akt pathway is upregulated in multiple human cancers, including that of the prostate. Substantial evidence points to a prominent role for abnormal PI3K/Akt signaling in prostatic malignancy and establishes it as a relevant and attractive target for therapeutic intervention.

This section of the review focuses on components of the PI3K/Akt signaling pathway. It is organized by molecular target and includes overviews of the corresponding pathways, their relevance to prostate cancer, and descriptions of new agents directed at these molecules that are currently being developed and evaluated. Agents that have been evaluated clinically in prostate cancer patients are emphasized. Information on clinical trials was gathered from the NCI clinical trials website (http://www.cancer.gov/search/clinical_trials/), unless otherwise indicated.

PI3K/Akt Signaling Pathway

The PI3K/Akt signaling cascade occupies a well-documented, central role in promoting cell survival and proliferation downstream of various extracellular stimuli,[19,20] commonly those transduced by receptor tyrosine kinases (RTKs). Signaling through this pathway is initiated by RTK-mediated activation of PI3K, which catalyzes the phosphorylation of plasma membrane lipids to form phosphatidylinositol-3,4-bisphosphate [PI(3,4)P$_2$] and PI-3,4,5-triphosphate (PIP$_3$). Signaling proteins containing pleckstrin homology (PH) domains, such as Akt and phosphoinositide-dependent kinase-1 (PDK-1), directly bind to these lipid products resulting in their co-localization at the plasma membrane, where Akt is phosphorylated at Thr308 by PDK-1 and at Ser473 by an undefined mechanism.[21–23] Phosphorylation at both sites fully stimulates Akt's kinase activity. Activated Akt conveys pro-survival signals by phosphorylating multiple substrates involved in the regulation of apoptosis and cell proliferation.[20,24,25] Proapoptotic and growth inhibitory substrates that are inactivated by Akt include the proapoptotic proteins, BAD and procaspase 9, transcriptional factors of the forkhead family, which support transcription of Fas ligand and the cyclin-dependent kinase inhibitor p27[kip1], and glycogen synthase kinase 3 (GSK3), which inhibits cyclin D1. Substrates activated by Akt include IκB-kinase-α (IKKα), which frees NF-κB to induce gene expression.[26] Negative regulation of PI3K/Akt signaling can be achieved by two phosphatases, phosphatase and tensin homologue deleted on chromosome ten (PTEN) and protein phosphatase 2A (PP2A). Through its lipid phosphatase activity, PTEN dephosphorylates PIP_3 at the 3-position, thereby countering the action of PI3K and inhibiting activation of Akt. PP2A opposes the activity of PDK-1 by directly dephosphorylating activated Akt.

Substantial evidence indicates that the PI3K/Akt signaling pathway is accentuated in cancer cells. Activation of the pathway occurs indirectly via inactivation of PTEN, the product of one of the most commonly mutated tumor suppressor genes in human cancers.[27,28] The functional loss of PTEN leading to overactive phosphoinositide signaling and subsequent Akt phosphorylation is a feature of prostate cancer, particularly in advanced disease.[29–34] Functional activation of this pathway also occurs as PI3K/Akt propagates signals from many of the RTKs involved in growth factor signaling known to be aberrantly upregulated in prostate cancer.[35] Indeed, elevated levels of phosphorylated Akt and Akt activity have been demonstrated in prostate cancer cell lines and human tumor specimens in association with corresponding changes in downstream signaling components, such as p27[kip1] and BAD.[36–39] Recently, in patient-matched normal epithelium, PIN, and invasive carcinoma, Paweletz *et al.*[38] combined laser capture microdissection and protein microarray analysis to show that disease progression was marked by significant elevations in phospho-Akt levels, which were directly correlated with decreased apoptosis; thereby linking suppression of apoptosis with activated Akt. Evidence of an oncogenic role for dysregulated signaling through PI3K/Akt in prostate cancer is derived from transgenic mouse models. *Pten* heterozygous mice (*Pten*+/−) and mice with prostate-specific overexpression of Akt exhibit phenotypic overlap in the development of PIN.[40,41] While a *Pten*+/− background accelerates prostate tumorigenesis in TRAMP mice and mice with inactivating mutations of the homeobox gene *Nkx3.1* or the gene for p27[kip1],[40,42,43] prostate-specific biallelic inactivation of *Pten* alone is sufficient to initiate early onset prostate tumorigenesis and metastasis.[44,45] In addition to oncogenesis, Akt is important for endothelial cell survival and angiogenesis,[46] and is a determinant of chemotherapeutic resistance in multiple cancers.[36,47–57]

Together, these clinical and experimental findings underscore the prominent role of aberrant PI3K/Akt signaling in prostatic malignancy. This, along with its position as a convergence point for multiple signaling pathways, establishes PI3K/Akt signaling as a relevant and attractive target for therapeutic intervention.

Receptor Tyrosine Kinases

Receptor tyrosine kinases are transmembrane receptors that are activated by a wide variety of ligands. High affinity ligand binding triggers dimerization of receptors resulting in the close apposition of the intracellular tyrosine kinase domains and subsequent tyrosine autophosphorylation. The activated receptors provide docking sites for other intracellular signaling molecules, which are in turn activated by phosphorylation or conformational changes thereby initiating signaling cascades that ultimately alter the transcription of genes regulating proliferation, apoptosis, and differentiation.[58] Aberrant up-regulation of signaling through RTKs and its subsequent activation of the PI3K/Akt pathway is a frequent defect in many cancers, including prostate cancer.[35,59] Mechanisms that have been shown to up-regulate RTK activity include receptor overexpression, activating mutations or chromosomal rearrangements, and overproduction of ligands.[60] The frequent implication of dysregulated growth factor-RTK pathways in prostate carcinogenesis and androgen-independent progression represents a rationale for directing therapeutic approaches against RTK signaling in this disease. Thus far, two approaches for the direct inhibition of RTKs have achieved degrees of clinical success: (a) Targeting the extracellular ligand binding domains with monoclonal antibodies (Fig. 1, site 1), and (b) targeting the intracellular ATP-binding sites with small molecules (Fig. 1, site 2).

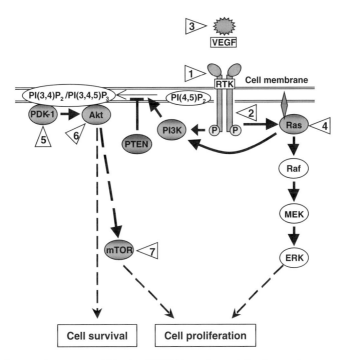

Fig. 1. Therapeutic targets within the PI3K/Akt pathway. The figure shows a schematic representation of the PI3K/Akt signaling pathway and its components that are targeted by the investigational agents discussed in this chapter. The numbered triangles identify sites of action of these agents which are described in the text: (1) ectodomain of receptor tyrosine kinases (targeted by monoclonal antibodies), (2) ATP-binding site of receptor tyrosine kinases (small molecule inhibitors), (3) vascular endothelial growth factor (monoclonal antibody), (4) Ras (farnesyl transferase inhibitors and antisense agents), (5) PDK-1 (small molecule inhibitors), (6) Akt (phospholipid analogs), and (7) mTOR (rapamycin analogs). mTOR, mammalian target of rapamycin; PDK-1, phosphoinositide-dependent kinase-1, PI3K, phosphatidylinositol-3-kinase; PI(4,5)P$_2$, phosphatidylinositol-4, 5-bisphosphate; PI(3,4,5)P$_3$, phosphatidylinositol-3,4,5-triphosphate; PTEN, phosphatase and tensin homologue deleted on chromosome 10; RTK, receptor tyrosine kinase; VEGF, vascular endothelial growth factor.

Epidermal Growth Factor Receptor (EGFR) Family

The EGFR superfamily is composed of four structurally related RTKs: HER1 (erbB1, EGFR), HER2 (neu, erbB2), HER3 (erbB3) and HER4 (erbB4). Of these, both HER1 and HER2 have been implicated in prostate cancer progression to androgen-independence. HER1 was expressed in nearly 90% of the androgen-independent metastases examined, in addition to evidence of a shift to an autocrine mechanism of receptor activation in these refractory metastatic tumor specimens.[61] In addition, a mutant HER1 carrying a deletion in the extracellular domain was shown to be constitutively active in the absence of ligand and to be highly expressed in malignant prostate tissue. Moreover, the level of expression of this variant increased in parallel with progression to malignancy.[62]

The case for HER2's role in prostate cancer biology has been considered less definitive. This uncertainty stems from highly variable data on expression levels of the receptor in HRPC tissues, and the absence of HER2 gene amplification as occurs in a subset of breast cancer patients,[3,63] in whom dramatic clinical success was achieved with HER2 inhibition. On the other hand, two independent groups reported nearly identical findings showing that the frequency of HER2 overexpression increased with progression from androgen-dependent to androgen-independent cancer,[64,65] suggesting a role for HER2 in the acquisition of hormone-independence. Supporting this contention is data from experimental systems which show that signaling through HER2 activates two parallel cascades, the Akt and MAPK pathways, which converge to phosphorylate and activate AR in a ligand-independent manner.[66,67]

In light of the likely importance of HER1 and HER2 in prostate cancer progression, therapeutic strategies for the direct suppression of these RTKs have been developed. Cetuximab (C225, Erbitux; ImClone) and ABX-EGF (Abgenix) are monoclonal antibodies directed against the extracellular ligand-binding domain of HER1. These antibodies block native ligand binding, HER1 autophosphorylation, and activation of the RTK.[68] Cetuximab has completed Phase I/II evaluation in which disease stabilization was achieved in combination with doxorubicin for androgen-independent prostate cancer.[59] Phase II evaluation of the fully humanized ABX-EGF in patients with HER1-overexpressing, hormone-resistant prostate tumors is underway. Trastuzumab (Herceptin, Genentech), a humanized monoclonal antibody directed against HER2, is clinically effective in women with HER2-overexpressing breast tumors. Against prostate cancer, it displayed antitumor activity in both androgen-dependent and -independent human prostate cancer xenograft models in combination with paclitaxel. As a single agent, however, androgen-independent tumors were unaffected by treatment.[69] The results of a recent Phase II study revealed a lack of efficacy in prostate cancer patients that did not overexpress HER2. In addition, difficulties in collecting metastatic tumor tissue thwarted identification of potentially responsive, HER2-overexpressing patients.[70] Another humanized monoclonal antibody directed against the HER2 ectodomain is 2C4 (pertuzumab; Genentech), which hinders the recruitment of HER2 into heterodimers with other HER receptors.[71] 2C4 inhibited androgen-independent prostate tumor growth in the 22Rv1 xenograft model[72] and will be evaluated in HRPC patients in a recently initiated Phase II trial.

A second strategy for therapeutic targeting of HER1 and HER2 signaling is the inhibition of tyrosine kinase activity using membrane-permeable small molecules. These compounds interfere with the ATP binding site in the intracellular domain thereby preventing ligand-induced receptor activation. Gefitinib (ZD1839; Iressa; AstraZeneca) is a highly selective HER1 tyrosine kinase inhibitor with a broad spectrum of antitumor activity against multiple types of human tumor xenografts, including prostate tumors. Combinations of gefitinib with conventional cytotoxic agents displayed additive and supra-additive effects in suppressing tumor growth.[73] Promising Phase I results in patients with a variety of solid tumors that express HER1, including advanced prostate cancer, has led to current Phase II studies in patients with HRPC and other malignancies.[74] Other small molecule inhibitors include the HER1/HER2 dual tyrosine kinase inhibitor, PKI-166 (Novartis), which exhibited antitumor activity against both androgen-dependent and androgen-independent prostate cancer xenografts.[75]

Platelet-Derived Growth Factor Receptor (PDGFR) Family

PDGFRs are RTKs that occur as α-homodimers (PDGFRα) or β-homodimers (PDGFRβ). Their ligands are PDGFs, which compose a family of disulfide-bonded dimeric isoforms. Four different PDGF chains have been identified: PDGF-A, -B, -C and -D, which exist as AA, BB, AB, CC and DD dimers. Ligand-induced receptor activation results in signaling through phosphoinositide-3-kinase (PI3K), phospholipase C and Ras/Raf/mitogen-activated protein kinase (MAPK) pathways.[76–78] PDGFs typically target connective tissue cell types, like fibroblasts and smooth muscle cells, to influence their growth, survival and function.[78]

The co-expression of PDGF and PDGFRs has been shown in numerous human malignancies, including prostate cancer,[79] suggesting a role in autocrine/paracrine growth stimulation. Furthermore, the PDGF-A chain and PDGFRα were preferentially expressed over the B chain and β-receptor in prostate tumors cells as determined by immunohistochemistry, but could not be detected in the normal cells surrounding the lesion.[79] Similarly, these two proteins were expressed in prostatic intraepithelial neoplasia (PIN) and in the tumor cells of prostate cancer bone metastases, but not in the adjacent normal bone stroma.[80,81] More recently, PDGFR was detected immunohistochemically in ≥80% of primary and metastatic prostate tumors.[82] These observations suggest that PDGFR expression is a feature of prostate cancer cells, occurs early in carcinogenesis, and is maintained throughout progression.

Small molecule inhibitors of PDGFR kinase activity that interfere with the ATP-binding pocket have been evaluated preclinically and in early clinical trials for efficacy against prostate cancer. Leflunomide (SU101; SUGEN Pharmaceuticals) is a potent inhibitor of PDGFR kinase activity *in vitro* and possesses antitumor activity against PDGFR-driven growth of xenograft tumors, including those derived from prostate cancer.[83] Phase II evaluation of leflunomide in pretreated patients with HRPC exhibited only modest clinical benefits, despite the immunohistochemical detection of PDGFR in ≥80% of primary and metastatic prostate tumors. This modest activity was attributed in part to the lability of the drug *in vivo*.[82] Imatinib mesylate (Gleevec, Novartis), the well known inhibitor of the Bcr-abl and c-kit tyrosine kinases, is an equally potent inhibitor of PDGFR kinase activity *in vitro*.[84] In a nude mouse xenograft model of bone metastasis, systemic treatment with imatinib mesylate reduced bone destruction caused by growth of prostate cancer cells after intratibial implantation. This effect was enhanced by co-treatment with paclitaxel and correlated with decreased levels of phosphorylated PDGFR. Notably, in untreated animals, strong expression of PDGFs and PDGFRs were detected in tumor cells within bone, but not in those growing outside the bone.[85] The findings support the clinical utility of PDGFR inhibition in the context of metastatic prostate cancer, and identify differences in tumor microenvironment as a factor that could influence the efficacy of RTK inhibitors.

Tropomyosin Receptor Kinase (trk) Family

Members of the trk family of RTKs, a subtype of the neurotrophin receptor family, are activated by the neurotrophin ligands: nerve growth factor (NGF), brain-derived neurotrophic factor (BDNF) and neurotrophins (NT)-3 and -4. Activation of trk receptors leads to downstream signaling through the Ras/Raf/MEK/MAPK and PI3K/Akt pathways.[86] The functional relevance of the trk receptor-neurotrophin axis to prostate carcinogenesis and progression is evident in the changes in the expression patterns of trk receptor types and neurotrophin ligands that occur during these processes. Specifically, in the normal prostate epithelium, a stromal-to-epithelial directed NGF-trkA paracrine axis exists, upon which the epithelial cells are not critically dependent for survival. During progression to adenocarcinoma, however, cancer cells acquire the ectopic expression of neurotrophins BDNT and NT-3, and their cognate receptors, trkB and trkC, thereby establishing a functional autocrine pathway. Also, cancer cells lose expression of p75NTR, which is a low affinity NT receptor that, in the appropriate context, can suppress trkA activity and induce apoptosis. Notably, tumor cells acquire a unique dependence on these acquired neurotrophin-trk pathways for survival.[87] Thus, neurotrophin-trk signaling represents a rational target for therapeutic intervention in HRPC.

Small molecule indolocarbazole analogs, designated CEP-751 and CEP-701 (Cephalon), are potent inhibitors of the tyrosine kinase activity of trk receptors. In a series of very careful studies, these compounds exhibited significant antitumor and antimetastatic activities in Dunning rat prostate cancer models, as well as human tumor xenografts through induction of apoptosis. By inhibiting trk activities, these agents blocked signaling through both pathways, Ras/Raf/MEK/MAPK and PI3K/Akt, with the latter pathway identified as the critical survival pathway emanating from ligand-activated trk receptors.[88–90] Currently, oral CEP-701 is being evaluated in a Phase II trial for patients with HRPC (www.hopkinskimmel-cancercenter.org/clinicaltrials/).

Vascular Endothelial Growth Factor Receptors (VEGFR)

Tumor growth requires new blood vessel formation, i.e. angiogenesis, which is dependent upon the paracrine action of proangiogenic molecules that are produced by tumor cells and act on the vascular endothelium. Among the proangiogenic factors that have been identified, VEGF (VEGF-A) plays a central role in tumor angiogenesis.[91] Other members of the VEGF family include VEGF-B, -C, -D and -E. VEGF induces angiogenesis by stimulating the proliferation, differentiation, migration and survival of endothelial cells through activation of the RTK, VEGFR-2 (Flk-1, KDR).[92,93] In prostate cancer, tumor growth and metastasis are dependent upon angiogenesis, and intratumoral vascular density is positively correlated with invasiveness and poor prognosis.[91,94] Moreover, established human prostate cancer cells lines, as well as human prostate cancer tissue specimens, can express functional VEGFRs.[95,96] These latter findings suggest the existence of an autocrine pathway through which prostate cancer cells themselves serve as a target for the stimulatory actions of VEGF. Thus, VEGF-induced signaling through VEGFRs is a logical therapeutic target in prostate cancer.

In the preclinical setting, the immunoneutralization of VEGF with monoclonal antibodies (Fig. 1, site 3) has been a successful strategy for the inhibition of angiogenesis and prostate tumor growth in animal models.[97–99] Bevacizumab (Avastin; Genentech), the recombinant humanized anti-VEGF monoclonal antibody, completed initial Phase I trials[100] and is currently being evaluated in numerous Phase II/III clinical trials for a variety of malignancies. Updated findings of a Phase III trial for patients with HRPC who received bevacizumab in combination with docetaxel and estramustine revealed high rates for PSA response (79%), measurable response (42%) and stable disease for 6 weeks or more (32%). Survival data from this study is not yet mature.[101]

ZD6474 (AstraZeneca), an orally available small molecule designed to be an inhibitor of the VEGFR family tyrosine kinase domain, caused profound regression of established PC-3 xenograft tumors in mice.[102] Interestingly, this compound also inhibits HER1 signaling which may add to its therapeutic efficacy.[103] It is currently being evaluated in a series of active Phase II trials for non-prostate cancers. SU5416 (semaxanib; Sugen) is another small molecule antiangiogenic agent that is a selective inhibitor of VEGFR-2 tyrosine kinase activity. Despite promising results from preclinical *in vivo* studies in prostate cancer models[104] and Phase I/II trials,[105] development of the agent was halted at Phase III.[106]

Ras

The Ras family of small GTP-binding proteins mediates signal transduction between the membrane and the nucleus. Its activation is a downstream component of signaling pathways emanating largely from a variety of RTKs which ultimately affect cell proliferation, differentiation, and survival. In order for Ras to function in signal transduction, it must be localized to the cell membrane. This is accomplished by the covalent addition of a farnesyl moiety to the C-terminal Cys of Ras by the enzyme farnesyl transferase.[107] Ras is inactive when bound to GDP. Ras activation occurs through its association with son of sevenless (SOS), which is bound to the activated RTK via the adaptor protein, Grb2. The subsequent conformational change in Ras permits the exchange of GTP for the GDP. Active, GTP-bound Ras then engages a variety of effectors that initiate a multitude of downstream signaling cascades of which the best characterized are the PI3K/Akt and Raf/MEK/MAPK pathways.[108] In the latter pathway, active Ras recruits Raf to the membrane, and then activates it. Raf in turn phosphorylates and activates MAPK kinases (MEK1/2), which then phosphorylate and activate MAPKs (extracellular signal-regulated kinases [ERK1/2]). ERK1/2 phosphorylate a number of substrates, including transcription factors, which can result in mitogenesis.

Activating mutations of Ras are common defects in human cancers;[109] however, such mutations are infrequent in prostate cancers.[110–112] Nonetheless, accumulating evidence supports the contention that wild-type Ras can be chronically activated by the aberrant autocrine/paracrine growth factor signaling that is characteristic of advanced prostate cancer[35] and implicates signaling through Ras/Raf/MAPK in prostate cancer progression to androgen-independence.[113,114] Thus, multiple components of this pathway appear to be potential targets for therapeutic intervention in this disease. For the purposes of this chapter, however, cross-talk between the PI3K/Akt and Ras/Raf/MEK/MAPK pathways at the level of Ras-induced activation of PI3K[108] identifies Ras as a therapeutic target for inhibiting PI3K/Akt signaling (Fig. 1, site 4).

The antisense compound, ISIS 2503 (Isis Pharmaceuticals), selectively inhibits the expression of H-Ras, and has been reported to inhibit cancer cell growth and to suppress H-Ras protein levels both *in vitro* and in xenograft models.[115] Notably, ISIS 2503 was shown to be effective even in cell lines with mutated K-Ras, as well as those without *ras* mutations, indicating a spectrum of activity not limited to cancers with mutated H-*ras*.[116] Although the results of Phase I trials were promising, patients with prostate cancer were not included in these studies,[116,117] or in any current Phase II trial evaluating this drug. Interestingly, ISIS 5132 (Isis Pharmaceuticals), an antisense drug targeting the downstream kinase, c-Raf, exhibited significant antitumor activity against a broad range of cancer cell types, including prostate cancer, in preclinical models,[118,119] leading to recent Phase I and II trials in patients with HRPC.[120] The farnesylation and subsequent localization of Ras to the cell membrane is a prerequisite for its ability to engage its partners and participate in signaling. Thus, the development of small molecule farnesyl transferase inhibitors (FTI) has been a focus for the therapeutic targeting of this signaling molecule.[121] Preclinically, FT inhibition has proven to be an effective strategy for growth suppression of prostate cancer cells *in vitro* and in prostate xenograft tumors *in vivo*.[122–126] The nonpeptidomimetic FTI, tipifarnib (R115777; Zarnestra; Johnson & Johnson) is undergoing evaluation in a number of clinical trials including a Phase II trial in HRPC patients. However, preliminary findings indicated no significant antitumor activity in these HRPC patients with the dose and schedule used, despite partial inhibition of FT activity and evidence of protein prenylation.[127] Other FTIs that have reached clinical trials, lonafarnib (SCH66336; Sarasar; Schering-Plough), BMS-214662 (Bristol-Myers Squibb), and L-778,123 (Merck) have not been evaluated in patients with prostate cancer.

PDK-1/Akt

The roles of PDK-1 and Akt in PI3K signaling and the importance of the pathway to prostate carcinogenesis and disease progression have been discussed. Despite the potential value of inhibiting PDK-1/Akt signaling, there exists a relative lack of clinically available agents directed at these molecules, in contrast to drugs targeting RTKs and the more downstream component of the pathway, mTOR (mammalian target of rapamycin; discussed below). Thus, the development of specific and effective small molecule inhibitors of PDK-1 and Akt (Fig. 1, sites 5 and 6, respectively) would fulfill a need in the development of therapies targeting this pathway. Industry efforts to develop drugs against the proximal components of the PI3K pathway include agents in preclinical studies targeting PI3K (Lilly, Iconix, Echelon-ComGenex), Akt (Kinetek, Celgene, Abbott, Kinacia), and integrin-linked kinase (ILK), a PDK-2 candidate (Kinetek).[128]

Despite industrial and academic efforts, no direct, small molecule inhibitor of Akt is available. Worth noting, however, is recent preclinical work demonstrating the efficacy of a novel alkylphospholipid, perifosine, against PTEN-null human PC-3 prostate cancer cells in which Akt is identified as an important target of perifosine action.[129] Perifosine inhibited PC-3 cell growth at low micromolar concentrations and caused rapid loss of Akt phosphorylation and activity in association with induction of p21. This phospholipid analog had no direct effects on PI3K, PDK-1, or Akt activities, but decreased membrane localization of Akt. Myristoylated-Akt abrogated these drug-induced effects, leading the authors to hypothesize that perifosine targets Akt by interacting with its PH-domain, thereby inhibiting its recruitment to the cell membrane by 3'-phosphorylated products of PI3K. Currently, two Phase II clinical trials are evaluating perifosine in prostate cancer patients with recurrent hormone-sensitive, and metastatic androgen-independent disease.

The only inhibitor of PDK-1, the upstream, activating kinase of Akt, currently in clinical trials is UCN-01 (7-hydroxystaurosporine; Kyowa Hakko Kogyo). However, this agent is not specific, having been shown to inhibit multiple kinases, including PDK-1, PKC, and cyclin-dependent kinases.[130,131] The apparent basis for this lack of specificity is its interaction with the ATP binding site, a mechanism associated with the broad-spectrum kinase inhibition that characterizes other competitive inhibitors of ATP binding, such as flavopiridol.[132] Nonetheless, Phase I evaluation of UCN-01 as monotherapy in patients with resistant solid tumors has been completed with some promising results in non-prostate cancer patients, and active Phase I trials are evaluating alternative dosing schedules and combinations with other chemotherapeutics.[132]

Another class of novel small molecule inhibitors of PDK-1/Akt signaling is being developed by the authors of this chapter. Although not yet in clinical trials, the lead compound, OSU-03012, is in preclinical development as part of the NCI's Rapid Access to Intervention Development (RAID) program and will be described briefly. Development of OSU-03012 evolved from mechanistic studies on the antitumor effects of the cyclooxygenase-2 (COX-2) inhibitor, celecoxib, in prostate cancer cells, which demonstrated that the two pharmacological effects of celecoxib (COX-2 inhibition and apoptosis induction) were separable, and which identified the structural requirements for each of these activities.[133,134] Moreover, blocking Akt activation through the inhibition of PDK-1 was shown to be a major COX-2-independent, antitumor target for celecoxib in prostate cancer cells.[135] These findings permitted the structure-based optimization of celecoxib to generate novel potent PDK-1 inhibitors that are devoid of COX-2-inhibitory activity. PDK-1 inhibition by these agents is achieved through interaction with the ATP binding site on the enzyme. OSU-03012 exhibits low micromolar IC_{50} values for PDK-1 inhibition, Akt dephosphorylation, and apoptosis induction in PC-3 cells. Moreover, the drug suppresses the growth of established PC-3 xenograft tumors after oral administration (C.S. Chen, unpublished findings).

mTOR

mTOR (also called FRAP and RAFT-6) is a serine-threonine kinase that is a downstream component in the PI3K/Akt signaling pathway.[136,137] Activation of mTOR by phosphorylation stimulates the translation of proteins important for cell cycle progression, such as cyclin D1, thereby coupling growth stimuli mediated by the PI3K/Akt pathway to cell proliferation. Specifically, mTOR phosphorylates two regulators of translation, the 40S ribosomal protein S6 kinase (p70^{S6K}) and eukaryotic initiation factor 4E-binding protein-1 (4E-BP1). Activated p70^{S6K} is important for ribosome biogenesis, while 4E-BP1, a repressor of mRNA translation, is inactivated by phosphorylation causing the release of active eukaryotic initiation factor 4E (eIF-4E). As a component of the translation initiation complex, eIF-4E promotes ribosome recruitment to mRNA and stimulates the translation of proteins essential for cell cycle progression from G1 to S phase.[63,138,139] The importance of dysregulated PI3K/Akt signaling in prostate cancer, particularly in advanced disease, as described above, suggests that mTOR is a relevant target for therapeutic intervention (Fig. 1, site 7). Indeed, both *in vitro* and *in vivo* studies, including those using prostate cancer cells, demonstrated that PTEN-inactive cells were preferentially sensitive to the growth inhibitory effects of mTOR inhibition.[140–143] These findings suggest that patients with tumors characterized by elevated PI3K/Akt signaling, such as HRPC, may represent a population responsive to mTOR-targeted therapies.

Currently, two investigational drugs that inhibit mTOR are in clinical trials as anticancer agents. Both of these agents, CCI-779 (Wyeth) and RAD001 (everolimus; Novartis), are soluble ester derivatives of the macrolide rapamycin, which is currently approved as an immunosuppressant for organ transplant patients (Rapamune; sirolimus; Wyeth). Rapamycin and its derivatives inhibit mTOR by binding to the immunophilin, FK506-binding protein 12 (FKBP12). This complex subsequently binds mTOR and inhibits its activation, thereby suppressing phosphorylation of downstream targets and cell proliferation.[144] Preclinically, pharmacological inhibition of mTOR has been shown to suppress cancer cell growth and to overcome chemotherapeutic resistance conferred by PTEN inactivation in both *in vitro* and *in vivo* models of prostate cancer.[140,145–149] CCI-779 has completed phase I studies without dose-limiting toxicity and with partial responses in some solid tumors (non-prostate).[63,139] It is currently being evaluated in two Phase II trials in prostate cancer patients; an open trial in the neoadjuvant setting and a closed trial in patients with androgen-independent metastatic tumors. RAD001 is currently in Phase I trials.[150]

Conclusions

Enthusiasm for the development of molecularly targeted agents has been spurred by the clinical successes of trastuzumab and imatinib mesylate, and the more recent approvals of gefitinib, cetuximab, and bevacizumab. One of the lessons learned from the development of these agents is the importance of target selection. Appropriate targets are the aberrant pathways or molecules upon which the cancer cell is critically dependent. The challenge here is whether targeting a single pathway or molecule will impact tumor burden given the redundancies in signaling pathways and the molecular heterogeneity inherent in the tumor cell population. In light of this problem, an approach that might prove effective is the targeting of convergence points of multiple signaling pathways, such as Akt. Modulation of such targets may provide more complete inhibition than those farther upstream, such as cell surface receptors. Of course, the potential benefits of such an approach will have to be balanced by careful evaluation of potential toxicities, as such points of signaling confluence are utilized in multiple cellular functions, including those in normal cell populations. Nevertheless, given the importance of signaling through PI3K/Akt in prostate cancer, targeting components of this pathway, either alone or in combination with cytotoxic agents or other targeted therapeutics, holds substantial promise.

Molecularly targeted agents that alter pathways critical to cancer cell survival and progression will undoubtedly compose, either alone or in combination, the foundation for future chemotherapeutic strategies for HRPC. The rate at which these strategies can mature and be translated to the clinical setting will rely in part on the identification and validation of appropriate targets, the consideration of more global signaling profiles or signatures in tumor cells that will facilitate the identification of critical pathways that can be targeted in combination, utilization of modern drug discovery/medicinal chemistry resources, access of clinician-scientists to new investigational agents developed by these resources, development of innovative means to identify patients who harbor a relevant target, and to assess drug responses in these patients, and on substantive and informative interactions among basic scientists and clinicians.

References

1. Oefelein MG, Resnick MI (2003) Effective testosterone suppression for patients with prostate cancer: Is there a best castration? *Urology* 62:207–213.
2. Goktas S, Crawford ED (1999) Optimal hormonal therapy for advanced prostatic carcinoma. *Semin Oncol* 26:162–173.
3. David AK, Khwaja R, Hudes GR (2003) Treatments for improving survival of patients with prostate cancer. *Drugs Aging* 20:683–699.
4. Small EJ, Vogelzang NJ (1997) Second-line hormonal therapy for advanced prostate cancer: A shifting paradigm. *J Clin Oncol* 15:382–388.
5. Roth BJ (1999) Androgen-independent prostate cancer: Not so chemorefractory after all. *Semin Oncol* 26:43–50.
6. Scherr D, Swindle PW, Scardino PT (2003) National Comprehensive Cancer Network guidelines for the management of prostate cancer. *Urology* 61: 14–24.
7. Smaletz O, Scher HI, Small EJ, *et al.* (2002) Nomogram for overall survival of patients with progressive metastatic prostate cancer after castration. *J Clin Oncol* 20:3972–3982.
8. Kamradt JM, Pienta KJ (2001) Prostate cancer chemotherapy: Closing out a century and opening a new one. In: Chung LWK, Isaacs WB, Simons JW, eds. *Prostate Cancer: Biology, Genetics and the New Therapeutics.* Human Press, Inc., Totowa, NJ, pp. 415–431.
9. Goodin S, Rao KV, DiPaola RS (2002) State-of-the-art treatment of metastatic hormone-refractory prostate cancer. *Oncologist* 7:360–370.
10. Solit DB, Kelly WK (2002) Chemotherapy for androgen-independent prostate cancer. In: Kantoff PW, Carroll PR, D'Amico AV, eds. *Prostate Cancer: Principles and Practice.* Lippincott, Williams and Wilkins, Philadelphia, PA, pp. 665–681.
11. Martel CL, Gumerlock PH, Meyers FJ, Lara PN (2003) Current strategies in the management of hormone refractory prostate cancer. *Cancer Treat Rev* 29:171 187.
12. Trump D, Lau YK (2003) Chemotherapy of prostate cancer: Present and future. *Curr Urol Rep* 4:229–232.
13. Stearns ME, Tew KD (1988) Estramustine binds MAP-2 to inhibit microtubule assembly *in vitro. J Cell Sci* 89(Pt 3):331–342.
14. Tew KD, Glusker JP, Hartley-Asp B, Hudes G, Speicher LA (1992) Preclinical and clinical perspectives on the use of estramustine as an antimitotic drug. *Pharmacol Ther* 56:323–339.

15. Obasaju C, Hudes GR (2001) Paclitaxel and docetaxel in prostate cancer. *Hematol Oncol Clin North Am* 15:525–545.
16. Slamon DJ, Leyland-Jones B, Shak S, *et al.* (2001) Use of chemotherapy plus a monoclonal antibody against HER2 for metastatic breast cancer that over-expresses HER2. *N Engl J Med* 344:783–792.
17. Druker BJ, Sawyers CL, Kantarjian H, *et al.* (2001) Activity of a specific inhibitor of the BCR-ABL tyrosine kinase in the blast crisis of chronic myeloid leukemia and acute lymphoblastic leukemia with the Philadelphia chromosome. *N Engl J Med* 344:1038–1042.
18. Joensuu H, Roberts PJ, Sarlomo-Rikala M, *et al.* (2001) Effect of the tyrosine kinase inhibitor STI571 in a patient with a metastatic gastrointestinal stromal tumor. *N Engl J Med* 344:1052–1056.
19. Chan TO, Rittenhouse SE, Tsichlis PN (1999) AKT/PKB and other D3 phosphoinositide-regulated kinases: Kinase activation by phosphoinositide-dependent phosphorylation. *Annu Rev Biochem* 68:965–1014.
20. Datta SR, Brunet A, Greenberg ME (1999) Cellular survival: A play in three Akts. *Genes Dev* 13:2905–2927.
21. Toker A, Cantley LC (1997) Signalling through the lipid products of phosphoinositide-3-OH kinase. *Nature* 387:673–676.
22. Storz P, Toker A (2002) 3'-phosphoinositide-dependent kinase-1 (PDK-1) in PI 3-kinase signaling. *Front Biosci* 7:886–902.
23. Scheid MP, Woodgett JR (2003) Unravelling the activation mechanisms of protein kinase B/Akt. *FEBS Lett* 546:108–112.
24. Cantley LC (2002) The phosphoinositide 3-kinase pathway. *Science* 296:1655–1657.
25. Hill MM, Hemmings BA (2002) Inhibition of protein kinase B/Akt. Implications for cancer therapy. *Pharmacol Therap* 93:243–251.
26. Ozes ON, Mayo LD, Gustin JA, Pfeffer SR, Pfeffer LM, Donner DB (1999) NF-kappaB activation by tumour necrosis factor requires the Akt serine-threonine kinase. *Nature* 401:82–85.
27. Cantley LC, Neel BG (1999) New insights into tumor suppression: PTEN suppresses tumor formation by restraining the phosphoinositide 3-kinase/AKT pathway. *Proc Natl Acad Sci USA* 96:4240–4245.
28. Di Cristofano A, Pandolfi PP (2000) The multiple roles of PTEN in tumor suppression. *Cell* 100:387–390.
29. Wang SI, Parsons R, Ittmann M (1998) Homozygous deletion of the PTEN tumor suppressor gene in a subset of prostate adenocarcinomas. *Clin Cancer Res* 4:811–815.

30. Whang YE, Wu X, Suzuki H, *et al.* (1998) Inactivation of the tumor suppressor PTEN/MMAC1 in advanced human prostate cancer through loss of expression. *Proc Natl Acad Sci USA* 95:5246–5250.

31. McMenamin ME, Soung P, Perera S, Kaplan I, Loda M, Sellers WR (1999) Loss of PTEN expression in paraffin-embedded primary prostate cancer correlates with high Gleason score and advanced stage. *Cancer Res* 59: 4291–4296.

32. Vlietstra RJ, van Alewijk DC, Hermans KG, van Steenbrugge GJ, Trapman J (1998) Frequent inactivation of PTEN in prostate cancer cell lines and xenografts. *Cancer Res* 58:2720–2723.

33. Abate-Shen C, Shen MM (2000) Molecular genetics of prostate cancer. *Genes Dev* 14:2410–2434.

34. DeMarzo AM, Nelson WG, Isaacs WB, Epstein JI (2003) Pathological and molecular aspects of prostate cancer. *Lancet* 361:955–964.

35. Djakiew D (2000) Dysregulated expression of growth factors and their receptors in the development of prostate cancer. *Prostate* 42:150–160.

36. Page C, Lin HJ, Jin Y, *et al.* (2000) Overexpression of Akt/AKT can modulate chemotherapy-induced apoptosis. *Anticancer Res* 20:407–416.

37. Graff JR, Konicek BW, McNulty AM, *et al.* (2000) Increased AKT activity contributes to prostate cancer progression by dramatically accelerating prostate tumor growth and diminishing p27Kip1 expression. *J Biol Chem* 275:24500–24505.

38. Paweletz CP, Charboneau L, Bichsel VE, *et al.* (2001) Reverse phase protein microarrays which capture disease progression show activation of pro-survival pathways at the cancer invasion front. *Oncogene* 20: 1981–1989.

39. Malik SN, Brattain M, Ghosh PM, *et al.* (2002) Immunohistochemical demonstration of phospho-Akt in high Gleason grade prostate cancer. *Clin Cancer Res* 8:1168–1171.

40. Di Cristofano A, De Acetis M, Koff A, Cordon-Cardo C, Pandolfi PP (2001) Pten and p27KIP1 cooperate in prostate cancer tumor suppression in the mouse. *Nat Genet* 27:222–224.

41. Majumder PK, Yeh JJ, George DJ, *et al.* (2003) Prostate intraepithelial neoplasia induced by prostate restricted Akt activation: The MPAKT model. *Proc Natl Acad Sci USA* 100:7841–7846.

42. Kwabi-Addo B, Giri D, Schmidt K, *et al.* (2001) Haploinsufficiency of the Pten tumor suppressor gene promotes prostate cancer progression. *Proc Natl Acad Sci USA* 98:11563–11568.

43. Kim MJ, Cardiff RD, Desai N, *et al.* (2002) Cooperativity of Nkx3.1 and Pten loss of function in a mouse model of prostate carcinogenesis. *Proc Natl Acad Sci USA* 99:2884–2889.
44. Backman SA, Ghazarian D, So K, *et al.* (2004) Early onset of neoplasia in the prostate and skin of mice with tissue-specific deletion of Pten. *Proc Natl Acad Sci USA* 101:1725–1730.
45. Wang S, Gao J, Lei Q, *et al.* (2003) Prostate-specific deletion of the murine Pten tumor suppressor gene leads to metastatic prostate cancer. *Cancer Cell* 4:209–221.
46. Dimmeler S, Zeiher AM (2000) Akt takes center stage in angiogenesis signaling. *Circ Res* 86:4–5.
47. Clark AS, West K, Streicher S, Dennis PA (2002) Constitutive and inducible Akt activity promotes resistance to chemotherapy, trastuzumab, or tamoxifen in breast cancer cells. *Mol Cancer Ther* 1:707–717.
48. Wu K, Wang C, D'Amico M, *et al.* (2002) Flavopiridol and trastuzumab synergistically inhibit proliferation of breast cancer cells: Association with selective cooperative inhibition of cyclin D1-dependent kinase and Akt signaling pathways. *Mol Cancer Ther* 1:695–706.
49. Hayakawa J, Ohmichi M, Kurachi H, *et al.* (2000) Inhibition of BAD phosphorylation either at serine 112 via extracellular signal-regulated protein kinase cascade or at serine 136 via Akt cascade sensitizes human ovarian cancer cells to cisplatin. *Cancer Res* 60:5988–5994.
50. Mabuchi S, Ohmichi M, Kimura A, *et al.* (2002) Inhibition of phosphorylation of BAD and Raf-1 by Akt sensitizes human ovarian cancer cells to paclitaxel. *J Biol Chem* 277:33490–33500.
51. Yip-Schneider MT, Wiesenauer CA, Schmidt CM (2003) Inhibition of the phosphatidylinositol 3'-kinase signaling pathway increases the responsiveness of pancreatic carcinoma cells to sulindac. *J Gastrointest Surg* 7:354–363.
52. Kraus AC, Ferber I, Bachmann SO, *et al.* (2002) *In vitro* chemo- and radio-resistance in small cell lung cancer correlates with cell adhesion and constitutive activation of AKT and MAP kinase pathways. *Oncogene* 21:8683–8695.
53. Krystal GW, Sulanke G, Litz J (2002) Inhibition of phosphatidylinositol 3-kinase-Akt signaling blocks growth, promotes apoptosis, and enhances sensitivity of small cell lung cancer cells to chemotherapy. *Mol Cancer Ther* 1:913–922.
54. O'Gorman DM, McKenna SL, McGahon AJ, Knox KA, Cotter TG (2000) Sensitisation of HL60 human leukaemic cells to cytotoxic drug-induced apoptosis by inhibition of PI3-kinase survival signals. *Leukemia* 14:602–611.

55. Neri LM, Borgatti P, Tazzari PL, *et al.* (2003) The phosphoinositide 3-kinase/ AKT1 pathway involvement in drug and all-trans-retinoic acid resistance of leukemia cells. *Mol Cancer Res* 1:234–246.

56. Beresford SA, Davies MA, Gallick GE, Donato NJ (2001) Differential effects of phosphatidylinositol-3/Akt-kinase inhibition on apoptotic sensitization to cytokines in LNCaP and PCc-3 prostate cancer cells. *J Interferon Cytokine Res* 21:313–322.

57. West KA, Sianna Castillo S, Dennis PA (2002) Activation of the PI3K/Akt pathway and chemotherapeutic resistance. *Drug Resist Updat* 5:234–248.

58. Schlessinger J (2000) Cell signaling by receptor tyrosine kinases. *Cell* 103: 211–225.

59. Barton J, Blackledge G, Wakeling A (2001) Growth factors and their receptors: New targets for prostate cancer therapy. *Urology* 58:114–122.

60. Fabbro D, Parkinson D, Matter A (2002) Protein tyrosine kinase inhibitors: New treatment modalities? *Curr Opin Pharmacol* 2:374–381.

61. Scher HI, Sarkis A, Reuter V, *et al.* (1995) Changing pattern of expression of the epidermal growth factor receptor and transforming growth factor alpha in the progression of prostatic neoplasms. *Clin Cancer Res* 1:545–550.

62. Olapade-Olaopa EO, Moscatello DK, MacKay EH, *et al.* (2000) Evidence for the differential expression of a variant EGF receptor protein in human prostate cancer. *Br J Cancer* 82:186–194.

63. Hudes GR (2002) Signaling inhibitors in the treatment of prostate cancer. *Invest New Drugs* 20:159–172.

64. Signoretti S, Montironi R, Manola J, *et al.* (2000) Her-2-neu expression and progression toward androgen independence in human prostate cancer. *J Natl Cancer Inst* 92:1918–1925.

65. Osman I, Scher HI, Drobnjak M, *et al.* (2001) HER-2/neu (p185neu) protein expression in the natural or treated history of prostate cancer. *Clin Cancer Res* 7:2643–2647.

66. Yeh S, Lin HK, Kang HY, Thin TH, Lin MF, Chang C (1999) From HER2/ Neu signal cascade to androgen receptor and its coactivators: A novel pathway by induction of androgen target genes through MAP kinase in prostate cancer cells. *Proc Natl Acad Sci USA* 96:5458–5463.

67. Wen Y, Hu MC, Makino K, *et al.* (2000) HER-2/neu promotes androgen-independent survival and growth of prostate cancer cells through the Akt pathway. *Cancer Res* 60:6841–6845.

68. Ratan HL, Gescher A, Steward WP, Mellon JK (2003) ErbB receptors: Possible therapeutic targets in prostate cancer? *BJU Int* 92:890–895.

69. Agus DB, Scher HI, Higgins B, *et al.* (1999) Response of prostate cancer to anti-Her-2/neu antibody in androgen-dependent and -independent human xenograft models. *Cancer Res* 59:4761–4764.
70. Morris MJ, Reuter VE, Kelly WK, *et al.* (2002) HER-2 profiling and targeting in prostate carcinoma. *Cancer* 94:980–986.
71. Albanell J, Codony J, Rovira A, Mellado B, Gascon P (2003) Mechanism of action of anti-HER2 monoclonal antibodies: Scientific update on trastuzumab and 2C4. *Adv Exp Med Biol* 532:253–268.
72. Mendoza N, Phillips GL, Silva J, Schwall R, Wickramasinghe D (2002) Inhibition of ligand-mediated HER2 activation in androgen-independent prostate cancer. *Cancer Res* 62:5485–5488.
73. Sirotnak FM, Zakowski MF, Miller VA, Scher HI, Kris MG (2000) Efficacy of cytotoxic agents against human tumor xenografts is markedly enhanced by coadministration of ZD1839 (Iressa), an inhibitor of EGFR tyrosine kinase. *Clin Cancer Res* 6:4885–4892.
74. Lorusso PM (2003) Phase I studies of ZD1839 in patients with common solid tumors. *Semin Oncol* 30:21–29.
75. Mellinghoff IK, Tran C, Sawyers CL (2002) Growth inhibitory effects of the dual ErbB1/ErbB2 tyrosine kinase inhibitor PKI-166 on human prostate cancer xenografts. *Cancer Res* 62:5254–5259.
76. Bergsten E, Uutela M, Li X, *et al.* (2001) PDGF-D is a specific, protease-activated ligand for the PDGF beta-receptor. *Nat Cell Biol* 3:512–516.
77. LaRochelle WJ, Jeffers M, McDonald WF, *et al.* (2001) PDGF-D, a new protease-activated growth factor. *Nat Cell Biol* 3:517–521.
78. Heldin CH, Westermark B (1999) Mechanism of action and *in vivo* role of platelet-derived growth factor. *Physiol Rev* 79:1283–1316.
79. Fudge K, Wang CY, Stearns ME (1994) Immunohistochemistry analysis of platelet-derived growth factor A and B chains and platelet-derived growth factor alpha and beta receptor expression in benign prostatic hyperplasias and Gleason-graded human prostate adenocarcinomas. *Mod Pathol* 7: 549–554.
80. Chott A, Sun Z, Morganstern D, *et al.* (1999) Tyrosine kinases expressed *in vivo* by human prostate cancer bone marrow metastases and loss of the type 1 insulin-like growth factor receptor. *Am J Pathol* 155:1271–1279.
81. Fudge K, Bostwick DG, Stearns ME (1996) Platelet-derived growth factor A and B chains and the alpha and beta receptors in prostatic intraepithelial neoplasia. *Prostate* 29:282–286.
82. Ko YJ, Small EJ, Kabbinavar F, *et al.* (2001) A multi-institutional phase ii study of SU101, a platelet-derived growth factor receptor inhibitor, for

patients with hormone-refractory prostate cancer. *Clin Cancer Res* 7: 800–805.

83. Shawver LK, Schwartz DP, Mann E, *et al.* (1997) Inhibition of platelet-derived growth factor-mediated signal transduction and tumor growth by N-[4-(trifluoromethyl)-phenyl]5-methylisoxazole-4-carboxamide. *Clin Cancer Res* 3:1167–1177.

84. Buchdunger E, Cioffi CL, Law N, *et al.* (2000) Abl protein-tyrosine kinase inhibitor STI571 inhibits *in vitro* signal transduction mediated by c-kit and platelet-derived growth factor receptors. *J Pharmacol Exp Ther* 295: 139–145.

85. Uehara H, Kim SJ, Karashima T, *et al.* (2003) Effects of blocking platelet-derived growth factor-receptor signaling in a mouse model of experimental prostate cancer bone metastases. *J Natl Cancer Inst* 95:458–470.

86. Kaplan DR, Miller FD (1997) Signal transduction by the neurotrophin receptors. *Curr Opin Cell Biol* 9:213–221.

87. Weeraratna AT, Arnold JT, George DJ, DeMarzo A, Isaacs JT (2000) Rational basis for Trk inhibition therapy for prostate cancer. *Prostate* 45:140–148.

88. Dionne CA, Camoratto AM, Jani JP, *et al.* (1998) Cell cycle-independent death of prostate adenocarcinoma is induced by the trk tyrosine kinase inhibitor CEP-751 (KT6587). *Clin Cancer Res* 4:1887–1898.

89. George DJ, Dionne CA, Jani J, *et al.* (1999) Sustained *in vivo* regression of Dunning H rat prostate cancers treated with combinations of androgen ablation and Trk tyrosine kinase inhibitors, CEP-751 (KT-6587) or CEP-701 (KT-5555). *Cancer Res* 59:2395–2401.

90. Weeraratna AT, Dalrymple SL, Lamb JC, *et al.* (2001) Pan-trk inhibition decreases metastasis and enhances host survival in experimental models as a result of its selective induction of apoptosis of prostate cancer cells. *Clin Cancer Res* 7:2237–2245.

91. Choy M, Rafii S (2001) Role of angiogenesis in the progression and treatment of prostate cancer. *Cancer Invest* 19:181–191.

92. Cross MJ, Dixelius J, Matsumoto T, Claesson-Welsh L (2003) VEGF-receptor signal transduction. *Trends Biochem Sci* 28:488–494.

93. Gerber HP, McMurtrey A, Kowalski J, *et al.* (1998) Vascular endothelial growth factor regulates endothelial cell survival through the phosphatidyli-nositol 3′-kinase/Akt signal transduction pathway. Requirement for Flk-1/KDR activation. *J Biol Chem* 273:30336–30343.

94. Weidner N, Carroll PR, Flax J, Blumenfeld W, Folkman J (1993) Tumor angiogenesis correlates with metastasis in invasive prostate carcinoma. *Am J Pathol* 143:401–409.

95. Ferrer FA, Miller LJ, Lindquist R, *et al.* (1999) Expression of vascular endothelial growth factor receptors in human prostate cancer. *Urology* 54:567–572.
96. Chevalier S, Defoy I, Lacoste J, *et al.* (2002) Vascular endothelial growth factor and signaling in the prostate: More than angiogenesis. *Mol Cell Endocrinol* 189:169–179.
97. Borgstrom P, Bourdon MA, Hillan KJ, Sriramarao P, Ferrara N (1998) Neutralizing anti-vascular endothelial growth factor antibody completely inhibits angiogenesis and growth of human prostate carcinoma micro tumors *in vivo. Prostate* 35:1–10.
98. Melnyk O, Zimmerman M, Kim KJ, Shuman M (1999) Neutralizing anti-vascular endothelial growth factor antibody inhibits further growth of established prostate cancer and metastases in a pre-clinical model. *J Urol* 161:960–963.
99. Fox WD, Higgins B, Maiese KM, *et al.* (2002) Antibody to vascular endothelial growth factor slows growth of an androgen-independent xenograft model of prostate cancer. *Clin Cancer Res* 8:3226–3231.
100. Gordon MS, Margolin K, Talpaz M, *et al.* (2001) Phase I safety and pharmacokinetic study of recombinant human anti-vascular endothelial growth factor in patients with advanced cancer. *J Clin Oncol* 19:843–850.
101. Picus J (2004) Docetaxel/Bevacizumab (avastin) in prostate cancer. *Cancer Invest* 22(Suppl 1):60 (Abstract 46).
102. Wedge SR, Ogilvie DJ, Dukes M, *et al.* (2002) ZD6474 inhibits vascular endothelial growth factor signaling, angiogenesis, and tumor growth following oral administration. *Cancer Res* 62:4645–4655.
103. Ciardiello F, Caputo R, Damiano V, *et al.* (2003) Antitumor effects of ZD6474, a small molecule vascular endothelial growth factor receptor tyrosine kinase inhibitor, with additional activity against epidermal growth factor receptor tyrosine kinase. *Clin Cancer Res* 9:1546–1556.
104. Fong TA, Shawver LK, Sun L, *et al.* (1999) SU5416 is a potent and selective inhibitor of the vascular endothelial growth factor receptor (Flk-1/KDR) that inhibits tyrosine kinase catalysis, tumor vascularization, and growth of multiple tumor types. *Cancer Res* 59:99–106.
105. Rothenberg ML, Berlin JD, Cropp GF, *et al.* (2001) Phase I/II study of SU5416 in combination with irinotecan/5-FU/LV (IFL) in patients with metastatic colorectal cancer. *Proc Am Soc Clin Oncol* 20:75a (Abstract 298).
106. Unknown (2002) Trials terminated (News Update). *Appl Clin Trials* 11:16.
107. Hancock JF (2003) Ras proteins: Different signals from different locations. *Nat Rev Mol Cell Biol* 4:373–384.

108. Shields JM, Pruitt K, McFall A, Shaub A, Der CJ (2000) Understanding Ras: 'It ain't over 'til it's over'. *Trends Cell Biol* 10:147–154.
109. Bos JL (1989) ras oncogenes in human cancer: A review. *Cancer Res* 49: 4682–4689.
110. Carter BS, Epstein JI, Isaacs WB (1990) ras gene mutations in human prostate cancer. *Cancer Res* 50:6830–6832.
111. Gumerlock PH, Poonamallee UR, Meyers FJ, deVere White RW (1991) Activated ras alleles in human carcinoma of the prostate are rare. *Cancer Res* 51:1632–1637.
112. Moul JW, Friedrichs PA, Lance RS, Theune SM, Chang EH (1992) Infrequent RAS oncogene mutations in human prostate cancer. *Prostate* 20:327–338.
113. Gioeli D, Mandell JW, Petroni GR, Frierson HF Jr, Weber MJ (1999) Activation of mitogen-activated protein kinase associated with prostate cancer progression. *Cancer Res* 59:279–284.
114. Bakin RE, Gioeli D, Sikes RA, Bissonette EA, Weber MJ (2003) Constitutive activation of the Ras/mitogen-activated protein kinase signaling pathway promotes androgen hypersensitivity in LNCaP prostate cancer cells. *Cancer Res* 63:1981–1989.
115. Holmlund JT, Monia BP, Kwoh TJ, Dorr FA (1999) Toward antisense oligonucleotide therapy for cancer: ISIS compounds in clinical development. *Curr Opin Mol Ther* 1:372–385.
116. Cunningham CC, Holmlund JT, Geary RS, et al. (2001) A Phase I trial of H-ras antisense oligonucleotide ISIS 2503 administered as a continuous intravenous infusion in patients with advanced carcinoma. *Cancer* 92:1265–1271.
117. Adjei AA, Dy GK, Erlichman C, et al. (2003) A phase I trial of ISIS 2503, an antisense inhibitor of H-ras, in combination with gemcitabine in patients with advanced cancer. *Clin Cancer Res* 9:115–123.
118. Monia BP, Johnston JF, Sasmor H, Cummins LL (1996) Nuclease resistance and antisense activity of modified oligonucleotides targeted to Ha-ras. *J Biol Chem* 271:14533–14540.
119. Geiger T, Muller M, Monia BP, Fabbro D (1997) Antitumor activity of a C-raf antisense oligonucleotide in combination with standard chemotherapeutic agents against various human tumors transplanted subcutaneously into nude mice. *Clin Cancer Res* 3:1179–1185.
120. Tolcher AW, Reyno L, Venner PM, et al. (2002) A randomized phase II and pharmacokinetic study of the antisense oligonucleotides ISIS 3521 and ISIS 5132 in patients with hormone-refractory prostate cancer. *Clin Cancer Res* 8:2530–2535.

121. Kohl NE (1999) Farnesyltransferase inhibitors. Preclinical development. *Ann N Y Acad Sci* 886:91–102.
122. Sepp-Lorenzino L, Tjaden G, Moasser MM, *et al.* (2001) Farnesyl: Protein transferase inhibitors as potential agents for the management of human prostate cancer. *Prostate Cancer Prostatic Dis* 4:33–43.
123. Shi B, Yaremko B, Hajian G, *et al.* (2000) The farnesyl protein transferase inhibitor SCH66336 synergizes with taxanes *in vitro* and enhances their antitumor activity *in vivo. Cancer Chemother Pharmacol* 46:387–393.
124. Liu M, Bryant MS, Chen J, *et al.* (1998) Antitumor activity of SCH 66336, an orally bioavailable tricyclic inhibitor of farnesyl protein transferase, in human tumor xenograft models and wap-ras transgenic mice. *Cancer Res* 58:4947–4956.
125. Nielsen LL, Shi B, Hajian G, *et al.* (1999) Combination therapy with the farnesyl protein transferase inhibitor SCH66336 and SCH58500 (p53 adenovirus) in preclinical cancer models. *Cancer Res* 59:5896–5901.
126. Sirotnak FM, Sepp-Lorenzino L, Kohl NE, Rosen N, Scher HI (2000) A peptidomimetic inhibitor of ras functionality markedly suppresses growth of human prostate tumor xenografts in mice. Prospects for long-term clinical utility. *Cancer Chemother Pharmacol* 46:79–83.
127. Haas N, Peereboom D, Rangnanathan S, Thistle A, Greenberg R (2002) Phase II trial of R115777, an inhibitor of farnesyltransferase, in patients with hormone refractory prostate cancer. *Proc Am Soc Clin Oncol* 21:181a (Abstract 721).
128. Mills GB, Kohn E, Lu Y, *et al.* (2003) Linking molecular diagnostics to molecular therapeutics: Targeting the PI3K pathway in breast cancer. *Semin Oncol* 30:93–104.
129. Kondapaka SB, Singh SS, Dasmahapatra GP, Sausville EA, Roy KK (2003) Perifosine, a novel alkylphospholipid, inhibits protein kinase B activation. *Mol Cancer Ther* 2:1093–1103.
130. Sato S, Fujita N, Tsuruo T (2002) Interference with PDK1-Akt survival signaling pathway by UCN-01 (7-hydroxystaurosporine). *Oncogene* 21:1727–1738.
131. Shao RG, Shimizu T, Pommier Y (1997) 7-Hydroxystaurosporine (UCN-01) induces apoptosis in human colon carcinoma and leukemia cells independently of p53. *Exp Cell Res* 234:388–397.
132. Senderowicz AM (2002) The cell cycle as a target for cancer therapy: Basic and clinical findings with the small molecule inhibitors flavopiridol and UCN-01. *Oncologist* 7(Suppl 3):12–19.

133. Song X, Lin HP, Johnson AJ, *et al.* (2002) Cyclooxygenase-2, player or spectator in cyclooxygenase-2 inhibitor-induced apoptosis in prostate cancer cells. *J Natl Cancer Inst* 94:585–591.
134. Zhu J, Song X, Lin HP, *et al.* (2002) Using cyclooxygenase-2 inhibitors as molecular platforms to develop a new class of apoptosis-inducing agents. *J Natl Cancer Inst* 94:1745–1757.
135. Kulp SK, Yang YT, Hung CC, *et al.* (2004) 3-phosphoinositide-dependent protein kinase-1/Akt signaling represents a major cyclooxygenase-2-independent target for celecoxib in prostate cancer cells. *Cancer Res* 64: 1444–1451.
136. Scott PH, Brunn GJ, Kohn AD, Roth RA, Lawrence JC Jr (1998) Evidence of insulin-stimulated phosphorylation and activation of the mammalian target of rapamycin mediated by a protein kinase B signaling pathway. *Proc Natl Acad Sci USA* 95:7772–7777.
137. Nave BT, Ouwens M, Withers DJ, Alessi DR, Shepherd PR (1999) Mammalian target of rapamycin is a direct target for protein kinase B: Identification of a convergence point for opposing effects of insulin and amino-acid deficiency on protein translation. *Biochem J* 344(Pt 2): 427–431.
138. Dutcher JP (2004) Mammalian target of rapamycin (mTOR) inhibitors. *Curr Oncol Rep* 6:111–115.
139. Tolcher AW (2004) Novel therapeutic molecular targets for prostate cancer: The mTOR signaling pathway and epidermal growth factor receptor. *J Urol* 171:S41–43 (discussion S44).
140. Neshat MS, Mellinghoff IK, Tran C, *et al.* (2001) Enhanced sensitivity of PTEN-deficient tumors to inhibition of FRAP/mTOR. *Proc Natl Acad Sci USA* 98:10314–10319.
141. Podsypanina K, Lee RT, Politis C, *et al.* (2001) An inhibitor of mTOR reduces neoplasia and normalizes p70/S6 kinase activity in Pten+/− mice. *Proc Natl Acad Sci USA* 98:10320–10325.
142. Shi Y, Gera J, Hu L, *et al.* (2002) Enhanced sensitivity of multiple myeloma cells containing PTEN mutations to CCI-779. *Cancer Res* 62: 5027–5034.
143. Yu K, Toral-Barza L, Discafani C, *et al.* (2001) mTOR, a novel target in breast cancer: The effect of CCI-779, an mTOR inhibitor, in preclinical models of breast cancer. *Endocr Relat Cancer* 8:249–258.
144. Hidalgo M, Rowinsky EK (2000) The rapamycin-sensitive signal transduction pathway as a target for cancer therapy. *Oncogene* 19:6680–6686.

145. Mousses S, Wagner U, Chen Y, *et al.* (2001) Failure of hormone therapy in prostate cancer involves systematic restoration of androgen responsive genes and activation of rapamycin sensitive signaling. *Oncogene* 20: 6718–6723.
146. Grunwald V, DeGraffenried L, Russel D, Friedrichs WE, Ray RB, Hidalgo M (2002) Inhibitors of mTOR reverse doxorubicin resistance conferred by PTEN status in prostate cancer cells. *Cancer Res* 62:6141–6145.
147. van der Poel HG, Hanrahan C, Zhong H, Simons JW (2003) Rapamycin induces Smad activity in prostate cancer cell lines. *Urol Res* 30:380–386.
148. Gao N, Zhang Z, Jiang BH, Shi X (2003) Role of PI3K/AKT/mTOR signaling in the cell cycle progression of human prostate cancer. *Biochem Biophys Res Commun* 310:1124–1132.
149. Gera JF, Mellinghoff IK, Shi Y, *et al.* (2004) AKT activity determines sensitivity to mammalian target of rapamycin (mTOR) inhibitors by regulating cyclin D1 and c-myc expression. *J Biol Chem* 279:2737–2746.
150. Huang S, Houghton PJ (2003) Targeting mTOR signaling for cancer therapy. *Curr Opin Pharmacol* 3:371–377.

6

CHEMOPREVENTION FOR PROSTATE CANCER

Noahiro Fujimoto

Department of Urology
University of Occupational and Environmental Health
Iseigaoka, Yahatanishiku, Kitakyushu, 807–8555, Japan

Introduction

Chemoprevention is defined as the use of specific agents to suppress or reverse carcinogenesis and to prevent the development of cancer.[1] Chemoprevention trials are ongoing for various cancers including prostate cancer. There are significant epidemiological differences related to the higher incidence of clinical prostate cancer observed in Western compared to Asian countries. However, the incidence of occult prostate cancer is very similar between Western and Asian countries. The development of prostate cancer is a long-term process involving multiple steps. Normal epithelia may require 10–30 years to develop into local clinical cancer and another 10–20 years to metastasize (Fig. 1).[2] Sex steroids, especially androgens, influence the development of prostate cancer. These findings provide multiple opportunities for preventing prostate cancer and investigation of chemoprevention is very attractive. The goal of prostate cancer chemoprevention is to find agents that modulate the progression from normal epithelium to clinically significant and localized cancer, and also prevent the progression from localized cancer to locally advanced, then to metastatic, and finally to hormone refractory cancer (Fig. 2).

The development of chemoprevention strategies against prostate cancer would have great overall impact both medically and economically. Various phase I–III chemoprevention trials were conducted by National Cancer Institute (NCI)[3] and several other trials are ongoing (Table 1).

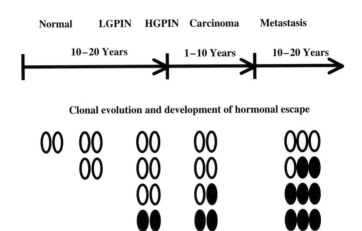

Fig. 1. Natural history of prostate carcinogenesis.[2] Early stages are androgen dependent. However, as disease progresses over time, androgen-dependent clones emerge, either *de novo* or in response to androgen deprivation therapy and clonal selection. Clear circles represent androgen-dependent or sensitive cells, filled circles represent androgen-independent or resistant cells. LGPIN: Low-grade prostatic intraepithelial neoplasia, HGPIN: high-grade prostatic intraepithelial neoplasia.

Chemopreventive Agents, Rationale and Clinical Trials

There are many candidate treatment strategies for prostate cancer prevention (Table 2).[4] Here we will focus on several chemopreventive agents and clinical trials.

Sex Steroid Signaling: Antiandrogens and Antiestrogens

It is well known that sex hormones influence the development of prostate cancer. Thus, the strategies altering sex steroid signaling may be useful tools for preventing prostate cancer.

5-α Reductase Inhibitor (Finasteride)

Finasteride is an inhibitor of 5-α reductase, the enzyme that converts testosterone to the more potent androgen, dihydrotestosterone (DHT) and

Preclinical stage

Clinically significant stage

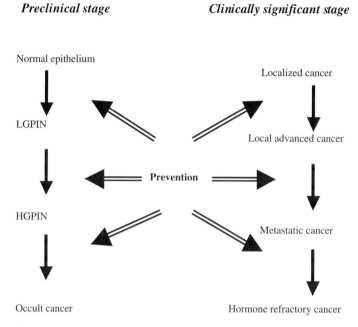

Fig. 2. Chemoprevention in the multiple-step process of prostate cancer progression. LGPIN: Low-grade prostatic intraepithelial neoplasia, HGPIN: high-grade prostatic intraepithelial neoplasia.

can lower the androgen level in the prostate. Thus, it was anticipated that finasteride would reduce the risk of prostate cancer. In 1993, The Prostate Cancer Prevention Trial (PCPT) was initiated and funded by the NCI to investigate chemoprevention of prostate cancer with finasteride. The PCPT was the first large-scale prospective phase III trial and demonstrated that finasteride significantly reduced the period-prevalence of prostate cancer. In this trial, 18,882 men, aged 55 years and older, with PSA level of 3.0 ng/ml or lower, and normal digital rectal examination, were randomized to treatment with finasteride (5 mg/day) or placebo for 7 years. In 2003, the PCPT was stopped and the results were published.[5] Prostate cancer was detected in 803 of the 4,368 men in the finasteride group (18.4%), and in 1,147 of the 4,692 men in the placebo group (24.4%), for a 24.8% reduction in prevalence over the seven-year-period (p ≤ 0.001). The difference in the incidence of prostate cancer between the two groups was observed early, and continued through late in the follow-up period. The early

Table 1. Ongoing Prostate Cancer Prevention Trials (National Cancer Institute)

Title of Trial	Protocol IDs
Phase I Randomized Study of Neoadjuvant Celecoxib Followed by Prostatectomy in Patients with Localized Prostate Cancer	JHOC-J0007, JHOC-00030801, NCI-N01-95129, NCI-P01-0186
Phase I Study of Lycopene for the Chemoprevention of Prostate Cancer	UIC-H-99-058, NCI-P00-0143, UIC-N01-CN-85081
Phase II Randomized Prevention Study of Fat- and/or Flaxseed-Modified Diets in Patients with Newly Diagnosed Prostate Cancer	CCUM-0202, DUMC-1385-02-7R3ER, NCI-P02-0235, UMCC-0202
Phase II Randomized Study of Dietary Soy in Patients with Elevated PSA Levels	CALGB-79806, NCI-P02-0207
Phase II Randomized Study of Doxercalciferol in Patients with Localized Prostate Cancer	WCCC-CO-99802, NCI-N01-CN-95130, NCI-P01-0188, WCCC-CO-2000169
Phase II Randomized Study of the Effects of a Low Fat, High Fiber Diet on Serum Factors in Patients with Prostate Cancer	UCLA-0001030, NCI-G01-1973
Phase II Randomized Study of Toremifene Followed by Radical Prostatectomy in Patients with Stage I or II Adenocarcinoma of the Prostate	PCI-00-105, NCI-P01-0181, PCI-N01-CN-75018
Phase II Randomized Study of Vitamin E, Selenium and Soy Protein Isolate in Patients with High-Grade Prostatic Intraepithelial Neoplasia	CAN-NCIC-PRP1
Phase IIB Randomized Chemoprevention Study of Eflornithine (DFMO) in Patients at High Genetic Risk for Prostate Cancer	UCIRVINE-97-18, NCI-P00-0164, UCIRVINE-U01-CA-81886-01
Phase III Randomized Study of Selenium and Vitamin E for the Prevention of Prostate Cancer (SELECT Trial)	SWOG-S0000, CALGB-S0000, CAN-NCIC-S0000, ECOG-S0000, NCCAM, NCI-P00-0172
Phase III Randomized Study of Selenium as Chemoprevention of prostate Cancer in Patients with High Grade Prostatic Intraepithelial Neoplasia	SWOG-S9917, CALGB-SWOG-S9917, ECOG-SWOG-S9917, NCI-P02-0203

Table 1 (*Continued*)

Title of Trial	Protocol IDs
Randomized Pilot Study of Isoflavones versus Lycopene Prior to Radical Prostatectomy in Patients with Localized Prostate Cancer	MCC-0105, NCI-3811, NCI-P02-0216
Randomized Study of Isoflavones in Reducing Risk Factors in Patients with Stage I or II Prostate Cancer	MCC-0002, NCI-4031, NCI-P01-0195

difference suggests that finasteride may have treated subclinical, microscopical cancer early in the study, and the fact that the difference continued to increase suggests that it prevented or delayed the onset of cancer.

However, the high-grade tumors (Gleason scores 7–10) were significantly common in the finasteride group. The high-grade tumors were noted in 6.4% of the men in the finasteride group, as compared with 5.1% of those in the placebo group. Possible explanations for this difference were (1) grading bias; histologic changes that mimic those of high grade disease are caused by androgen-deprivation therapy, and (2) finasteride might promote an environment that favors high-grade tumors, because there is clinical evidence that hypogonadal patients tend to have higher grade and more aggressive prostate cancers than patients with normal testicular function.[6-8] Finasteride may select for high-grade tumors by selectively inhibiting low-grade tumors. Long-term follow-up is needed to elucidate the association between finasteride and high-grade prostate cancer. Sexual side effects were more common, but urinary symptoms were less common in finasteride-treated men.

In summary, finasteride prevents or delays the appearance of prostate cancer, but this possible benefit and a reduced risk of urinary problems must be weighed against sexual side effects and the increased risk of high-grade prostate cancer.

Antiestrogen and Selective Estrogen Receptor Modulators (SERMs)

Shibata *et al.* reported that an age-dependent decrease in DHT, with an increase in the estradiol/DHT ratio in the aging prostate, leads to a

Table 2. Candidates of Chemopreventive Agents for Prostate Cancer[4]

Sex steroid signaling	5α Reductase inhibitors (finasteride)
	Antiandrogens (receptor antagonist)
	Selective estrogen receptor modulators (SERMs)
Differentiation/antiproliferation	Retinoids (RAR, RXR, selective agonists)
	Vitamin D analogs
	Ornithine decarboxylase inhibitors (DMFO)
Growth signaling pathways (angiogenesis)	PDGF receptor antagonists
	VEGF receptor antagonists
	Famestyl-protein transferase inhibitors
	Protein tyrosine kinase inhibitors (soy isoflavones)
Arachinoid acid-associated signaling (proapoptosis)	Nonselective cyclooxygenase inhibitors (NSAIDs)
	Selective cyclooxygenase-2 inhibitors (celecoxib, rofecoxib)
	5-Lipoxygenase inhibitors
	Other anti-inflammatory agents (R-flurbiprofen)
	PPAR modulators (sulindac sulfone)
Gene therapy	Genetically modified vaccines
	In situ delivery of immunostimulatory genes
	In situ delivery of cytotoxic genes
	Replication-restricted cytolytic viruses
Growth factors	Endothelin-1 antagonists
	Matrix metalloproteinase inhibitors
	IGF-1 pathway inhibitors
	PSA protease inhibitors
	PPARγ modulators (glitazones)
Antioxidants	Vitamin E
	Selenium
	Carotenoids
	Others (green tea polyphenols)

relatively estrogen dominant environment.[9] African-Americans have the highest levels of serum estrone and estradiol, whereas Japanese man have the lowest, which parallels their risk for prostate cancer.[10] Rising estrogens appear to increase sensitivity of the prostate tissue to androgens by up-regulation of the androgen receptor (AR).[11–13] Estradiol, in the presence of androgens, has been shown to stimulate carcinoma in situ and adenocarcinoma of the prostate in Noble rats.[14–17] Estradiol can induce high-grade prostatic intraepithelial neoplasia (PIN) and prostate cancer in the aging dog.[18,19] Those observations suggest that estrogenic stimulation with decreasing androgen levels contributes to the genesis of prostatic dysplasia and subsequent prostate cancer.

Phytoestrogens

Phytoestrogens, such as isoflavonoids and lignans, have weak estrogenic activity. Soybean is a major source of isoflavonoids mainly in the form called genistein. Large amounts of soy are consumed in China and Japan, where the incidence of prostate cancer is low.[20] A direct inverse correlation was observed between serum isoflavonoids levels and prostate cancer incidence.[21] Possible mechanisms of phytoestrogens' chemoprevention of prostate cancer are lowering the 5α-reductase activity, increasing sex hormone binding globlin, lowering free testosterone, decreasing tyrosine specific protein kinase activity, and reducing p450 aromatase activity.[21] Phytoestrogens are thought to prevent prostate cancer and are being investigated in NCI clinical trials.

SERMs

SERMs are nonsteroidal compounds that are generally considered to be weak estrogens and also possess cancer-suppressing activity. Toremifen is a chlorinated derivative of tamoxifen, widely used to treat breast cancer. In the transgenic adenocarcinoma of mouse prostate model, toremifene suppressed the development of high-grade PIN, decreased prostate cancer incidence, and increased survival. The molecular mechanism of toremifene's chemopreventive effects appears to be through estrogen receptor (ER)-α and to be androgen-independent.[22] Estrogen stimulates cellular proliferation by inducing local production of stimulatory growth factors such as transforming growth factor (TGF)-α, insulin-like growth factor, and epidermal growth factor, and by suppressing inhibitory effects of factors such as TGF-β.[23,24] Thus, SERMs would be expected to decrease the levels of stimulatory growth factors and augment the production of

TGFβ. The antiproliferative effects of SERMs may also be mediated by binding and sequestration of calmodulin,[25] inhibition of protein kinase C,[26] and induction of p21.[27] In addition, SERMs can bind to ER and the formation of SERM-ER complexes results in the inactivation of the estrogen-regulated genes, thereby decreasing cellular proliferation. Toremifene has been evaluated in a phase II exploratory trial in men with high-grade PIN. A four-month toremifene treatment regimen significantly reduced high-grade PIN[28] and the chemopreventive effect of toremifene is being investigated by placebo controlled, randomized, dose-finding phase II–III clinical trials. Raloxifen, one of the SERMs, has been shown to induce apoptosis in androgen-independent prostate cancer cell lines[29] and could be a candidate agent for prostate cancer chemoprevention.

Antiproliferation/Differentiation

Difluoromethylornithine (DFMO)

As polyamines are ubiquitous and essential for cell survival, limiting or inhibiting polyamine synthesis results in reduced cycling of highly proliferative cancer cells. DFMO is an irreversible inhibitor of ornithine decarboxylase (ODC), and is involved in the synthesis of polyamines and, consequently, related to cell proliferation. DFMO has been demonstrated to inhibit carcinogenesis in animal models of epithelial cancers including urinary bladder, colon, skin and breast. The concentrations of some polyamines such as spermine and spermidine are higher in the prostate than in most other tissues. Heston *et al.* demonstrated that DFMO inhibited tumor growth in the prostate.[30] Because a significant limiting side effect of DFMO is ototoxicity, optimal doses must be determined. Thus, DFMO and other inhibitors of polyamine synthesis are thought to be chemopreventive agents of prostate cancer.

Vitamin A and Related Compounds

Vitamin A and metabolites (retinoids) possess a close relationship with important cellular functions such as morphogenesis, proliferation and differentiation. Peehl *et al.*[31] demonstrated that clonal growth of prostatic epithelial cells was inhibited by retinoic acid (RA). The cellular changes provided evidence that the retinoids play a role in prostate cell apoptosis and differentiation. Many vitamin A metabolites bind nonspecifically to both retinoic acid receptor (RAR) and retinoid X receptor (RXR). The receptor dimers, such as RXR-RAR, RXR-peroxisome proliferator activated receptor (PPAR), and RXR-vitamin D receptor (VDR), are known to induce differentiation when activated. Several retinoids, such as 9-cis retinoic acid (a pan-agonist for retinoic acid receptor and RXR) and an RXR selective agonist, are under investigation for treatment of prostate cancer.

Short-Chain Fatty Acids

This class of differentiating agents includes the bioactively stable analogs of sodium butyrate, phenylbutyrate (PB) and phenylacetate (PA). Samid *et al.*[32] found that PA-treated human prostate cancer cells (PC-3, DU145, LNCaP) lost their ability to invade a basement membrane and showed diminished ability to form tumors when transplanted into athymic mice. Because a Phase I study did not show a benefit of PA, the focus of investigation turned to PB. PB is 1.5 to 2.5 times more active at inhibiting growth and inducing apoptosis than PA.[33,34] The mechanisms of action for short-chain fatty acids are most likely not mutually exclusive. Two acceptable mechanisms of action are inhibition of histone deacetylase and activation of the PPAR nuclear receptor.[34] A Phase I study suggested that PB delayed the progression of heavily pretreated androgen-independent prostate cancer.[35] The activities and low toxicity profile make PB attractive for further investigation as a chemopreventive agent.

Arachidonic Acid Signaling/Proapoptotics

Anti-inflammatory Drugs, COX Inhibitors

Epidemiologic studies, preclinical models, and randomized clinical trials support an association between nonsteroidal anti-inflammatory drugs (NSAIDs) and decreased incidence of cancers, such as colon and prostate. NSAIDs are potent inhibitors of cyclooxygenases, enzymes that catalyze the synthesis of prostaglandins from arachidonic acid. Cyclooxygenase 2 (COX2) is a key enzyme in the synthesis of proinflammatory prostaglandins (prostaglandin E2, PGE2). In humans, COX2 is upregulated in precancer and in prostatic carcinomas. NSAIDs were initially developed to suppress inflammation and pain by inhibiting the production of PGE2 and its metabolites. NSAIDs are active against prostate cancer in laboratory and clinical studies. Inhibition of COX2 by celecoxib, the first COX2-selective drug, inhibits carcinogenesis and suppresses tumor growth.[36,37] In addition, celecoxib is effective at inhibiting angiogenesis induced by basic fibroblast growth factor. Exisulind (sulindac sulfone) is a potent inhibitor of both COX1 and COX2. Anti-tumor activity was proven in clinical trials to treat familial adenomatous polyposis.[38,39] Exisulind has proven to be active in rodent models of chemical carcinogenesis against breast, colon, lung and bladder.[40–44] In mouse xenograft models of prostate cancer, exisulind induced apoptosis of cancer cells and showed anticancer activity.[45,46]

Antioxidants

Epidemiological studies have provided evidence for an inverse association between exposure to antioxidant nutrients (e.g. lycopene, soy isoflavones, selenium, vitamin E, green tea polyphenols) and prostate cancer incidence and mortality.

Selenium

Selenium is a nonmetallic trace element recognized as a nutrient essential to human health. Selenium inhibits tumorigenesis in a variety of experimental models. Many animal models, including prostate cancer models, have shown reductions in tumor incidence in response to selenium supplementation.[47,48] Possible mechanisms of selenium antitumorigenic effects are antioxidant effects, enhancement of immune function, induction of apoptosis, inhibition of cell proliferation, alteration of carcinogen metabolism, cytotoxicity of metabolites formed under high-selenium conditions, and an influence on testosterone production.[49–55] Two large, randomized trials have demonstrated that selenium supplementation could reduce overall cancer mortality, as well as mortality from stomach and esophageal cancers.[56,57] In addition, a case-control study demonstrated that the highest selenium status tested reduced the risk of advanced prostate cancer.[58] A large scale, randomized study demonstrated the chemopreventive effect of selenium.[59] In this study, 1,312 subjects with a prior history of skin cancer were randomized to receive selenium or placebo, and followed for an average of 4.5 years. While no difference was found in rate of recurrence of skin cancer, prostate cancer incidence was reduced by two thirds among those in the selenium-supplemented group.

Vitamin E (α-Tocopherol)

Vitamin E functions as the major lipid-soluble antioxidant in cell membranes: it is a chain-breaking, free-radical scavenger and specifically inhibits lipid peroxidation, the biologic activity relevant to carcinogen-induced DNA damage.[60] α-Tocopherol is the most active form of vitamin E and may influence the development of cancer through several mechanisms such as antioxidation,[61] inhibition of protein kinase C,[62,63] inducion of the detoxification enzyme NADHP, and inhibition of arachadonic acid and prostaglandin metabolism.[64,65] A study of 2,974 subjects, over 17-year follow-up period, found low α-tocopherol to be associated with higher prostate cancer risk.[66] A large-scale, randomized, placebo-controlled trial also suggested that vitamin E is effective for chemoprevention of prostate cancer. This trial, the Alpha-Tocopherol, Beta-Carotene Cancer Prevention Trial (ATBC), was conducted in Finland.[67] In this trial, 29,133 men, aged 50–69 years, were randomized and the median follow-up period was 6.1 years. A statistically significant 32% reduction in prostate cancer was observed in the α-tocopherol group.

As selenium and vitamin E are thought to be promising candidates for prostate cancer prevention, a new randomized, prospective, double-blind study was initiated in 2001.[68] This trial is called SELECT, the Selenium and Vitamin E Cancer Prevention Trial. SELECT was designed to determine whether selenium and vitamin E can reduce the risk of prostate cancer among healthy men, and the final results are anticipated in 2013.

Lycopene

Lycopene is a carotenoid naturally present in tomatoes and other fruits, is a potent antioxidant, and is the most significant free radical scavenger in the carotenoid family.[69] Mills *et al.* reported that tomato consumption was most strongly associated with reduced prostate cancer risk.[70] A nested case-control study within the context of the Health Professional Follow-up study showed that individuals consuming more than 10 servings per week of tomato-based products had an adjusted odds ratio of 0.65 for developing advanced/aggressive prostate cancers.[71] These observations suggest that lycopene supplementation may be beneficial in preventing the progression of prostate cancer.

Others

Protein tyrosine kinase inhibitors, pan-inhibitors of platelet-derived growth factor, vascular endothelial growth factor, and fibroblast growth factor, endothelin-1 antagonist and matrix metalloproteinase inhibitors are candidate prostate cancer chemopreventive agents and are under investigation.

Conclusions

For prostate cancer prevention, Lieberman[72] proposed a dual strategy; a public health approach and a cost effective pharmacologic, medically oriented, translational science strategy. A public health approach includes (1) changes in dietary practices with increased fruits and vegetables, decreased carbohydrates and charbroiled meat, (2) caloric restriction/ obesity control, (3) increased physical activity and stress reduction, and (4) early detection of precancerous lesions. A pharmacologic, medically oriented, translational science strategy includes (1) identification of individuals at risk using clinical, histologic, genetic and proteomic profiles, (2) risk reduction by using chemopreventive agents to modulate surrogate endpoints, (3) suppression/reversal of promoter methylation in target genes and (4) suppression/reversal of signature protein patterns of early prostate cancer to delay the onset of clinically active prostate cancer.

As mentioned above, there are many candidate chemopreventive agents, and some clinical trials demonstrated promising results in the prevention of carcinogenesis and progression of prostate cancer. Large-scale, prospective, randomized trials are absolutely necessary to obtain useful strategies to prevent prostate cancer. However, we still need to overcome or better understand several issues. For example, which populations are optimal targets? When the target population is a low-risk group (general population), targets are easily definable, readily available, and results are widely applicable, but large study population and long follow-up periods are required. In contrast, when high-risk groups such as populations with HGPIN, are targeted, sample size and duration can be reduced, but the diagnosis is subjective, and sampling errors will occur, and results are not widely applicable. We also must consider when chemoprevention should be introduced and how long it should be continued. Are combinations of agents or strategies more useful than single ones? Furthermore, the principles of combination of various agents must be considered, including, (1) using two or more agents with different mechanisms of action, (2) using agents with non-overlapping toxicity and (3) reducing the dose of each agent.

The economic aspect of clinical trials should also be considered. To run a Phase III clinical trial in EORTC, the average cost per patient involved is between $1,000 and $2,000 USD. When a sample size is 30,000 men, $20–$40 million are needed.

In addition, it is necessary to evaluate multi-organ systems for effectiveness of any agent, because each agent may prevent cancer in one organ but may promote cancer in others. For example, tamoxifen reduced the risk of invasive breast cancer by 49%, but increased invasive endometrial cancer (2.53 times greater risk compared to placebo group).[73]

Active basic and clinical research regarding the chemoprevention of prostate cancer is ongoing and will provide effective and safe strategies that result in clinical benefit.

References

1. Greenwald P, Kelloff GJ (1996) The role of chemoprevention in cancer control. Principles of chemoprevention. In: Stewart BW, McGregor D, Kleihues P, eds.

Principles of Chemoprevention. IARC Scientific Publication No.139, Lyon, IARC, pp. 13–22.

2. Liebarman R (2001) Androgen deprivation therapy for prostate cancer chemoprevention: Current status and future directions for agent development. *Urology* 58(Suppl 2A):83–90.

3. Lieberman R (2002) Chemoprevention of prostate cancer: Current status and future directions. *Cancer Metastasis Rev* 21:279–309.

4. Lieberman R, Nelson WG (2001) Executive summary of the National Cancer Institute workshop: Highlights and recommendation. *Urology* 57(Suppl 1): 4–27.

5. Thompson IM, Goodman PJ (2003) The influence of finasteride on the development of prostate cancer. *N Engl J Med* 349:215–224.

6. Ishikawa S, Soloway MS, van der Zwaag R, Todd B (1989) Prognostic factors in survival free progression after androgen deprivation therapy for treatment of prostate cancer. *J Urol* 141:1139–1142.

7. Hoffman MA, DeWolf WC, Morgentaler A (2000) Is low serum free testosterone a marker for high grade prostate cancer? *J Urol* 163:824–827.

8. Schatzl G, Madersbacher S, Haitel A, Gsur A, Preyer M, Haidinger G, Gassner C, Ochsner M, Marberger M (2003) Association of serum testosterone with microvessel density, androgen receptor gene polymorphism in prostate cancer. *J Urol* 169:1312–1315.

9. Shibata Y, Ito K, Suzuki K, Nakano K, Fukabori Y, Suzuki R, Kawabe Y, Honma S, Yamanaka H (2000) Changes in the endocrine environment of the human prostate transition zone with aging: Simultaneous quantitative analysis of prostatic sex steroids and comparison with human prostatic histological composition. *Prostate* 42:25–55.

10. Ross R, Bernstein L, Judd H, Hanisch R, Pike M, Henderson B (1986) Serum testosterone levels in healthy young black and white men. *J Natl Cancer Inst* 76:45–48.

11. Moore RJ, Gazac JM, Wilson JD (1979) Regulation of cytoplasmic dihydrotestosterone binding in dog prostate by 17β-estradiol. *J Clin Invest* 63:351–357.

12. Mobbs BG, Johnson IE, Connolly JG, Thompson J (1983) Concentration and cellular distribution of androgen receptor in human prostatic neoplasia: Can estrogen treatment increase androgen receptor content? *J Steroid Biochem* 19:1279–1290.

13. Blanchere M, Berthaut I, Portois MC, Mestayer C, Mowszowicz I (1998) Hormonal regulation of the androgen receptor expression in human prostatic cells in culture. *J Steroid Biochem Mol Biol* 66:319–326.

14. Leav I, Ho SM, Ofner P, Merk FB, Kwan PW, Damassa D (1988) Biochemical alterations in sex hormone-induced hyperplasia and dysplasia of the dorsolateral prostates of Noble rats. *J Natl Cancer Inst* 80:1045–1053.

15. Leave I, Merk FB, Kwan PW, Ho SM (1989) Androgen-supported estrogen-enhanced epithelial proliferation in the prostates of intact Noble rats. *Prostate* 15:23–40.

16. Ofner P, Bosl MC, Vena RL (1992) Differential effects of diethylstilbesterol and estradiol-17β in combination with testosterone on rat prostate lobes. *Toxicol Appl Pharmacol* 112:300–309.

17. Lau K, Leav I, Ho SM (1998) Rat estrogen receptor-α and -β and progesterone receptor mRNA expression in various prostatic lobes and microdissected normal and dysplastic epithelial tissues of the Noble rats. *Endocrinology* 139:424–427.

18. Ho SM, Lee KF. Lane K (1997) Neoplastic transformation of the prostate. In: Naz RK, ed. *Prostate: Basic and Clinical Aspects*. CRC Press, New York, pp. 74–114.

19. Waters DJ, Bostwick DG (1997) The canine prostate is a spontaneous model of intraepithelial neoplasia and prostate cancer progression. *Anticancer Res* 17:1467–1470.

20. Price KR, Fenwick GR (1985) Naturally occurring oestrogens in foods: A review. *Food Addit Contam* 2:73–106.

21. Denis L, Morton MS, Griffiths K (1999) Diet and its preventive role in prostatic disease. *Eur Urol* 35:377–387.

22. Raghow S, Hooshdaran MZ, Katiyar S, Steiner MS (2002) Toremifene prevents prostate cancer in the transgenic adenocarcinoma of mouse model. *Cancer Res* 62:1370–1376.

23. Steiner MS (1993) The role of peptide growth factors in the prostate: A review. *Urology* 42:99–110.

24. Steiner MS (1995) Review of peptide growth factors in benign prostatic hyperplasia and urologic malignancy. *J Urol* 153:1085–1096.

25. Lam HY (1984) Tamoxifen is a calmodulin antagonist in the activation of cAMP phosphodiesterase. *Biochem Biophys Res Commun* 118:27–32.

26. O'Brein CA, Liskamp RM, Solomon DH (1985) Inhibition of protein kinase C by tamoxifen. *Cancer Res* 45:2462–2465.

27. Rohlff C, Blagosklonny MV, Kyle E, Kesari A, Kim IY, Zelner DJ, Hakim F, Trepel J, Bergan RC (1998) Prostate cancer cell growth inhibition of protein kinase C and induction of p21(waf1/cip1). *Prostate* 37:51–59.

28. Steiner MS, Pound CR, Gingrich JR, Patterson AI, Wake RW, Conrad LW, Kisber RH, McSwain M, Shelton T (2002) Acapodene (GTx-006) reduces

high grade prostate intraepithelial neoplasia (HGPIN) in phase 2 clinical trial. Program and abstracts from the *American Society of Clinical Oncology 38th Annual Meeting*, 18–21, Orlando (Abstract 719).

29. Kim IY, Kim BC, Seong DH, Lee DK, Seo JM, Hong YJ, Kim HT, Morton RA, Kim SJ (2002) Raloxifen, a mixed estrogen agonist/antagonist, induces apoptosis in androgen-independent human prostate cancer cell lines. *Cancer Res* 62:5365–5369.

30. Heston WD, Kadmon D, Lazan DW, Fair WR (1982) Copenhagen rat prostatic tumor ornithine decarboxylase activity (ODC) and the effect of the ODC inhibitor alpha-difluoromethulornithine. *Prostate* 3:383–389.

31. Peehl DM, Wong ST, Stamey TA (1993) Vitamin A regulates proliferation and differentiation of human prostatic epithelial cells. *Prostate* 23:69–78.

32. Samid D, Shack S, Myers CE (1993) *J Clin Invest* 91:2288–2295.

33. Carducci MA, Nelson JB, Chan-Tack KM, Ayyagari SR, Sweatt WH, Campbell PA, Nelson WG, Simons JW, Carducci MA, Nelson JB, Chan-Tack KM (1996) Selective growth arrest and phenotypic reversion of prostate cancer cells *in vitro* by nontoxic pharmacological concentrations of phenylacetate. *Clin Cancer Res* 2:379–387.

34. Pineau T, Hudgins WR, Liu L, Chen LC, Sher T, Gonzalez FJ, Samid D (1996) Activation of a human peroxisome proliferator-activated receptor by the antitumor agent phenylacetate and its analogs. *Biochem Pharmacol* 52:659–667.

35. Carducci MA, Bowling MK, Eisenberger M (1997) Phenylbutyrate (PB) for refractory solid tumors: Phase 1 clinical and pharmacologic evaluation of intravenous and oral PB. Phenylbutyrate (PB) for refractory solid tumors: Phase 1 clinical and pharmacologic evaluation of intravenous and oral PB. *Anticancer Res* 17:3972a (Abstract 103).

36. Reddy BS, Hirose Y, Lubet R, Steele V, Kelloff G, Paulson S, Seibert K, Rao CV (2000) Chemoprevention of colon cancer by specific cyclooxygenase-2 inhibitor, celecoxib, administrated during different stages of carcinogenesis. *Cancer Res* 60:293–297.

37. Kawamori T, Rao CV, Seibert K, Reddy BS (1998) Chemopreventive activity of celecoxib, a specific cyclooxygenase-2 inhibitor, against colon carcinogenesis. *Cancer Res* 58:409–412.

38. Burke C, van Stolk R, Arber N (2000) Exislund prevents adenoma formation in familial adenomatous polyposis (FAP). *Gastroenterology* 118(4 Suppl 2): A657 (Abstract 3604).

39. Burke C, Arber N, Phillips R (2000) Exislund continues to prevent colonic adenoma formation in familial adenomatous polyposis (FAP) patients treated for 18 months. *Gastroenterology* 118(4 Suppl 2):A657 (Abstract 3605).

40. Thompson HJ, Briggs S, Paranka NS (1995) Sulfone metabolite of sulindac inhibits mammary carcinogenesis. *J Natl Cancer Inst* 85:1259–1261.

41. Thompson HJ, Jiang C, Lu J, Mehta RG, Piazza GA, Paranka NS, Pamukcu R (1997) Sulfone metabolite of sulindac inhibits mammary carcinogenesis. *Cancer Res* 57:267–271.

42. Piazza GA, Alberts DS, Hixson LJ, Paranka NS, Li H, Finn T, Bogert C, Guillen JM, Brendel K, Gross PH, Sperl G, Ritchie J, Burt RW, Ellsworth L, Ahnen DJ, Pamukcu R (1997) Sulindac sulfone inhibits azoxymethane-induced colon carcinogenesis in rats without reducing prostaglandin levels. *Cancer Res* 57:2909–2915.

43. Malkinson AM, Koski KM, Dwyer-Nield LD, Rice PL, Rioux N, Castonguay A, Ahnen DJ, Thompson H, Pamukcu R, Piazza GA (1998) Inhibition of 4-(methylnitrosoamino)-1-(3-pyridyl)-1-butanone-induced mouse lung tumor formation by FGN-1 (sulindac sulfone). *Carcinogenesis* 8:1353–1356.

44. Piazza GA, Pamukcu R, Thompson WJ, Alila DL, Hill I, Grubbs CJ, Horsham PA, Birmingham LA (2000) Inhibition of urinary bladder tumorgenesis in rats by exisulind (Aptosyn). *J Urol* 163(Suppl 4):122.

45. Lim JT, Piazza GA, Han EK, Delohery TM, Li H, Finn TS, Buttyan R, Yamamoto H, Sperl GJ, Brendel K, Gross PH, Pamukcu R, Weinstein IB (1999) Sulindac derivatives inhibit growth and induce apoptosis in human prostate cancer cell lines. *Biochem Pharmacol* 58:1097–1107.

46. Goluboff ET, Shabsigh A, Saidi JA, Weinstein IB, Mitra N, Heitjan D, Piazza GA, Pamukcu R, Buttyan R, Olsson CA (1997) Exisulind (sulindac sulfone) suppresses growth of human prostate cancer in a nude mouse xenograft model by increasing apoptosis. *Urology* 53:440–445.

47. Nakamura A, Shirai T, Takahashi S, Ogawa K, Hirose M, Ito N (1991) Lack of modification by naturally occurring antioxidants of 3, 2'-dimethyl-4-aminobiphenyl initiated rate prostate carcinogenesis. *Cancer Lett* 58:241–246.

48. Webber MM, Perez-Ripoli EA, James GT (1985) Inhibitory effects of selenium on the growth of DU145 human prostate carcinoma cells *in vitro*. *Biochem Biophys Res Comm* 130:603–609.

49. Ip C, Medina D (1987). In: Medina D, Kidwell W, Heppner G, Anderson EP, eds. *Current Concept of Selenium and Mammary Tumorigenesis. Cellular and Molecular Biology of Breast Cancer.* Plenum Press, New York, p. 479.

50. Kiremindjian-Scheumacher L, Stotzky G (1987) Review: Selenium and immune response. *Env Res* 42:277–303.

51. Thompson HJ, Wilson A, Lu J, Singh M, Jiang C, Upadhyaya P, El-Bayoumy K, Ip C (1994) Comparison of the effects of an organic and an inorganic form of selenium on a mammary carcinoma cell line. *Carcinogenesis* 15:183–186.

52. Redman C, Scott JA, Baines AT, Basye JL, Clark LC, Calley C, Roe D, Payne CM, Nelson MA (1998) Inhibitory effect of selenomethionine on the growth of three selected human tumor cell lines. *Cancer Lett* 125:103–110.

53. Shimada T, El-Bayoumy K, Upadhyaya P, Sutter TR, Guengerich FP, Yamazaki H (1997) Inhibition of human cytochrome P450-catalyzed oxidations of xenobiotics and procarcinogens by synthetic organoselenium compounds. *Cancer Res* 57:4757–4764.

54. El-Bayoumy K (1991) The role of selenium in cancer prevention. In: DeVita, VT, Hellman S, Rosenberg SS, eds. *Practice of Oncology.* Lippincott, Philadelphia, pp. 1–15.

55. Bedwal RS, Nair N, Sharma MP, Mathurk RS (1993) Selenium: Its biological perspectives. *Med Hyp* 41:150–159.

56. Blot WJ, Li JY, Taylor PR, Guo W, Dawsey S, Wang GQ, Yang CS, Zheng SF, Gail M, Li GY, Yu Y, Liu BQ, Tangrea J, Sun YH, Liu F, Fraumeni Jr JF, Zhang YH, Li B (1999) Nutrition intervention trials in Linxian, China: Supplementation with specific vitamin/mineral combination, cancer incidence, and disease-specific mortality in the general population. *J Natl Cancer Inst* 85:1483–1492.

57. Li JY, Taylor PR, Li B, Dawsey S, Wang GQ, Ershow AG, Guo W, Li SF, Yang CS, Shen Q, Wang W, Mark SD, Zuo XN, Greenwald P, Wu YP, Blot WJ (1999) Nutrition intervention trial in Linxian, China: Multiple vitamin/mineral supplementation, cancer incidence, and disease-specific mortality among adults with esophageal dysplasia. *J Natl Cancer Inst* 85: 1492–1498.

58. Yoshizawa K, Willett WC, Morris SJ, Stampfer MJ, Spiegelman D, Rimm EB, Giovannucci E (1998) Study of prediagnostic selenium level in toenails and the risk of advanced prostate cancer. *J Natl Cancer Inst* 90:1219–1224.

59. Clark LC, Combs GF Jr, Turnbull BW, Slate EH, Chalker DK, Chow J, Davis LS, Glover RA, Graham GF, Gross EG, Krongrad A, Lesher JL Jr, Park HK, Sanders BB Jr, Smith CL, Taylor JR (1996) Effects of selenium supplementation for cancer prevention in patients with carcinoma of the skin. A randomized controlled trial. Nutritional Prevention of Cancer Study Group. *JAMA* 276:1957–1963.

60. Barton GW, Ingold KU (1981) Autoxidation of biological molecules. 1. The antioxidant activity of vitamin E and related chain-breaking phenolic antioxidants *in vitro. J Am Chem Soc* 103:6472.

61. Fleshner NE, Kucuk O (2001) Antioxidant dietary supplements: Rationale and current status as chemopreventive agents for prostate cancer. *Urology* 57(Suppl 4A):90–94.

62. Mahoney CW, Azzi A (1998) Vitamin E inhibits protein kinase C activity. *Biochem Biophys Res Commun* 154:694–697.
63. Chatelain E, Boscoboinik DO, Bartoli GM, Kagan VE, Gey FK, Packer L, Azzi A (1993) Inhibition of smooth muscle cell proliferation and protein kinase C activity by tocopherols and tocotrienols. *Biochem Biophys Acta* 117:83–89.
64. Wang W, Higuchi CM (1995) Induction of NAD(P)H: Quinone reductase by vitamins A, E and C in Colo205 colon cancer cells. *Cancer Lett* 98:63–69.
65. Traber MG, Packer L (1995) Vitamin E: Beyond antioxidant function. *Am J Clin Nutr* 62:1501–1509.
66. Hsing AW, Comstock GW, Abbey H, Polk BF (1990) Serologic precursors of cancer retinol, carotenoids, and tocopherol and risk of prostate cancer. *J Natl Cancer Inst* 82:941–946.
67. Heinonen OP, Albanes D, Virtamo J, Taylor PR, Huttunen JK, Hartman AM, Haapakoski J, Malila N, Rautalahti M, Ripatti S, Maenpaa H, Teerenhovi L, Koss L, Virolainen M, Edwards BK, Heinonen OP, Albanes D, Huttunen JK (1998) Prostate cancer and supplementation with α-tocopherol and β-carotene: Incidence and mortality in a controlled trial. *J Natl Cancer Inst* 90:440–446.
68. Klein EA, Thompson IM, Lippman SM, Goodman PJ, Albanes D, Taylor PR, Coltman C (2001) SELECT: The next prostate cancer prevention trial. *J Urol* 166:1311–1315.
69. Stahl W, Nicolai S, Briviba K, Hanusch M, Broszeit G, Peters M, Martin HD, Sies H, Stahl W, Nicolai S, Briviba K (1997) Biological activities of natural and synthetic carotenoids: Induction of gap junctional communication and singlet oxygen quenching. *Carcinogenesis* 18:89–92.
70. Mills PK, Beeson WL, Phillips RL, Fraser GE (1989) Cohort study of diet, lifestyle and prostate cancer in Adventist men. *Cancer* 64:598–604.
71. Giovannucci E, Ascherio A, Rimm EB, Stampfer MJ, Colditz GA, Willett WC (1995) Intake of carotenoids and retinol in relationship to risk of prostate cancer. *J Natl Cancer Inst* 87:1767–1776.
72. Lieberman R (2003) Evolving strategies for prostate cancer chemoprevention trials. *World J Urol* 21:3–8.
73. Fisher B, Costantino JP, Wickerham DL, Redmond CK, Kavanah M, Cronin WM, Vogel V, Robidoux A, Dimitrov N, Atkins J, Daly M, Wieand S, Tan-Chiu E, Ford L, Wolmark N (1998) Tamoxifen for prevention of breast cancer: Report of the National Surgical Adjuvant Breast and Bowel Project P-1 Study. *J Natl Cancer Inst* 90:1371–1288.

7

NEUROENDOCRINE DIFFERENTIATION AND ANDROGEN-INDEPENDENCE IN PROSTATE CANCER

Sonal J. Desai, Clifford G. Tepper and Hsing-Jien Kung

Department of Biological Chemistry and Cancer Center
University of California at Davis
Sacramento, CA 95817, USA

Introduction

One of the most troubling aspects of prostate cancer (PCa) is the emergence of hormone-refractory cells, which currently defy treatment.[1,2] Increasing evidence suggests that a majority of hormone-refractory PCa cells, while androgen-independent, retain the expression and activity of the androgen receptor (AR).[3] In fact, the level of AR or its coactivators in these tumors may actually be higher,[4,5] suggesting that the receptor is activated by amplification or other cellular factors, independent of the action of androgen (or in the presence of castrate levels of androgen).[6] Understanding these factors is the key to the identification of targets and the development of intervention therapy for androgen-independent tumors. Among the factors accompanying the progression of PCa to an androgen-independent state, are the appearance of an increased number of neuroendocrine (NE) cells and the increased serum level of chromogranin A (CgA), IL-6, and IL-8, soluble factors relevant to neuroendocrine differentiation (NED). In this chapter, we will describe the molecular pathways leading to NED and to androgen-independence, and their potential causal relationship. There have been excellent reviews on the subject of either NED or androgen-independence. The readers are referred to those publications[2,7-14] for more details.

As discussed above, an association of increased NED as well as high serum concentrations of growth factors, cytokines, and neuropeptides has been frequently observed in androgen-independent tumors. Interestingly, growing evidence suggests androgen-withdrawal itself (and by implication androgen-ablation therapy)[15] or in combination with circulating factors such as IL-6,[16–19] epinephrine,[20,21] or stromal factors such as HB-EGF,[22,23] induces NED in the prostate. These differentiated cells become growth arrested, but are strongly resistant to apoptosis and at some point begin secreting factors (e.g., neuropeptides) that elicit signals that contribute to the survival and growth of surrounding, undifferentiated PCa cells, which would have otherwise died under androgen-deprived conditions. These surviving cells, upon further genetic aberrations evolve to become androgen-independent, untreatable clones. This is the central hypothesis of this chapter (Fig. 1) and we will elaborate on the current understanding of the molecular and cellular details of these processes.

PCa Disease Progression Model

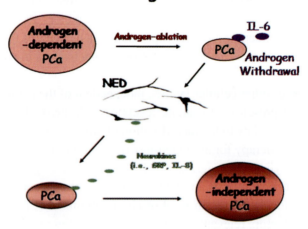

Fig. 1. PCa disease progression model. Initial occurrence of PCa is as an androgen-dependent tumor. Androgen-ablation therapy causes the tumor to regress, but, by itself or in combination with other soluble factors also induces NED of some cells. These NED cells then secrete neurokines that act on surrounding non-NED cells to promote androgen-independent growth of the tumor.

Neuroendocrine Differentiation

NE cells are terminally differentiated, postmitotic cells. They are characterized by the presence of neuritic outgrowths and neurosecretory granules as well as by the expression and secretion of neuron-specific proteins.[13] NE cells are present in all regions of the prostate at birth, but soon disappear from the peripheral regions. At the onset of puberty, NE cells reappear and increase to a low but apparently optimum level.[1,24-26] The origin of NE cells is unclear. Based on cell line studies described in the next section, interconversion (or trans-differentiation) between prostate epithelial cells and prostate NE cells can occur. A current model is that the three cell types comprising the prostate epithelium (epithelial, basal, and NE) originate from a common endodermal pluripotent stem cell. The epithelial cells are androgen-dependent while the basal and NE cells are androgen-independent.[24,25] Little is known about the function of NE cells in the prostate, but they appear to be essential for growth and differentiation as well as homeostatic regulation of the secretory processes in the mature prostate. Tumor cell populations have been reported to become enriched for NE cells and are correlated with elevated levels of NE markers.[1,19,27] While the occurrence of purely NE, or small cell carcinoma and carcinoid or carcinoid-like tumors, is rare (1% of all prostate cancers),[28,29] an increase in the number of cells in the prostate with NE characteristics has been reported as a marker for the development of androgen-independence in PCa. Furthermore, overexpression of SV40 large T antigen in prostatic tissue of mice models intended for prostate carcinoma gives rise to NE tumors, again suggesting a kinship of these two cell types in prostate carcinogenesis.[30-32] There has been a great deal of research in characterizing NE cells and identifying markers that could be used in determining the prognosis and possible treatment of PCa.[33-42] However, the factors that induce these changes are relatively unknown. NE cells found in PCa posses phenotypic traits of both normal NE cells, such as the expression of NE markers (i.e., CgA and NSE) as well as epithelial characteristics, such as PSA, and secrete neuropeptides, such as neurotensin, serotonin, and the bombesin homologue gastrin-releasing peptide (GRP). One theory is that, due to its origin from a pluripotent stem cell, a malignant cancer cell can mobilize a mix of genes that are normally differentially expressed in basal, epithelial, or NE cells, which would explain the cell's ability to transform as well as the duality of characteristics within one cell and the ability of a usually postmitotic, terminally differentiated cell to proliferate. This would generate a cancer cell more adaptable to environmental changes, such as androgen depletion, and enhance its ability to respond to circulating aberrant growth signals.[1,24,25] A summary of the signaling pathways involved in NED, which we will discuss below, is presented in Fig. 2A.

Androgen-Withdrawal Induced Neuroendocrine Differentiation

An increase in the number of NED cells in the prostate as evidenced by chromogranin A (CgA) staining has been associated with androgen-ablation therapy.[43,44] The aggressive nature of these cells is underscored by the fact that while TUNEL staining demonstrated the occurrence of apoptosis in the exocrine cells of prostate tumors, CgA-positive NE cells were resistant to apoptosis.[45] This phenomenon was also seen in the canine prostate[46] and in human PCa xenograft PC-310[47,48] grown in nude mice subjected to castration or anti-androgen treatment. In addition, *in vitro* withdrawal of androgen from the androgen-dependent PCa cell line, LNCaP, results in cell cycle arrest[49] and NE trans-differentiation[15] characterized by distinctive morphological changes including rounding up of the cell bodies and the extension of neuritic processes (Fig. 3B). This is accompanied biochemically by an increase in the expression of NSE,[50] CgA,[41] GRP[34] and neurotensin.[51] Similar to *in vivo* observations, LNCaP cells are resistant to apoptosis when androgen is removed.[52] While apoptosis appears to be initiated, ascertained by the appearance of DNA fragmentation, it is not completed. Instead, the cells are growth arrested and mRNA expression of anti-apoptotic proteins is seen. Substantial evidence supports the fact that suppression of AR signaling is obligatory for NED.[53] AR serves as the pivotal effector of androgen deprivation, as elimination of its ligand essentially shuts down the AR pathway by simultaneously terminating signals emanating from the receptor and causing a marked down-regulation in AR protein levels.[54] Accordingly, NED of LNCaP can be induced by antagonism of AR function with the anti-androgen bicalutamide (Casodex)[49,55] or by AR silencing with siRNAs as evidenced by the appearance of the typical NE phenotype and expression of NE markers,

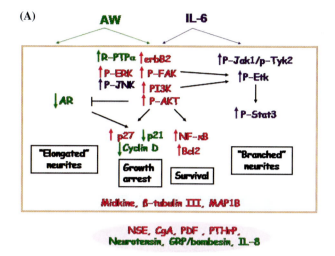

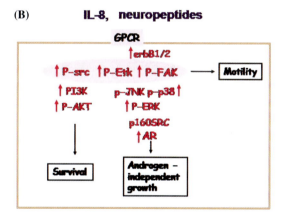

Fig. 2. (A) Signals associated with NED induced by androgen withdrawal (AW) or by IL-6. Molecules in red are activated (up arrow) or down-modulated (down arrow) by both AW and IL-6. Molecules in green are known to be modulated by AW only. Molecules in blue are modulated by IL-6 only. The phenotypes associated with individual signal pathways are indicated in boxes. Intracellular neuronal-related and secreted neurokines modulated by AW and IL-6 are indicated. **(B)** Signals associated with neuropeptides and IL-8 induced androgen-independent growth. Both IL-8 and neuropeptides engage G-protein-coupled receptors (GPCR). ErbB family receptor tyrosine kinases, erbB1 and erbB2, are activated. The trimeric tyrosine kinase complex of Src, Etk, and FAK is also activated. The signals are then transmitted from tyrosine kinases to PI-3 kinase (PI3K) and serine/threonine kinases (JNK, p38MAPK, ERK, and Akt). Activated or phosphorylated ERK (P-ERK) is known to phosphorylate steroid receptor coactivator (p160SRC), which is co-recruited with androgen receptor (AR) to androgen response elements.

(A) **Untreated**   (B) **Androgen-withdrawal**

(C) **+ IL-6**   (D) **+ Forskolin**

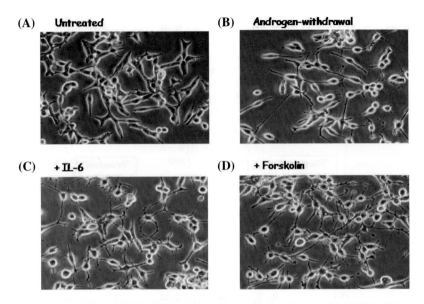

Fig. 3. Neuroendocrine differentiation in LNCaP cells. Cells were plated in RPMI 1640 supplemented with 2% FBS. The following day, cells were either **(A)** left untreated or treated with **(B)** androgen withdrawal (RPMI 1640 supplemented with 2% CDS-FBS), **(C)** IL-6 (50 ng/ml IL-6 in RPMI 1640 supplemented with 2% FBS), or **(D)** Forskolin (10 μM Forskolin in RPMI supplemented with 2% FBS). Photographs were taken 96 hours after treatment.

such as NSE and beta-tubulin III.[53] Conversely, addition of androgen to hormone-depleted media inhibited NED of LNCaP and could restore basal expression levels of NSE and neurotensin.[49] In contrast, while androgen deprivation for 4–7 days induces a terminal differentiation by morphological criteria, the cells retain the capacity to respond to androgen and overcome growth arrest (Desai, unpublished data).

Investigation into signaling events that occur upon androgen withdrawal in LNCaP cells have implicated kinases and cell cycle regulators in the process of growth arrest and resistance to apoptosis. Notably, PI3K signaling is deregulated and augmented in the LNCaP model as a consequence of mutational inactivation of the PTEN lipid phosphatase.[56,57] As a result, this aberrant signal poses as a dominant mediator of survival primarily through the resultant elevation in the basal level of active Akt/PKB,[58] a major PI3K target known to negatively regulate apoptosis via the phosphorylation and inactivation of pro-apoptotic molecules.[59,60] Akt emerged as a critical mediator of survival during androgen-deprivation by studies demonstrating its rapid hyper-activation observable within 8 hours of androgen withdrawal[49] and persisting for up to 60 days (Tepper, unpublished data). Although AR is a *bona fide* Akt substrate,[61,62] Akt-mediated phosphorylation paradoxically promotes AR instability by targeting it for Mdm2-mediated ubiquitination and subsequent proteasome-mediated degradation.[63] Similar to other PCa models, chronic androgen ablation of LNCaP results in the transition from an androgen-dependent to -independent state in which growth arrest is overcome.[49,64,65] In accord with elevated serum PSA serving as the clinical benchmark for the occurrence of hormone-refractory disease, reinstatement of the AR pathway (i.e., AR expression, PSA secretion) in experimental models is one hallmark of the transition to androgen-independence.[49,64–67] The reappearance of AR is due, at least in part, to enhanced stability of the receptor.[68] In late passage and androgen-independent LNCaP cell lines (e.g., LNCaP-AI, LNCaP-rf, LNCaP-cds)[49,64,67,69] this potentially involves a conversion of persistent PI3K/Akt activation from a degradation signal to an AR activator.[67]

Consistent with androgen withdrawal-induced Akt activation, treatment of LNCaP cells with R1881, a synthetic androgen, can decrease PI3K and Akt activation in both parental LNCaP and LNCaP-rf cell lines.[49] The mechanism by which this occurs is yet to be determined. The receptor tyrosine kinase erbB2, a member of the EGFR family, is an upstream activator of the PI3K pathway. ErbB2 is found expressed in NE cells of patients who have undergone radical prostatectomy[70] and is both upregulated and activated in androgen-deprived LNCaP cells (Tepper, unpublished data). However, it is unlikely that erbB2 is solely required for Akt activation by androgen withdrawal since functional knockout of erbB2, by its sequestration in the ER via expression of an erbB2-specific single chain antibody,[71] did not diminish Akt phosphorylation (Tepper, unpublished data). Therefore, multiple pathways for PI3K activation probably exist. ErbB2, a known activator of MAPK, could be responsible for constitutive activation of MAPK after androgen withdrawal (Desai, unpublished data).[72] RPTP-α also increases in androgen deprived NE differentiated LNCaP cells and contributes to MAPK activation.[50,55] One interesting possibility is that erbB2 and RPTP-α may cross-talk during the differentiation process leading to MAPK activation. The induction of

PI3K and Akt appears to be responsible for LNCaP resistance to apoptosis in the absence of androgen. Inhibiting PI3K either by treatment with pharmacological agents such as wortmannin or LY294002 or by overexpressing PTEN can selectively induce apoptosis in LNCaP cells during androgen deprivation.[49] This is accompanied by decreased Akt activation and triggering of the apoptotic proteolytic cascade, evidenced by caspase-3 activation. Short-term (3-day) androgen withdrawal prior to the addition of PI3K inhibitors further sensitizes LNCaP to apoptosis induced by PI3K inhibitors. PI3K inhibition might translate into enhanced apoptosis susceptibility via down-regulation of the anti-apoptotic protein Bcl-2, which increases upon androgen withdrawal.[73] In contrast, LNCaP-rf cells are remarkably resistant to treatment with PI3K inhibitors which might be explained by their markedly elevated levels of activated Akt and by Bcl-2 only being decreased by 50% upon treatment with the inhibitors (Tepper, unpublished data). Together, this suggests that immediate signaling stimuli are replaced by other factors as LNCaP cells progress to androgen-independence. These factors may be secreted by NE cells themselves, in a paracrine or autocrine fashion, allowing differentiated cells to eventually obtain signaling and growth autonomy.

PI3K signaling may contribute to overcoming growth arrest, in addition to suppressing apoptosis. Downstream effects of PI3K pathway dysregulation can certainly manifest as inappropriate progression through the Rb-mediated restriction point. Specifically, while cyclin-dependent kinase inhibitor p27^{kip1} and p16^{Ink4a} protein levels increased upon acute androgen withdrawal in LNCaP cells, they are significantly decreased in androgen-independent LNCaP and CWR22 cells and xenografts.[49,54,69] Although PI3K/Akt activation can suppress forkhead-mediated p27^{kip1} transcription,[74] the primary mechanism for p27^{kip1} protein down-regulation in this model was via increasing its rate of ubiquitin-mediated degradation,[75] as LY294002 treatment of androgen-independent LNCaP cells in the presence of the protein synthesis inhibitor cycloheximide markedly enhanced p27^{kip1} stability.[49] At present, it is rather unclear as to how androgen withdrawal augments p27^{kip1} expression level in the presence of PI3K/Akt activation. However, the expression of p27^{kip1} seems to be a determining factor for the growth arrest of NE cells. p21$^{Waf1/Cip1}$ exhibits the opposite expression pattern to p27^{kip1}, decreasing during acute androgen withdrawal followed by reinstatement in the refractory stage.[49] This seems to contradict the conventional role of p21[Wafl/Cip1] as an inducer of cell cycle arrest. However, it may be explained by recent findings that p21[Wafl/Cip1] can be either cell-cycle inhibitory or mitogenic, depending on its cellular localization.[76–78] In the nucleus, p21[Wafl/Cip1] binds to and inhibits cyclin/CDK activity, thereby blocking cell cycle progression.[79] Upon phosphorylation of p21[Wafl/Cip1] by Akt, p21[Wafl/Cip1] translocates to the cytoplasm, where it promotes cell growth.[80] In addition, p21[Wafl/Cip1] has been demonstrated to be critical for the assembly of cyclin D-cdk4 complexes.[81] Thus the restoration of p21[Wafl/Cip1] expression might be a pivotal event for the resumption of G1-S progression in the refractory stage. The AR and PI3K pathways play complimentary roles in positively regulating p21[Wafl/Cip1] expression. While androgen stimulates transcription of the p21[Wafl/Cip1] gene through AR binding to a consensus binding site in the p21[Wafl/Cip1] promoter,[82] Akt stabilizes the translated product by phosphorylation on residues Thr145 and Ser146.[83] Accordingly, inhibition of PI3K causes a decrease in p21[Wafl/Cip1]. Usurping p53-mediated growth arrest through mutational inactivation[84] or reduction in p53 expression[54,85] also figures as a prominent mechanism underlying androgen-independent growth. Recent data implicates PI3K as a potent suppressor of the p53 pathway as Akt-mediated phosphorylation of Mdm2 promotes its nuclear localization, high affinity binding to p53-p300 complexes, ubiquitination, and enhanced targeting of p53 for proteasome-mediated degradation.[80] However, the role of these cell cycle proteins and their requirements during NED has yet to be uncovered. Importantly, the theme of PI3K activation promoting hormone-refractory PCa appears to be conserved even in models that do not possess genetic defects in PI3K pathway regulation, such as CWR22. For instance, microarray analyses of CWR22 recurrent tumors demonstrated elevated expression of genes encoding growth factors (e.g., HGF, VEGFC, FGF2, PDGFA) known to stimulate PI3K/Akt.[86]

IL-6-Induced Neuroendocrine Differentiation

Another potential inducer of NED in PCa is Interleukin-6 (IL-6), a 212 amino acid glycoprotein that was first identified as a regulator of immune and inflammatory responses, but later shown to be involved in cell growth, differentiation, and metastasis.[87] IL-6 has been implicated as a driving factor in the progression of PCa and elevated serum IL-6 levels are often found in PCa patients.[88] The receptors for IL-6, an 80-kd IL-6 specific receptor subunit (alpha chain) and a 130-kd signal transducer called gp130,[87,89,90] are expressed in prostate carcinomas and the PCa cell lines LNCaP, PC-3, and DU145.[91] The androgen-independent PCa cell lines PC-3 and DU145 express IL-6, but LNCaP cells do not.[91] An antibody to either IL-6 or the 80-kd subunit IL-6 receptor can inhibit growth of PC-3 cells suggesting that IL-6 is part of an autocrine loop promoting the growth and androgen-independence of PC-3 cells.[92] In contrast, IL-6 treatment of LNCaP cells induces p27[kip1] and consequent growth arrest[18,19] and NED, as evidenced by morphological criteria (Fig. 3C) and the expression of NE markers NSE, CgA, and beta-tubulin III.[18,19,50,93] The receptors for IL-6 are found in cholesterol rich lipid rafts of the plasma membrane and the formation of these rafts appear to be required for IL-6 induced signaling and NED.[94] IL-6 stimulation of gp130 has been shown to interact with and activate erbB2 and erbB3 receptors in LNCaP cells. Under these conditions, erbB2 appears to be required for IL-6 induced mitogen activated protein kinase (MAPK) phosphorylation.[95] IL-6 also induces expression of erbB2 (Desai, unpublished data). The above properties are thus shared with androgen-deprived LNCaP cells. Signaling in LNCaP cells induced by IL-6 utilizes the customary JAK-STAT family as mediators of signal transduction.[96] The binding of IL-6 to its receptor complex results in the autophosphorylation and activation of JAK1, JAK2, and Tyk2, which in turn leads to the phosphorylation of and transcriptional activation by STAT3. STAT1, STAT5a, and STAT5b are expressed in LNCaP, but do not become activated by IL-6 signaling.[16] STAT3 appears to be the key player in NED induced by IL-6, as ectopic expression of a dominant-negative form of STAT3 in LNCaP cells abrogate their differentiation into NE cells and the expression of NSE and CgA.[93] IL-6 does not induce differentiation or NSE expression in PC-3 cells, which do not express STAT3. However, STAT3 overexpression in PC-3 cells results in an NED like morphology. Treatment with IL-6 does not further increase the NED phenotype, but does slightly induce NSE expression. Consistent with IL-6 induced NED, STAT3 overexpression in PC-3 cells leads to constitutive activation of STAT3 and growth inhibition of PC-3.[93]

IL-6 can also mediate PCa aggressiveness through antagonism of apoptosis. Similar to androgen withdrawal, IL-6 triggers the PI3K pathway. IL-6 has previously been reported to protect Hep3B hepatocarcinoma cells from TGF-β induced apoptosis through PI3K-Akt activation and by inhibiting caspase-3 activation.[17] Accordingly, inhibition of IL-6 signaling sensitizes PC-3 cells to etoposide-mediated cytotoxicity.[92] In LNCaP cells, IL-6 activates Etk, a member of the Btk tyrosine kinase family,[97] in a PI3K-dependent manner.[19] Etk overexpression protects LNCaP cells from apoptosis induced by oxidative stress or thapsigargin.[98] This protection was abolished by treatment with LY294002 prior to challenge with either stress. Indeed, Etk poses as a critical anti-apoptotic component of the IL6R-PI3K axis parallel to Akt signaling. IL-6 induced STAT3 activation has been implicated as an anti-apoptotic signal by virtue of affording protection to Hep3B cells,[17] and by gp130-STAT3-mediated induction of Bcl-2 in BAF-B03 mouse pro-B cells.[99] However, the role played by STAT3 in IL-6-treated LNCaP cells with respect to apoptosis has yet to be determined.

Etk appears to play a critical role in modulating the cytoskeletal changes that manifest as the characteristic NE morphology induced by IL-6. Treatment of LNCaP cells with IL-6 promotes the extension of short neuritic processes having a high level of branching complexity. While this can be recapitulated by overexpression of Etk in the absence of ligand, abrogation of Etk function using a dominant-negative approach alters the morphological changes to long, unbranched outgrowths[19] more typical of the response to androgen withdrawal. Consistent with these observations, we have been unable to detect Etk activation in the latter scenario (Desai, unpublished data) thereby implicating Etk as a strong effector of branching seen in IL-6 induced NED. Currently, the mechanism via which Etk activation translates into extension of neurites is speculative. The small GTPase RhoA, but not Rac1 or Cdc24, has recently been shown to be activated by Etk.[100] Since RhoA controls the organization of cytoskeletal actin and mediates the formation of stress fibers, RhoA activation by Etk would be consistent with the requirement of Etk in the IL-6 induced NED phenotype. Etk can also associate with focal adhesion kinase (FAK) in LNCaP cells.[101,102] FAK has been shown to promote neurite outgrowth in PC12 cells[103] and appears to be necessary for this process in LNCaP cells since expression of a dominant negative form of FAK prevents differentiation by

IL-6 stimulation or androgen withdrawal (Desai, unpublished data). As with nonmalignant cells, cellular morphology and the processes regulating cell shape have functional implications. This is exemplified by the Etk-FAK association also serving as a migration signal in response to GRP or integrin stimulation of LNCaP or HUVEC cells, respectively.[101,102] Interestingly, Etk is highly expressed in PC-3 cells, which have a greater migratory potential compared to LNCaP cells.[102] Etk has been shown to interact with Cas, a docking protein, and enhance the interaction of Cas with Crk.[104] The Cas/Crk complex is involved in regulating actin and cell motility and loss of Etk inhibits migration in COS-7 cells. Both Cas and Crk are also recruited by FAK, and it will be interesting to see whether an Etk/FAK/Cas/Crk complex is formed at the cellular membrane during IL-6 induced NED of LNCaP cells. This suggests that the final NE morphology and aggressiveness of the cell might be determined by levels of Etk, FAK, and the molecules with which they interact.

Other Factors Inducing Neuroendocrine Differentiation

While other factors have been shown to induce NED, less is known about the pathways involved. Inducers of cyclic AMP, such as epinephrine, forskolin (Fig. 3D), and PAPCA, can induce NED of LNCaP cells.[16,20,21,105,106] Cyclic AMP elevation leads to growth arrest and expression of NSE, CgA, PTHrP, neurotensin, and serotonin. PKA and MAPK activation are thought to be involved[16,20] and may lead to activation of the transcription factor CREB.[106] Contrary to IL-6 or androgen-withdrawal-induced differentiation, cAMP-induced differentiation does not appear to be terminal. Removal of cAMP inducers results in the loss of the NED phenotype and an increase in protein kinase activities.[21] Co-treatment of IL-6 with cAMP enhances the extent of NED suggesting that these agents may cooperate to induce differentiation in PCa.[16] HB-EGF, a prostate stromal-derived factor that promotes survival, can induce differentiation and increase NSE expression through MAPK activation.[23] In contrast to other NED inducers, HB-EGF does not induce cell cycle arrest,[23] but instead promotes androgen-independent growth of LNCaP cells and down-modulates AR.[22] IL-1β and IL-2,[107,108] and anticancer agents that induce growth arrest such as jolkinolide B,[109] the COX-2 inhibitor NS-398,[110] and silibinin[111] also induce NED and an increase in NSE and CgA expression in LNCaP cells suggesting that NED may be a default pathway in response to cellular stress in androgen-dependent cells.

As discussed above, a wealth of clinical and experimental data implicates NED as a common feature of hormone-refractory disease. Although NED can be induced by circulating cytokines or passively as a result of androgen ablative therapy, NE cells possess the potential to actively and potently drive the metastatic growth of PCa cells in the absence of androgens and/or in the presence of AR antagonists. This is primarily accomplished through the paracrine, and possibly autocrine, secretion of polypeptide factors such as neurotrophins and cytokines. Below, we will discuss the signaling pathways triggered by several of these polypeptide ligands and how they engender one or more of the vital components of androgen-independent growth such as reinstatement of AR signaling and stimulation of metastasis through enhanced motility, invasiveness, and angiogenesis. Since there is significant diversity in these ligands, the receptor-mediated signals they evoke, and their ultimate biological effects, the combinatorial outcome of "Neurokine" signaling might be sufficient to support androgen-independent growth. A summary of the signal pathways involved in neurokine-induced androgen-independence is presented in Fig. 2B.

Androgen-Independent Growth

The absence of androgen and subsequent down-regulation of AR during androgen-ablation therapy would suggest that AR is no longer required in androgen-independent tumors. However, AR is still expressed in almost all androgen-independent tumors[3] and this suggests that AR is involved in androgen-independent growth of PCa. Amplification of AR and its coactivators such as p160 SRCs[4-6] are also detected in relapsed and metastatic tumors. Androgen-independent LNCaP cell lines, which can grow in the absence of androgen, show an increased level of AR expression.[49,64,112] Mutations in AR can lead to the activation of AR by other steroids such as estrogens,[113] glucocorticoids,[114] and even nonsteroidal anti-androgens used to treat PCa.[115] However, the low frequency of mutations in androgen-independent tumors is leading investigators to investigate alternative mechanisms of AR activation, either being ligand-independent or in synergy with castrate levels of androgen.

Three classes of activators have been identified (1) circulating growth factors that bind to transmembrane receptor tyrosine kinases (EGF, IGF-1, and KGF); (2) neuropeptides (GRP and neurotensin) and chemokines (IL-8) secreted by neuroendocrine cells that activate G-protein-coupled receptors (GPCR); and (3) interleukins (e.g., IL-6) that bind to cytokine receptors. These factors, while differing in the detailed signal pathways they transmit, share certain common traits. For instance, they all induce phosphorylation cascades and activate tyrosine and serine/threonine kinases. It has been suggested that phosphorylation of AR, or its activators, facilitates the assembly of a transcriptional complex that mimics the recruitment by androgen-bound AR, and may be an alternate route to AR activation.[116] Since AR and its coactivators are known to be phosphorylated only at serines and threonines, serine/threonine kinases are thought to be immediate activators of the AR complex, whereas tyrosine kinases are the upstream activators of serine/threonine kinases. Phosphorylation and activation of AR by the serine/threonine kinases ERK,[117,118] Akt,[62] PKA,[119,120] PKC,[121,122] and CAK[123] have been reported. Examples of serine/threonine kinase activation of AR coactivators include ERK phosphorylation of SRC-1[64] and phosphorylation of SRC-2[4] by IL-6 and EGF stimulation, respectively. Most of these studies were based on *in vitro* studies or transient expression systems. The *in vivo* phosphorylation sites of AR have recently been identified,[124–126] and ironically none of the sites are consensus phosphorylation sites of ERK or Akt,[124] raising the possibility that other novel kinases are involved. Studies to identify protein kinases associated with or induced by AR have resulted in the discovery of several novel kinases, ANPK,[127] SPAK[128] MAK,[129] and PAK6.[130,131] These kinases modulate (ANPK, SPAK, and MAK activate, while PAK6 represses) AR activity by directly binding to AR, but do not seem to directly phosphorylate AR or affect cellular growth induced by androgen. Despite these new twists, it seems clear that AR activity can be enhanced by kinases. In the ensuing sections, we will review how soluble factors induce the activation of these kinases.

Growth Factors

Growth factors such as KGF, IGF-1, and EGF have been shown to activate AR in the absence of androgen,[132] via the activation of their respective receptor tyrosine kinases (FGF-R, IGF-R, and EGFR). ErbB2, when over-expressed, can induce PSA expression in an androgen-independent, but not AR-dependent manner.[117,118] All of the receptor tyrosine kinases are known to activate serine/threonine kinases, such as MAPK[117,118] and Akt,[62] which in turn activate AR activity as discussed above.

Neuropeptides

Of growing interest is elucidating the role of neuropeptides in the androgen-independent growth of PCa. Since neuropeptides are secreted by NE cells, the potential contribution of the prostate micro-environment to cancer growth becomes significant. As mentioned in the previous section, NE cells in the prostate and NE-differentiated LNCaP cells secrete neuropeptides such as GRP and neurotensin. Androgen-independent PCas and PCa cell lines also express GRP and neurotensin, as well as chemokines such as IL-8, that appear to be involved in an autocrine loop that stimulates growth. GRP receptors[133,134] and neurotensin receptors[135] are found in PCas and PCa cell lines. GRP and neurotensin have been shown to stimulate androgen-independent growth in PC-3, DU145, and LNCaP cells.[51,101,135–138] Conversely, GRP antagonists[139–142] and neurotensin antagonists[135] have been shown to inhibit PC-3 and DU145 growth. The majority of information about the mechanism mediating neuropeptide-induced growth of PCa pertains to GRP signaling. GRP binds to and activates GPCR proteins (Fig. 2B), which engage the heterotrimeric G proteins α, β, and γ, which in turn leads to sequential Ca^+ mobilization, PLC and PKC activation, and ultimately cellular proliferation.[143] The specific response in the cell is dependent on which G protein is activated and whether it is stimulatory or inhibitory. In the case of GRP, GRP-R has been shown to activate $G_{\alpha q}$, which activates the PLCβ pathway and $G_{\alpha 12}$, which activates the Rho pathway. However, activation of $G_{\alpha q}$ and $G_{\alpha 12}$ by GRP in PCa cells has not been verified. In PC-3 and DU145, cross-talk between GPCR proteins and receptor tyrosine kinases[144] has been demonstrated by the ability of GRP to transactivate EGFR and that it requires Src activation and Ca^+ mobilization. Once EGFR is activated it leads to Ras and MAPK activation and DNA synthesis. The transcription factor Elk-1, and immediate early genes *c-fos* and *c-myc* are also up-regulated by GRP presenting a possible pathway for growth induction.[145] Evidence for GRP as a progression factor is provided by its ability to up-regulate proangiogenic factors such as MMP-9,[146,147] VEGF, and IL-8,[148] the latter two being mediated through NF-κB. Furthermore, cross-talk between GRP signaling and β1 integrin results in enhanced processing of pro-MMP-9 into its active form as a result of Src and PI3K activation culminating in the up-regulation of membrane-bound uPA.[146] GRP activation of the PKC pathway in PC-3 cells leads to the activation of FAK and increased motility suggesting that GRP may also play an important role in tissue invasion, increasing the potential for metastasis.[149]

GRP and neurotensin have also been shown to activate AR and induce androgen-independent growth of LNCaP cells.[101] GRP can act synergistically with low levels of androgen to activate AR, leading to the possibility that residual circulating androgen present after androgen-ablation therapy could cooperate with GRP in achieving an androgen-independent state.[150] GRP-induced activation and complex formation of Etk, FAK, and Src are required for AR activation. Interestingly, Etk activation is dependent upon Src and FAK, but not on PI3K, as is the case with IL-6 stimulated Etk activation. Activation of AR supports the notion that neuropeptides might mediate the transition from an androgen-dependent to -independent state in PCa. Further indication that GRP may be a transition-promoting factor is the evidence that neutral endopeptidase (NEP), which cleaves neuropeptides, is down-regulated in androgen-independent tumors,[151] and is down-regulated by GRP in LNCaP.[152] Reintroduction of NEP in androgen-independent cells interferes with GRP signaling[153] and cellular migration.[154]

Chemokines

As mentioned above, the chemokine IL-8 is an angiogenic factor involved in the migration and invasion of cancer cells. Serum IL-8 levels are elevated in PCa patients[155] and IL-8 is overexpressed in PC-3 cells.[156] The

IL-8 receptors, CXCR1 and CXCR2, are expressed in DU145 and PC-3 cells[157] and antisense-mediated suppression of IL-8 expression reduces invasion and metastatic potential of PC-3 xenografts in nude mice.[158] Many studies have focused on the role of IL-8 in tissue invasion and metastasis.[158–160] However, a recent finding showed that IL-8 could stimulate the androgen-independent growth of LNCaP cells via recruitment of the AR transcription complex to the proximal region of the PSA promoter.[161] Analogous to GRP signaling, IL-8 induces Src, FAK, and MAPK activation (Fig. 2B) and promotes migration of LNCaP cells. Src and MAPK appear to be required for AR activity and LNCaP proliferation, while Src and FAK are required for LNCaP migration. Together, these data indicate that GRP and IL-8 may be progression factors of PCa contributing to the androgen-independence and metastatic potential of advanced cancers.

Cytokines

As described in the previous section, our work, as well as that of others, demonstrated that IL-6 treatment of LNCaP induced NED and growth arrest.[19,162] Paradoxically, IL-6 has also been found to induce growth of PCa cells, including LNCaP. When subjected to prolonged IL-6 treatment, eventual selection of proliferating LNCaP cells occured. While the molecular details of the genetic adaptation caused by IL-6 is not clear, once achieved, the cells become androgen-independent and can grow in the presence of IL-6. This may be related to the observation that in low-passage LNCaP cells, activated Akt down-modulates AR, whereas in high-passage LNCaP cells, it enhances AR activity.[67] In fact, a very interesting aspect of the pleiotropic influence of IL-6 upon the transition to androgen-independence is its ability to directly regulate AR.[163–167] Although IL-6 activation of AR can occur without androgen, IL-6 can also act synergistically with low levels of androgen.[163–165] The pathway of IL-6-mediated AR activation is complex and involves multiple signal transducers. Two reports demonstrated that JAK-STAT3 activation is the principal pathway responsible for AR activation via direct STAT3-AR interaction.[163,164] This was confirmed by inhibition of AR activation in the presence of over-expressed dominant negative STAT3. However, a third report implicated

MEK/MAPK, PKA, and PKC, since AR activation could be inhibited with pharmacological inhibition of each of these kinases.[165] Yet another paper showed that IL-6 activation of AR depends on ERK and p300.[167] One reason for this diversity may lie in differences in cellular milieu and the outcome of competition for cellular resources that can activate AR.[166] For instance, STAT3 is the dominant mediator of IL-6 signaling and AR activation in LNCaP cells, but PKA or PKC might predominate to activate ectopically-expressed AR in the STAT3-deficient cell line PC-3. An intriguing question is how IL-6 and AR cooperate under diverse conditions of NED. In contrast to down-regulation of AR activity and protein levels during androgen withdrawal, IL-6 might contribute to cell survival during androgen ablation therapy through its ability to activate the AR. This could result in maintenance of AR expression so that other growth factors are able to utilize AR to circumvent androgen dependence.

Summary

In summary, there is considerable evidence that NED represents an integral and potentially important part of prostate carcinogenesis. The propensity of prostate carcinoma cells to undergo NED under a variety of conditions including androgen withdrawal suggest that it is an innate property of prostate epithelial cells to survive and to overcome adverse conditions. Although the cellular signals involved in this trans-differentiation process vary with different inducing conditions, the differentiated cells have three common characteristics: resistance to apoptosis, growth arrest, and expression of neuronal phenotypes. The release by these cells of neurokines, which are survival and growth factors, is likely to have an impact on surrounding undifferentiated prostate cancer cells undergoing androgen-deprivation crisis. Accumulating evidence suggests that these neurokines are capable of activating AR, presumably via kinase signaling. This may be one way a fraction of PCas survive androgen ablation and eventually develop into androgen-independent clones. If true, targeting neurokines and the downstream protein kinases in conjunction with hormone therapy offers a new intervention strategy for treatment of prostate cancer and in particular, androgen-independent tumors. (This work from the authors' labs was supported by grants from the NIH and DOD.)

References

1. Abrahamsson PA (1999) Neuroendocrine differentiation and hormone-refractory prostate cancer. *Prostate* 6(Suppl):3–8.
2. Arnold JT, Isaacs JT (2002) Mechanisms involved in the progression of androgen-independent prostate cancers: It is not only the cancer cell's fault. *Endocr Relat Cancer* 9:61–73.
3. Culig Z, Hobisch A, Hittmair A, Peterziel H, Cato A, Bartsch G, Klocker H (1998) Expression, structure, and function of androgen receptor in advanced prostatic carcinoma. *Prostate* 35:63–70.
4. Gregory CW, Fei X, Ponguta LA, He B, Bill HM, French FS, Wilson EM (2004) Epidermal growth factor increases coactivation of the androgen receptor in recurrent prostate cancer. *J Biol Chem* 279:7119–7130.
5. Zhou G, Hashimoto Y, Kwak I, Tsai SY, Tsai MJ (2003) Role of the steroid receptor coactivator SRC-3 in cell growth. *Mol Cell Biol* 23: 7742–7755.
6. Chen CD, Welsbie DS, Tran C, Baek SH, Chen R, Vessella R, Rosenfeld MG, Sawyers CL (2004) Molecular determinants of resistance to antiandrogen therapy. *Nat Med* 10:33–39.
7. Hanson J, Abrahamsson PA (2001) Neuroendocrine pathogenesis in adeno-carcinoma of the prostate. *Ann Oncol* 12(Suppl 2):S145–152.
8. Bonkoff H (2001) Neuroendocrine differentiation in human prostate cancer. Morphogenesis, proliferation and androgen receptor status. *Ann Oncol* 12(Suppl 2):S141–144.
9. di Sant'Agnese PA (2001) Neuroendocrine differentiation in prostatic carci-noma: An update on recent developments. *Ann Oncol* 12(Suppl 2):S135–140.
10. Abrahamsson PA (1999) Neuroendocrine cell in tumor growth in the prostate. *Endocr Relat Cancer* 6:503–519.
11. di Sant'Agnese PA (1998) Neuroendocrine differentiation in prostatic carci-noma: An updatel. *Prostate* 8(Suppl):74–79.
12. Aprikian AG, Han K, Guy L, Landry F, Begin LR, Chevalier S (1998) Neuroendocrine differentiation and the bombesin/gastrin-releasing peptide family of neuropeptides in the progression of human prostate cancer. *Prostate* 8(Suppl):52–61.
13. di Sant'Agnese PA (1998) Neuroendocrine cell of the prostate and neuroen-docrine differentiation in prostatic carcinoma: A review of morphologic aspects. *Urology* 51:121–124.
14. Gkonos PJ, Krongrad A, Roos BA (1995) Neuroendocrine peptides in the prostate. *Urol Res* 23:81–87.

15. Burchardt T, Burchardt M, Chen MW, Cao Y, de la Taille A, Shabsigh A, Hayek O, Dorai T, Buttyan R (1999) Transdifferentiation of prostate cancer cell to a neuroendocrine cell phenotype *in vitro* and *in vivo*. *J Urol* 162:1800–1805.

16. Deeble PD, Murphy DJ, Parsons SJ, Cox ME (2001) Interleukin-6-and cyclic AMP mediated signaling potentiates NED of LNCaP prostate tumor cells. *Mol Cell Bio* 21:8471–8482.

17. Chen RH, Chang MC, Su YS, Tsai YT, Kuo ML (1999) Interleukin-6 inhibits transforming growth factor-beta-induced apoptosis through the phosphatidylinositol 3'-kinase/Atk and signal transducers and activators of transcription 3 pathway. *J Bio Chem* 274:23013–23019.

18. Mori S, Murakami-Mori K, Bonavida B (1999) Interleukin-6 induces G1 arrest through induction of p27Kip1, a cyclin-dependent kinase inhibitor, and neuron-like morphology in LNCaP prostate tumor cells. *Biochem Biophys Res Commun* 257:609–614.

19. Qui Y, Robinson D, Pretlow TG, Kung HJ (1998) Etk/Bmx, a tyrosine kinase with a pleckstrin-homology domain, is an effector of phosphatidylinositol 3'-kinase and is involved in interleukin 6-induced NED of PCa cells. *Proc Natl Acad Sci* 95:3644–3649.

20. Cox ME, Deeble PD, Bissonette EA, Parsons SJ (2000) Activated 3',5'-cyclic AMP-dependent protein kinase is sufficient to induce neuroendocrine-like differentiation of the LNCaP prostate tumor cell line. *J Biol Chem* 275:13812–13818.

21. Cox ME, Deeble PD, Lakhani S, Parsons SJ (1999) Acquisition of neuroendocrine characteristics by prostate tumor cells is reversible: Implications for prostate cancer progression. *Cancer Res* 59:3821–3830.

22. Adam RM, Kim J, Lin J, Orsola A, Zhuang L, Rice DC, Freeman MR (2002) Heparin-binding epidermal growth factor-like growth factor stimulates androgen-independent prostate tumor growth and antagonizes androgen receptor function. *Endocrinology* 143:4599–4608.

23. Kim J, Adam RM, Freeman MR (2002) Activation of the Erk mitogen-activated protein kinase pathway stimulates neuroendocrine differentiation in LNCaP cells independently of cell cycle withdrawal and STAT3 phosphorylation. *Cancer Res* 62:1549–1554.

24. Schalken JA, van Leenders G (2003) Cellular and molecular biology of the prostate: Stem cell biology. *Urology* 62:11–20.

25. Xue Y, Smedts F, Verhofstad A, Debruyne F, de la Rosette J, Schalken J (1998) Cell kinetics of prostate exocrine and neuroendocrine epithelium and their differential interrelationship: New perspectives. *Prostate* 8(Suppl):62–73.

26. Bonkhoff H, Remberger K (1996) Differentiation pathways and histogenetic aspects of normal and abnormal prostatic growth: A stem cell model. *Prostate* 22:98–106.

27. di Sant'Agnese PA, de Mesy Jensen KL (1987) Neuroendocrine differentiation in prostatic carcinoma. *Human Pathol* 18:849–856.

28. Helpap B, Kollermann J, Oehler U (1999) Neuroendocrine differentiation in prostatic carcinomas: Histogenesis, biology, clinical relevance and future therapeutical perspectives. *Urol Int* 62:133–138.

29. di Sant'Agnese PA (1992) Neuroendocrine differentiation in carcinoma of the prostate. Diagnostic, prognostic, and therapeutic implications. *Cancer* 70:254–268.

30. Hu Y, Ippolito JE, Garabedian EM, Humphrey PA, Gordon JI (2002) Molecular characterization of a metastatic neuroendocrine cell cancer arising in the prostates of transgenic mice. *J Biol Chem* 277:44462–44474.

31. Masumori N, Thomas TZ, Chaurand P, Case T, Paul M, Kasper S, PCarioli RM, Tsukamoto T, Shappell SB, Matusik RJ (2001) A probasin-large T antigen transgenic mouse line develops prostate adenocarcinoma and neuroendocrine carcinoma with metastatic potential. *Cancer Res* 61:2239–2249.

32. Garabedian EM, Humphrey PA, Gordon JI (1998) A transgenic mouse model of metastatic prostate cancer originating from neuroendocrine cells. *Proc Natl Acad Sci USA* 95:15382–15387.

33. Clegg N, Ferguson C, True LD, Arnold H, Moorman A, Quinn JA, Vessella RL, Nelson PS (2003) Molecular characterization of prostatic small-cell neuroendocrine carcinoma. *Prostate* 55:55–64.

34. Hvamstad T, Jordal A, Hekmat N, Paus E, Fossa SD (2003) Neuroendocrine serum tumour markers in hormone-resistant prostate cancer. *Eur Urol* 44: 215–221.

35. Kamiya N, Akakura K, Suzuki H, Isshiki S, Komiya A, Ueda T, Ito H (2003) Pretreatment serum level of neuron specific enolase (NSE) as a prognostic factor in metastatic prostate cancer patients treated with endocrine therapy. *Eur Urol* 44:309–314.

36. Berruti A, Dogliotti L, Mosca A, Gorzegno G, Bollito E, Mari M, Tarabuzzi R, Poggio M, Torta M, Fontana D, Angeli A (2001) Potential clinical value of circulating chromogranin A in patients with prostate carcinoma. *Ann Oncol* 12(Suppl 2):S153–157.

37. Bollito E, Berruti A, Bellina M, Mosca A, Leonardo E, Tarabuzzi R, Capia S, Ari MM, Tampellini M, Fontana D, Gubetta L, Angeli A, Dogliotti L (2001) Relationship between neuroendocrine features and prognostic parameters in human prostate adenocarcinoma. *Ann Oncol* 12(Suppl 2):S159–164.

38. Ferrero-Poüs M, Hersant AM, Pecking A, Brésard-Leroy M, Pichon MF (2001) Serum chromogranin-A in advanced prostate cancer. *BJU Int* 88:790–796.
39. Ather MH, Abbas F (2000) Prognostic significance of neuroendocrine differentiation in prostate cancer. *Eur Urol* 38:535–542.
40. Abrahamsson PA, Cockett ATK, di Sant'Agnese PA (1998) Prognostic significance of neuroendocrine differentiation in clinically localized prostatic carcinoma. *Prostate* 8(Suppl):37–42.
41. Deftos LJ (1998) Granin-A, parathyroid hormone-related protein, and calcitonin gene products in neuroendocrine prostate cancer. *Prostate* 8(Suppl):23–31.
42. Deftos LJ, Abrahamsson PA (1998) Granins and prostate cancer. *Urology* 51:141–145.
43. Jiborn T, Bjartell A, Abrahamsson P-A (1998) NED in prostatic carcinoma during hormonal treatment. *Urology* 51:585–589.
44. Tarle M, Ahel MZ, Kovacic K (2002) Aquired NE-positivity during maximal androgen blockade in prostate cancer patients. *Anticancer Res* 22:2525–2529.
45. Fixemer T, Remberger K, Bonkhoff H (2002) Apoptosis resistance of NE phenotypes in prostatic adenocarcinoma. *Prostate* 53:118–123.
46. Ismail A HR, Landry F, Aprikian AG, Chevalier S (2002) Androgen ablation promotes NE cell differentiation in dog and human prostate. *Prostate* 51:117–125.
47. Jongsma J, Oomen MH, Noordzij MA, van Weerden WM, Martens GJM, van der Kwast TH, Schröder FH, van Steenbrugge GJ (2000) Androgen deprivation of the prohormone convertase-310 human prostate cancer model system induces NED. *Cancer Res* 60:741–748.
48. Jongsma J, Oomen MH, Noordzij MA, van Weerden WM, Martens GJM, van der Kwast TH, Schröder FH, van Steenbrugge GJ (2002) Different profiles of NE cell differentiation evolve in the PC-310 human prostate cancer model during long-term androgen deprivation. *Prostate* 50:203–215.
49. Murillo H, Huang H, Schmidt LJ, Smith DI, Tindall DJ (2001) Role of PI3K signaling in survival and progression of LNCaP prostate cancer cells to the androgen refractory state. *Endocrinology* 142:4795–4805.
50. Zelivianski S, Verni M, Moore C, Kondrikov D, Taylor R, Lin M-F (2001) Multipathways for transdifferentiation of human prostate cancer cells into NE-like phenotype. *Biochim Biophys Acta* 1539:28–43.
51. Sehgal I, Powers S, Huntley B, Powis G, Pittelkow M, Maihle NJ (1994) Neurotensin is an autocrine trophic factor stimulated by androgen withdrawal in human prostate cancer. *Proc Natl Acad Sci USA* 91:4673–4677.

52. Saeed B, Zhang H, Ng SC (1997) Apoptotic program is initiated but not completed in LNCaP cells in response to growth in charcoal-stripped media. *Prostate* 31:145–152.
53. Wright ME, Tsai MJ, Aebersold R (2003) AR represses the NE transdifferentiation process in prostate cancer cells. *Mol Endocrinol* 17:1726–1737.
54. Agus DB, Cordon-Cardo C, Fox W, Drobnjak M, Koff A, Golde DW, Scher HI (1999) Prostate cancer cell cycle regulators: Response to androgen withdrawal and development of androgen independence. *J Natl Cancer Inst* 91:1869–1876.
55. Zhang XQ, Kondrikov D, Yuan TC, Lin FF, Hansen J, Lin MF (2003) Receptor protein tyrosine phosphatase alpha signaling is involved in androgen depletion-induced NED of androgen-sensitive LNCaP human prostate cancer cells. *Oncogene* 22:6704–6716.
56. Teng DH, Hu R, Lin H, Davis T, Iliev D, Frye C, Swedlund B, Hansen KL, Vinson VL, Gumpper KL, Ellis L, El-Naggar A, Frazier M, Jasser S, Langford LA, Lee J, Mills GB, Pershouse MA, Pollack RE, Tornos C, Troncoso P, Yung WK, Fujii G, Berson A, Steck PA (1997) MMAC1/PTEN mutations in primary tumor specimens and tumor cell lines. *Cancer Res* 57:5221–5225.
57. Carson JP, Kulik G, Weber MJ (1999) Antiapoptotic signaling in LNCaP prostate cancer cells: A survival signaling pathway independent of phosphatidylinositol 3′-kinase and Akt/protein kinase B. *Cancer ResI* 59:1449–1453.
58. Chan TO, Rittenhouse SE, Tsichlis PN (1999) AKT/PKB and other D3 phosphoinositide-regulated kinases: Kinase activation by phosphoinositide-dependent phosphorylation. *Annu Rev Biochem* 68:965–1014.
59. Lawlor MA, Alessi DR (2001) PKB/Akt: A key mediator of cell proliferation, survival and insulin responses? *J Cell Sci* 114:2903–2910.
60. Milburn CC, Deak M, Kelly SM, Price NC, Alessi DR, Van Aalten DM (2003) Binding of phosphatidylinositol 3,4,5-trisphosphate to the pleckstrin homology domain of protein kinase B induces a conformational change. *Biochem J* 375:531–538.
61. Lin IIK, Yeh S, Kang HY, Chang C (2001) Akt suppresses androgen-induced apoptosis by phosphorylating and inhibiting androgen receptor. *Proc Natl Acad Sci USA* 98:7200–7205.
62. Wen Y, Hu MC, Makino K, Spohn B, Bartholomeusz G, Yan DH, Hung MC (2000) HER-2/neu promotes androgen-independent survival and growth of prostate cancer cells through the Akt pathway. *Cancer Res* 60:6841–6845.
63. Lin HK, Wang L, Hu YC, Altuwaijri S, Chang C (2002) Phosphorylation-dependent ubiquitylation and degradation of androgen receptor by Akt require Mdm2 E3 ligase. *EMBO J* 21:4037–4048.

64. Shi XB, Ma AH, Tepper CG, Xia L, Gregg JP, Gandour-Edwards R, Mack PC, Kung HJ, de Vere White RW (2004) Molecular alterations associated with LNCaP cell progression to androgen independence. *Prostate,* in press.

65. Kokontis JM, Hay N, Liao S (1998) Progression of LNCaP prostate tumor cells during androgen deprivation: Hormone-independent growth, repression of proliferation by androgen, and role for p27Kip1 in androgen-induced cell cycle arrest. *Mol Endocrinol* 12:941–953.

66. Nagabhushan M, Miller CM, Pretlow TP, Giaconia JM, Edgehouse NL, Schwartz S, Kung HJ, de Vere White RW, Gumerlock PH, Resnick MI, Amini SB, Pretlow TG (1996) CWR22: The first human prostate cancer xenograft with strongly androgen-dependent and relapsed strains both *in vivo* and in soft agar. *Cancer Res* 56:3042–3046.

67. Lin HK, Hu YC, Yang L, Altuwaijri S, Chen YT, Kang HY, Chang C (2003) Suppression versus induction of androgen receptor functions by the phosphatidylinositol 3-kinase/Akt pathway in prostate cancer LNCaP cells with different passage numbers. *J Biol Chem* 278:50902–50907.

68. Gregory CW, Johnson RT Jr, Mohler JL, French FS, Wilson EM (2001) Androgen receptor stabilization in recurrent prostate cancer is associated with hypersensitivity to low androgen. *Cancer Res* 61:2892–2898.

69. Graff JR, Konicek BW, McNulty AM, Wang Z, Houck K, Allen S, Paul JD, Hbaiu A, Goode RG, Sandusky GE, Vessella RL, Neubauer BL (2000) Increased AKT activity contributes to prostate cancer progression by dramatically accelerating prostate tumor growth and diminishing p27Kip1 expression. *J Biol Chem* 275:24500–24505.

70. Iwamura M, Koshiba K, Cockett ATK (1998) Receptors for BPH growth factors are located in some NE cells. *Prostate* 8:14–17.

71. Beerli RR, Wels W, Hynes NE (1994) Intracellular expression of single chain antibodies reverts ErbB-2 transformation. *J Biol Chem* 269:23931–23936.

72. Gioeli D, Mandell JW, Petroni GR, Frierson HF Jr, Weber MJ (1999) Activation of mitogen-activated protein kinase associated with prostate cancer progression. *Cancer Res* 59:279–284.

73. Pugazhenthi S, Nesterova A, Sable C, Heidenreich KA, Boxer LM, Heasley LE, Reusch JE (2000) Akt/protein kinase B up-regulates Bcl-2 expression through cAMP-response element-binding protein. *J Biol Chem* 275:10761–10766.

74. Medema RH, Kops GJ, Bos JL, Burgering BM (2000) AFX-like Forkhead transcription factors mediate cell-cycle regulation by Ras and PKB through p27kip1. *Nature* 404:782–787.

75. Slingerland J, Pagano M (2000) Regulation of the cdk inhibitor p27 and its deregulation in cancer. *J Cell Physiol* 183:10–17.

76. Dong Y, Chi SL, Borowsky AD, Fan Y, Weiss RH (2004) Cytosolic p21Waf1/Cip1 increases cell cycle transit in vascular smooth muscle cells. *Cell Signal* 16:263–269.

77. Dupont J, Karas M, LeRoith D (2003) The cyclin-dependent kinase inhibitor p21CIP/WAF1 is a positive regulator of insulin-like growth factor I-induced cell proliferation in MCF-7 human breast cancer cells. *J Biol Chem* 278: 37256–37264.

78. Weiss RH (2003) p21Waf1/Cip1 as a therapeutic target in breast and other cancers. *Cancer Cell* 4:425–429.

79. Hengst L, Gopfert U, Lashuel HA, Reed SI (1998) Complete inhibition of Cdk/cyclin by on molecule of p21 (Cip1). *Genes Dev* 12:3882–3888.

80. Zhou BP, Liao Y, Xia W, Zou Y, Spohn B, Hung MC (2001) HER-2/neu induces p53 ubiquitination via Akt-mediated MDM2 phosphorylation. *Nat Cell Biol* 3:973–982.

81. Cheng M, Olivier P, Diehl JA, Fero M, Roussel MF, Roberts JM, Sherr CJ (1999) The p21(Cip1) and p27(Kip1) CDK 'inhibitors' are essential activators of cyclin D-dependent kinases in murine fibroblasts. *EMBO J* 18: 1571–1583.

82. Lu S, Liu M, Epner DE, Tsai SY, Tsai MJ (1999) Androgen regulation of the cyclin-dependent kinase inhibitor p21 gene through an androgen response element in the proximal promoter. *Mol Endocrinol* 13:376–384.

83. Li Y, Dowbenko D, Lasky LA (2002) AKT/PKB phosphorylation of p21Cip/WAF1 enhances protein stability of p21Cip/WAF1 and promotes cell survival. *J Biol Chem* 277:11352–11361.

84. Meyers FJ, Gumerlock PH, Chi SG, Borchers H, Deitch AD, deVere White RW (1998) Very frequent p53 mutations in metastatic prostate carcinoma and in matched primary tumors. *Cancer* 83:2534–2539.

85. Burchardt M, Burchardt T, Shabsigh A, Ghafar M, Chen MW, Anastasiadis A, de la Taille A, Kiss A, Buttyan R (2001) Reduction of wild type p53 function confers a hormone resistant phenotype on LNCaP prostate cancer cells. *Prostate* 48:225–230.

86. Mousses S, Wagner U, Chen Y, Kim JW, Bubendorf L, Bittner M, Pretlow T, Elkahloun AG, Trepel JB, Kallioniemi OP (2001) Failure of hormone therapy in prostate cancer involves systematic restoration of androgen responsive genes and activation of rapamycin sensitive signaling. *Oncogene* 20:6718–6723.

87. Bonkhoff H (1998) NE cells in benign and malignant prostate tissue: morphogenesis, proliferation, and AR status. *Prostate* 8(Suppl):18–22.

88. Twillie DA, Eisenberger MA, Carducci MA, Hseih WS, Kim WY, Simons JW (1995) Interleukin-6: A candidate mediator of human prostate cancer morbidity. *Urology* 45:542–549.

89. Hibi M, Murakami M, Saito M, Hirano T, Taga T, Kishimoto T, Hirata Y, Yamasaki K, Yasukawa K, Matsuda T (1990) Molecular cloning and expression of an IL-6 signal transducer, gp130. *Cell* 63:1149–1157.

90. Taga T, Hibi M, Hirata Y, Yamasaki K, Yasukawa K, Matsuda T, Hirano T, Kishimoto T (1989) Interleukin-6 triggers the association of its receptor with a possible signal transducer, gp130. *Cell* 58:573–581.

91. Lou W, Ni Z, Dyer K, Tweardy DJ, Gao AC (2000) Interleukin-6 induces prostate cancer cell growth accompanied by activation of Stat3 signaling pathway. *Prostate* 42:239–242.

92. Borsellino N, Bonavida B, Ciliberto G, Toniatti C, Travali S, D'Alessandro N (1999) Blocking signaling through the gp130 receptor chain by interleukin-6 and oncostatin M inhibits PC-3 cell growth and sensitizes the tumor cells to etoposide and cisplatin-mediated cytotoxicity. *Cancer* 85:134–144.

93. Spiotto MT, Chung TDK (2000) STAT3 mediates IL-6-induced NED in prostate cancer cells. *Prostate* 42:186–195.

94. Kim J, Adam RM, Solomon K, Freeman MR (2004) Involvement of cholesterol-rich lipid rafts in interleukine-6-induced NED of LNCaP prostate cancer cells. *Endocrinology* 145:613–619.

95. Qui Y, Ravi L, Kung HJ (1998) Requirement of ErbB2 for signaling by interleukin-6 in prostate carcinoma cells. *Nature* 393:83–85.

96. Heinrich PC, Behrmann I, Haan S, Hermanns HM, Muller-Newen G, Schaper F (2003) Principles of interleukin (IL)-6-type cytokine signaling and its regulation. *Biochem J* 374:1–20.

97. Qui Y, Kung HJ (2000) Signaling network of the Btk family kinases. *Oncogene* 19:5651–5661.

98. Xue LY, Qiu Y, He J, Kung HJ, Oleinick NL (1999) Etk/Bmx a PH-domain containing tyrosine kinase, protects prostate cancer cells from apoptosis induced by photodynamic therapy or thapsigargin. *Oncogene* 18: 3391–3398.

99. Fukada T, Hibi M, Yamanaka Y, Takahashi-Tezuka M, Fujitani Y, Yamaguchi Y, Nakajima K, Hirano T (1996) Two signals are necessary for cell proliferation induced by a cytokine receptor gp130: Involvement of STAT3 in anti-apoptosis. *Immunity* 5:449–460.

100. Kim O, Yang J, Qiu Y (2002) Selective activation of small GTPase RhoA by tyrosine kinase Etk through its pleckstrin homology domain. *J Biol Chem* 33:30066–30071.

101. Lee LF, Guan J, Qiu Y, Kung HJ (2001) Neuropeptide-induced androgen independence in prostate cancer cells: roles of nonreceptor tyrosine kinases Etk/Bmx, Src, and focal adhesion kinase. *Mol Cell Biol* 21:8385–8397.

102. Chen R, Kim O, Li M, Xiong X, Guan JL, Kung HJ, Chen H, Shimizu Y, Qiu Y (2001) Regulation of the PH-domain-containing tyrosine kinase Etk by focal adhesion kinase through the FERM domain. *Nat Cell Biol* 3:439–444.

103. Ivankovic-Dikic I, Grönroos E, Blaukat A, Barth BU, Dikic I (2000) Pyk2 and FAK regulate neurite outgrowth induced by growth factors and integrins. *Nature Cell Biol* 2:574–581.

104. Abassi YA, Rehn M, Ekman N, Alitalo K, Vuori K (2003) p130Cas couples the tyrosine kinase Bmx/Etk with regulation of the actin cytoskeleton and cell migration. *J Biol Chem* 278:35636–35643.

105. Bang YJ, Pirnia F, Fang WG, Kang WK, Sartor O, Whitesell L, Ha MJ, Tsokos M, Sheahan MD, Nguyen P, Niklinski WT, Myers CE, Trepel JB (1994) Terminal neuroendocrine differentiation of human prostate carcinoma cells in response to increased intracellular cyclic AMP. *Proc Natl Acad Sci USA* 91:5330–5334.

106. Farini D, Puglianiello A, Mammi C, Siracusa G, Moretti C (2003) Dual effect of pituitary adenylate cyclase activating polypeptide on prostate tumor LNCaP cells: Short- and long-term exposure affect proliferation and neuroendocrine differentiation. *Endocrinology* 144:1631–1643.

107. Diaz M, Abdul M, Hoosein N (1998) Modulation of neuroendocrine differentiation in prostate cancer by interleukin-1 and -2. *Prostate* 8(Suppl): 32–36.

108. Chiao JW, Hsieh TC, Xu W, Sklarew RJ, Kancherla R (1999) Development of human prostate cancer cells to neuroendocrine-like cells by interleukin-1. *Int J Oncol* 15:1033–1037.

109. Liu WK, Ho JC, Qin G, Che CT (2002) Jolkinolide B induces neuroendocrine differentiation of human prostate LNCaP cancer cell line. *Biochem Pharmacol* 63:951–957.

110. Meyer-Siegler K (2001) COX-2 specific inhibitor, NS-398, increases macrophage migration inhibitory factor expression and induces neuroendocrine differentiation in C4–2b prostate cancer cells. *Mol Med* 7:850–860.

111. Tyagi A, Agarwal C, Agarwal R (2002) Inhibition of retinoblastoma protein (Rb) phosphorylation at serine sites and an increase in Rb-E2F complex formation by silibinin in androgen-dependent human prostate carcinoma LNCaP cells: Role in prostate cancer prevention. *Mol Cancer Ther* 7:525–532.

112. Kokontis J, Takakura K, Hay N, Liao S (1994) Increased androgen receptor and altered c-myc expression in prostate cancer cells after long-term androgen deprivation. *Cancer Res* 54:1566–1573.

113. Yeh S, Miyamoto H, Shima H, Chang C (1998) From estrogen to androgen receptor: A new pathway for sex hormones in prostate. *Proc Natl Acad Sci USA* 95:5527–5532.

114. Zhao XY, Malloy PJ, Krishnan AV, Swami S, Navone NM, Peehl DM, Feldman D (2000) Glucocorticoids can promote androgen-independent growth of prostate cancer cells through a mutated androgen receptor. *Nat Med* 6:703–706.

115. Reid P, Kantoff P, Oh W (1999) Antiandrogens in prostate cancer. *Invest New Drugs* 17:271–289.

116. Denhardt DT (1996) Signal-transducing protein phosphorylation cascades mediated by Ras/Rho proteins in the mammalian cell: The potential for multiplex signaling. *Biochem J* 318:729–747.

117. Craft N, Shostak Y, Carey M, Sawyers CL (1999) A mechanism for hormone independent prostate cancer through modulation of androgen receptor signaling by the HER-2/neu tyrosine kinase. *Nat Med* 5:280–285.

118. Yeh S, Lin HK, Kang HY, Thin TH, Lin MF, Chang C (1999) From HER2/neu signal cascade to androgen receptor and its coactivators: A novel pathway by induction of androgen target genes through MAP kinase in prostate cancer cells. *Proc Natl Acad Sci USA* 96:5458–5463.

119. Rawlings DJ, Scharenberg AM, Park H, Wahl MI, Lin S, Kato RM, Fluckinger AC, Witte ON, Kiner JP (1996) Activation of BTK by a phosphorylation mechanism initiated by SRC family kinases. *Science* 271:822–825.

120. Sadar MD (1999) Androgen-independent induction of prostate-specific antigen gene expression via cross-talk between the androgen receptor and protein kinase A signal transduction pathways. *J Biol Chem* 274: 7777–7783.

121. Ikonen T, Palvimo JJ, Kallio PJ, Reinikainen P, Janne OA (1994) Stimulation of androgen-regulated transactivation by modulators of protein phosphorylation. *Endocrinology* 135:1359–1366.

122. de Ruiter PE, Teuwen R, Trapman J, Dijkema R, Brinkmann AO (1995) Synergism between androgens and protein kinase-C on androgen-regulated gene expression. *Mol Cell Endocrinol* 110:R1–6.

123. Lee DK, Duan HO, Chang C (2000) From androgen receptor to the general transcription factor TFIIH. Identification of cdk activation kinase (CAK) as an androgen receptor NH(2)-terminal associated coactivator. *J Biol Chem* 275:9308–9313.

124. Gioeli D, Ficarro SB, Kwiek JJ, Aaronson D, Hancock M, Catling AD, White FM, Christian RE, Settlage RE, Shabanowitz J, Hunt DF, Weber MJ (2002) Androgen receptor phosphorylation. Regulation and identification of the phosphorylation sites. *J Biol Chem* 277:29304–29314.

125. Zhu Z, Becklin RR, Desiderio DM, Dalton JT (2001) Identification of a novel phosphorylation site in human androgen receptor by mass spectrometry. *Biochem Biophys Res Commun* 284:836–844.

126. Zhou ZX, Kemppainen JA, Wilson EM (1995) Identification of three praline-directed phosphorylation sites in the human androgen receptor. *Mol Endocrinol* 9:605–615.

127. Moilanen AM, Poukka H, Karvonen U, Hakli M, Janne OA, Palvimo JJ (1998) Identification of a novel RING finger protein as a coregulator in steroid receptor-mediated gene transcription. *Mol Cell Biol* 18: 5128–5129.

128. Qi H, Labrie Y, Grenier J, Fournier A, Fillion C, Labrie C (2001) Androgens induce expression of SPAK, a STE20/SPS1-related kinase, in LNCaP human prostate cancer cells. *Mol Cell Endocrinol* 182:181–192.

129. Xia L, Robinson D, Ma AH, Chen HC, Wu F, Qui Y, Kung HJ (2002) Identification of human male germ cell-associated kinase, a kinase transcriptionally activated by androgen in prostate cancer cells. *J Biol Chem* 227:35422–35433.

130. Schrantz N, da Silva Correia J, Fowler B, Ge Q, Sun Z, Bokoch GM (2004) Mechanism of p21-activated kinase 6-mediated inhibition of androgen receptor signaling. *J Biol Chem* 279:1922–1931.

131. Schuur ER, Henderson GA, Kmetec LA, Miller JD, Lamparski HG, Henderson DR (1996) Prostate-specific antigen expression is regulated by an upstream enhancer. *J Biol Chem* 271:7043–7051.

132. Culig Z, Hobisch A, Cronauer MV, Radmayr C, Trapman J, Hittmair A, Bartsch G, Klocker H (1994) Androgen receptor activation in prostatic tumor cell lines by insulin-like growth factor-I, keratinocyte growth factor, and epidermal growth factor. *Cancer Res* 54:5474–5478.

133. Markwalder R, Reubi JC (1999) Gastrin-releasing peptide receptors in the human prostate: Relation to neoplastic transformation. *Cancer Res* 59: 1152–1159.

134. Reubi JC, Wenger S, Schmuckli-Maurer J, Schaer JC, Gugger M (2002) Bombesin receptor subtypes in human cancers: Detection with the universal radioligand ^{125}I-[D-TYR^6, β-ALA^{11}, PHE^{13}, NLE^{14}] bombesin (6–14) *Clin Cancer Res* 8:1139–1146.

135. Seethalakshmi L, Mitra SP, Dobner PR, Menon M, Carraway RE (1997) Neurotensin receptor expression in prostate cancer cell line and growth effect of NT at physiological concentrations. *Prostate* 31:183–192.

136. Jongsma J, Oomen MH, Noordzij MA, Romijn JC, van der Kwast TH, Schröder FH, van Steenbrugge GJ (2000) Androgen-independent growth is induced by neuropeptides in human prostate cancer cell lines. *Prostate* 42:34–44.

137. Bologna M, Festuccia C, Muzi P, Biordi L, Ciomei M (1989) Bombesin stimulates growth of human prostatic cancer cell *in vitro. Cancer* 63:1714–1720.

138. Pinski J, Schally AV, Halmos G, Szepeshazi K (1993) Effect of somatostatin analog RC-160 and bombesin/gastrin releasing peptide antagonist RC-3095 on growth of PC-3 human prostate-cancer xenografts in nude mice. *Int J Cancer* 55:963–967.

139. Milovanovic SR, Radulovic S, Groot K, Schally AV (1992) Inhibition of growth of PC-82 human prostate cancer line xenocrafts in nude mice by bombesin antagonist RC-3095 or combination of agonist [D-Trp6]-luteinizing hormone-releasing hormone and somatostatin analog RC-160. *Prostate* 20:269–280.

140. Plonowski A, Nagy A, Schally AV, Sun B, Groot K, Halmos G (2000) *In vivo* inhibition of PC-3 human androgen-independent prostate cancer by targeted cytotoxic bombesin analogue, AN-215. *Int J Cancer* 88:652–657.

141. Jungwirth A, Galvan G, Pinski J, Halmos G, Szepeshazi K, Cai RZ, Groot K, Schally AV (1997) Luteinizing hormone-releasing hormone antagonist cetrorelix (SB-75) and bombesin antagonist RC-3940-II inhibit the growth of androgen-independent PC-3 prostate cancer in nude mice. *Prostate* 32:164–172.

142. Jungwirth A, Pinski J, Galvan G, Halmos G, Szepeshazi K, Cai RZ, Groot K, Vadillo-Buenfil M, Schally AV (1997) Inhibition of growth of androgen-independent DU-145 prostate cancer *in vivo* by luteinizing hormone-releasing hormone antagonist cetrorelix and bombesin antagonists RC-3940-II and RC3950-II. *Eur J Cancer* 33:1141–1148.

143. Rozengurt E (1998) Signal transduction pathways in the mitogenic response to G protein-coupled neuropeptide receptor agonists. *J Cell Physiol* 177: 507–517.

144. Xiao D, Qu X, Webe HC (2003) Activation of extracellular signal-regulated kinase mediates bombesin-induced mitogenic responses in prostate cancer cells. *Cell Signal* 15:945–953.

145. Xiao D, Qu X, Webe HC (2002) GRP receptor-mediated immediate early gene expression and transcription factor Elk-1 activation in prostate cancer cells. *Regulatory Peptides* 109:141–148.

146. Festuccia C, Angelucci A, Gravina GL, Eleuterio E, Vicentini C, Bologna M (2002) Bombesin-dependent pro-MMP-9 activation in prostatic cancer cells requires β1 integrin engagement. *Exp Cell Res* 280:1–11.

147. Ishimaru H, Yukio K, Tetsuo H, Tetsuo N, Yoshinobu E, Kazunori K (2002) Expression of matrix metalloproteinase-9 and bombesin/gastrin-releasing peptide in human prostate cancer and their lymph node metastases. *Acta Oncol* 41:289–296.

148. Levine L, Lucci JA, Pazdrak B, Cheng JZ, Guo YS, Townsend Jr CM, Hellmich MR (2003) Bombesin stimulates nuclear factor κB activation and expression of proangiogenic factors in prostate cancer cells. *Cancer Res* 63:3495–3502.

149. Aprikian AG, Tremblay L, Han K, Chevalier S (1997) Bombesin stimulates the motility of human prostate-carcinoma cells through tyrosine phosphorylation of focal adhesion kinase and of integrin-associated proteins. *Int J Cancer* 72:498–504.

150. Dai J, Shen R, Sumitomo M, Stahl R, Navarro D, Gershengorn MC, Nanus DM (2002) Synergistic activation of the androgen receptor by bombesin and low-dose androgen. *Clin Cancer Res* 8:2399–2405.

151. Dai J, Shen R, Sumitomo M, Goldberg JS, Geng Y, Navarro D, Xu S, Koutcher JA, Garzotto M, Powell CT, Nanus DM (2001) Tumor-suppressive effects of neutral endopeptidase in androgen-independent prostate cancer cells. *Clin Cancer Res* 7:1370–1377.

152. Albrecht M, Doroszewicz J, Gillen S, Gomes I, Wilhelm B, Stief T, Aumüller G (2004) Proliferation of prostate cancer cells and activity of neutral endopeptidase is regulated by bombesin and IL-1β with IL-1β acting as a modulator of cellular differentiation. *Prostate* 58:82–94.

153. Sumitomo M, Milowsky MI, Shen R, Navarro D, Dai J, Asano T, Hayakawa M, Nanus DM (2001) Neutral endopeptidase inhibits neuropeptide-mediated transactivation of the insulin-like growth factor receptor-Akt cell survival pathway. *Cancer Res* 61:3294–3298.

154. Sumitomo M, Shen R, Walburg M, Dai J, Geng Y, Navarro D, Boileau G, Papandreou CN, Giancotti FG, Knudsen B, Nanus DM (2000) Neutral endopeptidase inhibits prostate cancer cell migration by blocking focal adhesion kinase signaling. *J Clin Invest* 106:1399–1407.

155. Veltri RW, Miller MC, Zhao G, Ng A, Marley GM, Wright GL Jr, Vessella RL, Ralph D (1999) Interleukin-8 serum levels in patients with benign prostatic hyperplasia and prostate cancer. *Urology* 53:139–147.

156. Moore BB, Arenberg DA, Stoy K, Morgan T, Addison CL, Morris SB, Glass M, Wilke C, Xue YY, Sitterding S, Kunkel SL, Burdick MD,

Strieter RM (1999) Distinct CXC chemokines mediate tumorigenicity of prostate cancer cells. *Am J Path* 162:5511–5518.

157. Reiland J, Furcht LT, McCarthy JB (1999) CXC-chemokines stimulate invasion and chemotaxis in prostate carcinoma cells through the CXCR2 receptor. *Prostate* 41:78–88.

158. Inoue K, Slaton JW, Eve BY, Kim SJ, Perrotte P, Balbay MD, Yano S, Bar-Eli M, Radinsky R, Pettaway CA, Dinney CPN (2000) Interleukin 8 expression regulates tumorigenicity and metastases in androgen-independent prostate cancer. *Clin Cancer Res* 6:2104–2119.

159. Greene GF, Kitadai Y, Pettaway CA, von Eschenbach AC, Bucana CD, Fidler IJ (1997) Correlation of metastasis-related gene expression with metastatic potential in human prostate carcinoma cells implanted in nude mice using an *in situ* messenger RNA hybridization technique. *Am J Pathol* 150:1571–1582.

160. Ferrer FA, Miller LJ, Andrawis RI, Kurtzman SH, Albertsen PC, Laudone VP, Kreutzer DL (1998) Angiogenesis and prostate cancer: *In vivo* and *in vitro* expression of angiogenesis factors by prostate cancer cells. *Urology* 51:161–167.

161. Lee LF, Louie MC, Desai SJ, Yang J, Chen HW, Evans CP, Kung HJ (2004) Interleukin-8 confers androgen-independent growth and migration of LNCaP: Differential effects of tyrosine kinases Src and FAK. *Oncogene* 23:2197–2205.

162. Culig Z, Bartsch G, Hobisch A (2002) Interleukin-6 regulates androgen receptor activity and prostate cancer cell growth. *Mol Cell Endocrinol* 197:231–238.

163. Ueda T, Bruchovsky N, Sadar MD (2001) Activation of the androgen receptor N-terminal domain by Interleukin-6 via MAPK and STAT3 signal transduction pathways. *J Biol Chem* 277:7076–7085.

164. Chen T, Wang LH, Farrar WL (2000) Interleukin 6 activates androgen receptor-mediated gene expression through a signal transducer and activator of transcription 3-dependent pathway in LNCaP prostate cancer cells. *Cancer Res* 60:2132–2135.

165. Hobisch A, Eder IE, Putz T, Horninger W, Bartsch G, Klocker H, Culig Z (1998) Interleukin-6 regulates prostate-specific protein expression in prostate carcinoma cells by activation of the androgen receptor. *Cancer Res* 58:4640–4645.

166. Yang L, Wang L, Lin HK, Kan PY, Xie S, Tsai MY, Wang PH, Chen YT, Chang C (2003) Interleukin-6 differentially regulates androgen receptor

transactivation via PI3K-Akt, STAT3, and MAPK, three distinct signal pathways in prostate cancer cells. *Biochem Biophys Res Commun* 305: 462–469.

167. Debes JD, Sebo TJ, Lohse CM, Murphy LM, Haugen de AL, Tindall DJ (2003) P300 in prostate cancer proliferation and progression. *Cancer Res* 63:7638–7640.

8

BIOLOGY OF PROSTATIC ACID PHOSPHATASE AND PROSTATE-SPECIFIC ANTIGEN AND THEIR APPLICATIONS IN PROSTATE CANCER

Suresh Veeramani*, Ta-Chun Yuan*, Siu-Ju Chen*
Fen-Fen Lin* and Ming-Fong Lin*[,†,‡]

*Department of Biochemistry and Molecular Biology
†Department of Surgery/Urology, College of Medicine and
‡Eppley Institute for Cancer Research
University of Nebraska Medical Center
Omaha, NE 68198, USA

Introduction

Prostatic acid phosphatase (PAcP) and prostate-specific antigen (PSA) are two well-known biomarkers of prostate epithelial cells and are of immense value historically in the detection of prostate cancer (PCa). Because both are elevated significantly in the circulation of patients with PCa, correlating with the stages of clinical PCa, PAcP is an old marker for PCa diagnosis and PSA is the new gold standard. Early detection of PCa has been accomplished in recent years utilizing PSA-based screening methods that have led to the early treatment of PCa and decreased incidence of PCa death. In this chapter, we focus our discussion on the recent advances in the biology of PAcP and PSA, and include a brief overview of the history of PAcP and PSA in PCa diagnosis. Various clinical tests based on PSA that have revolutionized the field of PCa diagnosis are beyond the scope of this chapter but are described elsewhere.[1–3] In the first section, we focus on the role of PAcP in androgen-regulation of cell proliferation and the tumorigenicity of PCa cells. In the second section, we discuss the biological function of PSA. The major impediment in the treatment of PCa is the development of hormone-refractory cancer, which is indicated by the rebound of the circulating PSA level. We focus our discussion, in the latter part of the chapter, on the possible mechanisms of androgen-independent PSA secretion by hormone-refractory PCa.

Historical Review — Discovery and Clinical Applications of PAcP and PSA

PCa has become the most predominant cancer in American men, with approximately 30,000 deaths each year.[4] With increased testing and screening programs, most PCa cases are diagnosed while they are still confined to the prostate.[1,2] Since the early 1930s, the quest for a suitable marker for the diagnosis of PCa has been the center of attraction. In 1936, Gutman and his colleagues made the seminal observations that the activity of PAcP is increased in the circulation of patients with PCa, especially those with bone metastasis, to a level higher than that in normal adult males.[5] Subsequent studies confirmed that secretory PAcP (sPAcP) activity correlates with prostate tumor progression and can serve as an indicator of treatment.[6] Since then, sPAcP had been studied extensively as a marker for PCa diagnosis and therapeutic efficacy until the usefulness of PSA was appreciated.[1,6]

PSA was discovered by Chu and associates in a major research effort in search of promising markers for PCa diagnosis.[7] Quantitative assessments of PSA in the early 1980s revealed that the level of PSA is elevated in the circulation of patients with PCa[1,8] and correlates with cancer stage. PSA is of immense value in predicting the survival rate of patients with advanced PCa.[9] Within a few years of its discovery, the clinical potential of PSA was fully appreciated and PSA test kits shortly became available. Those basic efforts have led to early diagnosis and decreased PCa death rates.[1]

Although there is a general concern that PSA may detect too many clinically insignificant tumors, it should be emphasized that with the available modifications to increase the specificity of PSA-based tests, the detection of organ-confined clinical cancer has increased 2-fold, with reduction in disseminated cancer between 1986 and 1992, and reduction in death rates from 34,902 to 31,078 in the years 1994 and 2000.[1,4] Hence, the introduction of PSA-based tests has not only led to the increased detection of early PCa but also led to timely therapeutic intervention resulting in reduced mortality rates.

PAcP

Biochemical Properties of PAcP

The active form of PAcP protein contains two subunits with a similar molecular size of approximately 50 kDa. The PAcP subunit was initially translated as a proprotein with 386 amino acids containing a 32-amino acid signal peptide.[10] Post-translational modifications in the endoplasmic reticulum are apparently required for the stability of PAcP protein because the expression of a signal peptide-null PAcP from a cDNA expression vector occurs at very low levels (X. Q. Zhang and M. F. Lin, unpublished observations). Post-translational processings generate several intermediate species of PAcP proteins.[11]

PAcP is the major acid phosphatase in normal, well-differentiated prostate epithelial cells.[12–14] There are two forms of PAcP: the cellular (cPAcP) and the sPAcP forms. Both forms of PAcP can hydrolyze a broad variety of small organic phosphomonoesters *in vitro* in acidic conditions.[12–15] Physiologically, cPAcP level is negligible before adolescence in males. In normal adults, cPAcP is found at a high level of approximately 0.5 mg/gm wet tissue.[12,16] sPAcP is secreted into seminal fluid at concentrations of approximately 1 mg/ml.[17] Thus, sPAcP may have a functional role in fertility. Interestingly, sPAcP might also exhibit amidolytic activity on seminal proteins.[18] Further studies are needed to clarify the roles of sPAcP.

PAcP — An Authentic Protein Tyrosine Phosphatase

PAcP efficiently hydrolyzes small organic compounds, including phosphoamino acids, with *Km* values at mM ranges.[19] Interestingly, PAcP preferably hydrolyzes aromatic compounds over aliphatic compounds.[20] PAcP was initially shown to be co-purified with the major protein tyrosine phosphatase (PTP) activity in non-cancerous prostatic cells.[21] Further studies revealed that biochemically, PAcP exhibits dual-specific protein phosphatase activity.[19,22,23] It has a very high affinity for the p-Tyr linkage in protein substrates with *Km* values in the nM range, which is over 50-fold higher than for p-Ser/p-Thr linkages and several orders of magnitude higher than for free phospho-amino acids.[19] Unexpectedly, a low *Vmax* is observed, which could be due to high affinity interactions between PAcP and p-Tyr protein substrates resulting in a delay in the release of the dephosphorylated substrate.

The PTP activity of PAcP has been demonstrated by various approaches.[24–29] The site-directed mutagenesis approach confirmed that PAcP indeed exhibits authentic PTP activity.[30] It is interesting to note that PAcP contains neither the characteristic signature motif of the PTP superfamily nor the signature motif of the dual-specific protein phosphatase.[10,31] Based on the three-dimensional structure of rat PAcP, it was proposed that the Cys^{183} residue of PAcP functions as the phosphate acceptor and participates in the dephosphorylation reaction.[32] The reactivity of Cys^{183} was confirmed by titration experiments.[33] Additionally, Asp^{258} is conserved in the PTP family.[32] Nevertheless, His^{12} and Asp^{258}, but not Cys^{183} or Cys^{281}, are required for the PTP activity of PAcP.[30] The results thus indicated that PAcP is a novel PTP and uses the same active site and catalytic mechanism of acid phosphatase (AcP) to execute its PTP activity.

ErbB-2/HER-2/Neu (ErbB-2) — An In Vivo Substrate of PacP

cPAcP is implicated to be the major PTP in non-cancerous prostate epithelial cells.[19,21] Using the autophosphorylated epidermal growth factor receptor as a substrate, p-Tyr dephosphorylation by PAcP was optimal at a neutral pH.[34] The putative substrate of cPAcP was established in the mid-1990s. Incorporation of PAcP protein into PAcP-null DU145 PCa cells showed decreased tyrosine phosphorylation of a 185 kDa phosphoprotein[35] that was later identified to be the ErbB-2 protein. Thus, PAcP interacts with ErbB-2 and dephosphorylates the p-Tyr linkage of ErbB-2.[36] Initial analyses showed that cPAcP dephosphorylates ErbB-2 protein primarily at the Tyr^{1248} residue[30] that interacts with $p52^{Shc}$ protein, which is involved in regulating androgen action.[37] ErbB-2 is a putative growth factor receptor with an intrinsic tyrosine kinase activity.[38] Thus, the low cPAcP activity in prostate carcinomas[29,39–41] may infer unregulated tyrosine phosphorylation of ErbB-2, leading to aberrant tyrosine phos-phorylation signaling.[29] The function of cPAcP in PCa cells is, at least in part, to cause p-Tyr dephosphorylation of ErbB-2 protein.[29,30,36]

Biological Activity of cPAcP

Effect of cPAcP on the Growth and the Tumorigenicity of PCa Cells

In PCa cells, the level of cPAcP inversely correlates with the proliferation rate and the tumorigenicity (Table 1).[42,43] For example, growth stimulation of LNCaP cells by various stimuli results in decreased cPAcP activity. Furthermore, the introduction of exogenous PAcP into PC-3 cells, by a cDNA expression vector, diminishes growth rates and tumorigenicity (Table 1).[26,29]

Table 1. Correlation of cPAcP with the Proliferation and the Tumorigenicity of PCa Cells

	C-33	C-51	C-81	LN-28	PC-3	PC-411
	20 →	33 →	80 → 125	and -40		and -416
Androgen Sensitivity	+++	++	+	++/+++	−	+
AR	+++	+++	+++	+++	+	+
cPAcP Expression	+++	++	+	++	−	+
pErbB-2 Level	+	++	+++	+	+++	+
ErbB-2 Protein	+++	+++	+++	+++	++	++
Cell Growth*	112	57	49	86	33	52
PSA Secretion (Steroid-Reduced Condition)	+	++	+++	+	N/A[†]	N/A[†]
Tumorigenicity[‡]	+	++	+++	+	++++	++/+++

*The doubling time in hours was estimated in the steroid-reduced condition.[36]
[†]Not applicable because PC-3 cells do not express PSA.
[‡]Tumorigenicity was analyzed utilizing xenograft animal models.[29]
Note: LNCaP C-33, C-51 and C-81 cells are LNCaP-FGC cells that have passage numbers between 20–33, 35–80 and 81–125, respectively. LN-28 and LN-40 cells are stable subclones of C-81 cells transfected with a PAcP cDNA expression vector, while PC-411 and PC-416 cells are stable subclones of PC-3 cells transfected with PAcP cDNA expression vector.[27,36] PAcP expression gradually decreases upon passage in LNCaP cells. This results in aberrant tyrosine phosphorylation of ErbB-2 protein lead-ing to increased cell growth, PSA secretion, and tumorigenicity even under androgen-depleted condi-tions. The LNCaP cell model closely resembles the observations in the clinical PCa specimens.

We have established an interesting cell model system using the LNCaP cell line, which recapitulates PCa progression in the clinic.[27,43] Prolonged passage of androgen-sensitive parental LNCaP C-33 cells (starting at passages 20–33) in regular culture conditions resulted in loss of androgen-sensitivity and development of androgen independence by passage 81 (LNCaP C-81) (Table 1). Although C-81 cells express a similar level of functional androgen receptor (AR) as their parental C-33 cells, they behave as androgen-independent cells, resembling the clinical progression to advanced hormone-refractory PCa.[43] Importantly, even in the absence of androgen, PSA secretion in C-81 cells is much higher than in C-33 cells.[43] Interestingly, C-81 cells showed decreased cPAcP expression, and increased proliferation rate and malignancy as compared to the C-33 cells.

Several lines of evidence show that cPAcP exhibits the characteristics of a tumor suppressor. First, the expression of cPAcP is decreased or absent in prostate carcinomas, correlating with cancer progression.[39–41] Second, the loss of cPAcP expression in PCa cells correlates with increased tumorigenicity.[29] Finally, ectopic expression of cPAcP directly suppresses tumor growth in xenograft animal models.[28,29] Collectively, decreased expression of cPAcP correlates with PCa progression, rapid tumor formation, and androgen-independent cell proliferation. Thus, the level of cPAcP may serve as a useful marker for predicting the metastatic potential of PCa cells.

Effect of cPAcP on Androgen Sensitivity of PCa Cells

In AR-positive PCa cells, the expression of cPAcP correlates with androgen sensitivity (Table 1). In AR-positive, androgen-independent PCa cells, ectopic expression of cPAcP restores androgen-stimulated proliferation.[27,44] One possible explanation of this phenomenon is that in AR-positive, cPAcP-expressing cells the cell growth is decreased, in part, due to ErbB-2 dephosphorylation (Fig. 1). Upon androgen stimulation, cPAcP activity decreases, resulting in increased tyrophosphorylation of ErbB-2 and subsequent promotion of cell proliferation.[25,26,44] In PAcP-null PCa cells, ErbB-2 is hyper-tyrophosphorylated, which promotes cell proliferation and decreases androgen dependence, despite the expression of functional AR.[27,44] These results provide an explanation of the clinical phenomenon of advanced

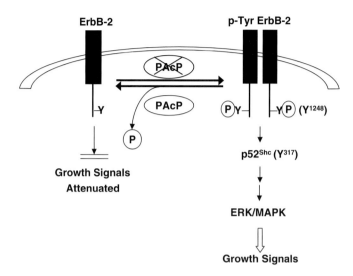

Fig. 1. Proposed roles of cPAcP and ErbB-2 in the regulation of prostate cell growth. cPAcP is involved in dephosphorylating the ErbB-2 protein, at least at Tyr^{1248}, thereby blocking the growth signals from ErbB-2. In the absence of or low levels of cPAcP, e.g., upon dihydroxytestosterone stimulation and in advanced PCa, ErbB-2 can be aberrantly tyrophosphorylated, which can transduce signals to the ERK/MAPK through $p52^{Shc}$, leading to growth promotion.

hormone-refractory PCa, in which AR is functional and the expression of cPAcP is decreased,[29,40] while the ErbB-2 gene is not amplified.[45] Nevertheless, the detailed molecular mechanism by which cPAcP and ErbB-2 regulate androgen-stimulated cell proliferation remains to be further elucidated.

PSA

Biological Activity of PSA

PSA, a member of kallikrein family, is a serine protease and exhibits activity and specificity similar to that of chymotrypsin.[46] PSA is predominantly expressed and secreted by prostate secretory epithelia at approximately 1 mg/ml in the seminal plasma of healthy men.[47] PSA is also expressed in a wide range of tissues.[48–51] In these tissues, PSA may be involved in growth regulation by steroid hormones.[52]

The synthesis and control of PSA expression in prostatic cells are well documented. Naïve translated PSA, or proPSA, is a 244-amino acid protein with a 17-amino acid leader sequence.[53] Several inactive truncated forms of PSA are found to be increased in benign prostatic hyperplasia (BPH).[54,55] The ratio of truncated PSA to total PSA (PSA index) aids in the discrimination between non-cancerous and cancerous prostate gland.[1] Serum PSA may form complexes with α-antichymotrypsin and α$_2$-macroglobulin[3] and circulate as complexed PSA.[1,2]

PSA may be involved in the proteolytic cleavage of seminal proteins. Semenogelin I/seminal plasma motility inhibitor (SPMI) precursor and its active product SPMI may be the substrates for PSA.[56,57] Other putative substrates of PSA include IGFBP-3,[58] PTHrP,[59] and extracellular matrix (ECM) proteins, such as fibronectin and laminin.[60] Since PSA can modulate *in vitro* interactions between IGF-I and IGFBP-3, PSA may play a role in regulating the growth of prostatic fibromuscular cells.[61]

Effect of PSA on Prostate Tumorigenicity

The highly invasive property of androgen-independent PCa cells could be due in part to the degradation of the ECM proteins by increased secretion of PSA, since a monoclonal antibody (mAb) against PSA blocked PCa invasion in a dose-dependent manner.[60] This is in parallel with the clinical observation that patients with metastatic PCa have elevated levels of serum PSA. On the contrary, PSA exhibits anti-angiogenic activity[62] and has a direct suppressive effect on new blood vessel formation in PCa.[63] Furthermore, recombinant PSA inhibits endothelial cell proliferation and tube formation, which are essential features of angiogenesis.[62] It is also suggested that anti-angiogenic drugs such as TNP-470 might act through increasing PSA secretion.[64] Future studies are needed to clarify the role of PSA in PCa metastasis.

Androgen-Independent PSA Secretion

Androgens are well documented as key factors regulating PSA gene expression.[65] Since PCa cells initially depend on androgens for proliferation, androgen ablation therapy is the mainstay of treatment for advanced PCa, and leads to a drop in circulating PSA. Unfortunately, cancer cells eventually escape from the steroid requirement and progress to androgen independence, which is indicated by the rebound of PSA levels in circulation.[66] The ability to treat these patients is limited. Interestingly, most of the hormone-refractory PCa cells express functional AR and PSA. The molecular mechanism of androgen-independent PSA secretion deserves careful analysis.

Biochemically, upon androgen binding, AR exhibits conformational changes, induced by modifications including phosphorylation and dimerization, for its activation.[67] It is proposed that in hormone-refractory cancers, in the absence of androgen, AR is also activated by phosphorylation.[68] Hence, a direct cross-talk between AR and cellular kinases may be an important factor involved in the elevation of androgen-independent PSA secretion. Our understanding of the cross-talk between AR and protein kinases is discussed briefly as follows.

ErbB-2/HER-2/Neu (ErbB-2) → ERK/MAPK Pathway

Data from our lab strongly indicate that ErbB-2 plays a critical role in hormone-refractory proliferation of PCa cells as well as in their enhanced androgen-independent PSA secretion, and are of clinical relevance (Fig. 2). This notion of ErbB-2 regulation is shown in ErbB-2 cDNA-transfected C-33 cells in which the growth rate and PSA secretion are elevated, even in the absence of androgen.[38,44,69] Conversely, in C-81 cells in which ErbB-2 is activated and PSA secretion is increased, the expression of a dominant-negative mutant of ErbB-2, or addition of ErbB-2 inhibitors, reduces the elevated androgen-independent PSA secretion.[38]

In androgen-deprived environments, ErbB-2, via the ERK/MAPK or Akt pathway, might activate AR by serine phosphorylation (Ser[514] for ERK/MAPK and Ser[791] for Akt).[69–71] Our data indicate that ERK/MAPK plays a key role in the early stage of androgen-independent PSA secretion, as well as in tumor progression. For example, in androgen-depleted conditions, elevated PSA secretion is decreased by MEK1 inhibitor, PD98059, in C-81 cells, while PSA secretion is increased by MEK1 cDNA transfection in C-33 cells.[38] Furthermore, in ErbB-2 cDNA-transfected C-33 cells,

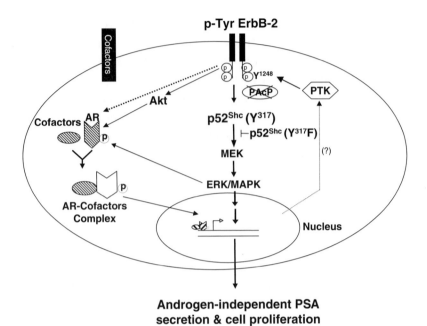

Fig. 2. Proposed model of regulation of PSA expression and secretion by ErbB-2 in hormone-refractory PCa. In androgen-independent human PCa cells, ErbB-2 is activated by hyper-tyrophosphorylation, in part, due to the loss of cPAcP expression. The activated ErbB-2 can transduce its signals *via* p52[Shc] to activate the downstream ERK/MAPK, which may lead to AR phosphorylation, resulting in an increase in androgen-independent expression and secretion of PSA, as well as cell proliferation. Activated ErbB-2 may also phosphorylate AR *via* Akt.

PD98059 effectively abolishes the increased PSA secretion in steroid-reduced conditions. This mechanism (Fig. 2) thus provides an explanation of the clinical observations of hormone-refractory prostate carcinomas in which cPAcP is decreased,[29,39–41] the ErbB-2 gene is not amplified, while the ErbB-2 protein could be either activated by tyrophosphorylation and/or elevated.[45,72] Subsequently, ERK/MAPKs are activated by phosphorylation,[73,74] leading to AR activation by phosphorylation,[75] as well as the rebound of PSA levels in the circulation of most patients.[1] Collectively, our data strongly indicate that the ErbB-2($\rightarrow$)ERK/MAPK pathway is crucial in androgen-independent PCa cell proliferation, as well as PSA secretion.

ErbB-2 can up-regulate PSA secretion at two levels: the transcriptional level and the post-translational level in the secretory pathway. In C-81 cells in which ErbB-2 is activated by hyper-tyrophosphorylation, the level of PSA mRNA is elevated in the steroid-reduced condition, compared to C-33 cells,[27,43] which may be due in part to the activation of the PSA promoter by ErbB-2 *via* ERK/MAPK and AR.[69] Alternatively, ErbB-2 may activate MEK1, leading to the up-regulation of a transcription factor(s) that subsequently activates the PSA promoter.[76] ErbB-2 may also activate the secretory pathway of PSA in those cells (M. S. Lee and M. F. Lin, unpublished observations). Nevertheless, further experiments are needed.

Akt Pathway

AR phosphorylation might also occur through the PI3K → Akt pathway in hormone-refractory PCa cells.[71] Androgen-responsive, low passage LNCaP cells have a lower Akt activity than the androgen-independent high passage cells,[77] which implies that this pathway could be important in later stages of advanced metastatic cancer, where PTEN mutation leads to constant Akt activation. Nevertheless, it should be noted that pathways other than PTEN could be involved in activating Akt in higher passage LNCaP cells because PTEN is also mutated in the lower passage LNCaP cells.[78,79] Interestingly, the anti-androgen flutamide blocks Akt-induced PSA secretion in IL-4-treated LNCaP cells,[80] while it stimulates the growth of LNCaP cells,[81] indicating the differential roles of Akt. Nevertheless, IGFBP-5 cDNA-transfected LNCaP cells express hyperactivated Akt and exhibit higher growth rates and PSA secretion levels in castrated mice than do control cells.[82] Further experiments are required to clarify the role of Akt in androgen-independent PSA secretion *vs.* hormone-refractory PCa cell proliferation and its clinical relevance.

Cytokine Pathway

Interleukin-6 (IL-6) has been proposed to play a role in the development of androgen-independence in PCa cells because IL-6 enhances the growth of LNCaP cells in androgen-depleted environment and serum IL-6 levels are found to be elevated in some patients with advanced PCa. Since androgen-independent LNCaP-IL-6+ cells, which were selected by continuous passage in media containing 5 ng/ml IL-6, are resistant to the cell cycle arrest mediated by IL-6,[83] it is inferred that IL-6 may contribute to PCa progression, and *via* the ErbB-2($\rightarrow$)ERK/MAPK pathway, stimulate androgen-independent PSA secretion.[84,85] IL-4 might also have a role in the androgen-independent, AR-mediated PSA secretion,[80] because IL-4 level is elevated in some PCa patients with hormone-refractory cancer.[86]

PKA Pathway

Forskolin, a PKA activator, can increase the activity of the PSA promoter in the absence of androgen.[87] The activation of PKA by forskolin also results in increased PSA expression in androgen-depleted LNCaP cells.[88] Butyrate, a differentiation agent, increased circulating PSA levels in castrated animals. Electromobility shift assay showed an increased AR-ARE complex formation in butyrate-treated LNCaP cells that is partially inhibited by a PKA blocker, indicating that butyrate action on LNCaP cells might, in part, involve the PKA pathway.[88]

Other Downstream Mechanisms

Protein phosphorylation may activate other regulatory factors, e.g., AR cofactors, leading to increased PSA secretion. Alternatively, aberrantly regulated transcriptional factors may play a role in this mode of regulation. For example, nuclear factor-Kappa B (NF-κB), which is increased in androgen-independent PCa cells, can activate PSA expression,[89] while the growth of those cells is inhibited by NF-κB inhibitors.[90] A 45-kDa cell-specific transcription factor (p45) has also been implicated in androgen-independent expression of the PSA gene.[91]

Future Perspectives

The decreased expression of cPAcP is implicated as a crucial step in carcinogenesis and/or progression of human PCa. More studies of the basic biology of PAcP may provide new insights into its potential roles in tumor suppression and potential uses for therapy of PCa. In xenograft animal models, a single intratumoral injection of an expression vector encoding the wild type PAcP resulted in the growth suppression of prostate tumors.[28] The restoration of cPAcP expression in PCa may provide a new avenue for treating patients with advanced PCa in which the expression of PAcP is lost.

Functional molecules involved in androgen-independent pathways may serve as potential targets for clinical therapy. Inhibitors of androgen-independent pathways such as ErbB-2 and ERK/MAPK blockers might prove valuable in the treatment of hormone-refractory PCa. Studies indicated that co-administration of the ERK/MAPK inhibitor PD98059 with docetaxel increases the apoptotic death of androgen-independent PCa cells.[92] Chemointerventions for hormone-refractory PCa might be made more useful with co-administration of these pathway blockers with the regular therapeutic regime.

Immunotherapy for PCa also has potential value. Phase I studies using PSA expressing vaccinia viral vectors indicated that T cells could be induced in the patients.[93] Vaccination with dendritic cells preloaded with PSA mRNA resulted in the reduction of circulating PSA levels in 80% of the patients.[94] Similar experiments with PAcP also showed some efficacy.[95] Future work is needed in the clinical utilization of PAcP and PSA as targets of immunotherapy against PCa.

The proteolytic property of PSA has been exploited in the development of therapeutic interventions for PCa. For example, peptide-conjugated - doxorubicin[96] and vinblastine,[97,98] which can be activated in prostate tissue by PSA, has shown some promising results. Similar strategies have been applied for PAcP (M. F. Lin, unpublished observations). Nevertheless, promotion of such strategies to clinical application requires further studies. In conclusion, due to the recent advances in understanding the biology of PAcP and PSA, as well as their functional roles in PCa progression and metastasis, new avenues through which to develop novel strategies for improving the efficacy of treating hormone-refractory PCa are expected.

Acknowledgments

This project is in part supported by NIH, NCI, CA88184, and UNMC Graduate Student Fellowship (T. C. Y; S. J. C). We thank all group members for their efforts toward conquering this cancer. We are also indebted to Dr. T. M. Chu and his colleagues for the discovery of PSA.

References

1. Chu TM, Lin MF (1998) PSA and acid phosphatase in the diagnosis of prostate cancer. *J Clin Ligand Assay* 21:24–34.
2. Chu TM (1997) Prostate-specific antigen (PSA) and early detection of prostate cancer. *Tumour Biol* 18:123–134.
3. Armbruster DA (1993) Prostate-specific antigen: biochemistry, analytical methods, and clinical application. *Clin Chem* 39:181–195.
4. Jemal A, Murray T, Samuels A, Ghafoor A, Ward E, Thun MJ (2003) Cancer Statistics 2003. *CA Cancer J Clin* 53:5–26.
5. Gutman EB, Sproul EE, Gutman AB (1936) Significance of increased phosphatase activity at the site of osteoplastic metastases secondary to carcinoma of the prostate gland. *Am J Cancer* 28:485–495.
6. Huggins C, Hodges CV (1941) Studies on prostatic cancer: the effect of castration, of estrogen and of androgen injection on serum phosphatases in metastatic carcinoma of the prostate. *Cancer Res* 1:293–297.
7. Wang MC, Valenzuela LA, Murphy GP, Chu TM (1979) Purification of a human prostate specific antigen. *Invest Urol* 17:159–163.
8. Kuriyama M, Wang MC, Lee CL, Killian CS, Papsidero LD, Inaji H, Loor RM, Lin MF, Nishiura T, Slack NH, Murphy GP, Chu TM (1982) Multiple marker evaluation in human prostate cancer with the use of tissue-specific antigens. *J Natl Cancer Inst* 68:99–105.
9. Kuriyama M, Wang MC, Lee CL, Papsidero LD, Killian CS, Inaji H, Slack NH, Nishiura T, Murphy CP, Chu TM (1981) Use of human prostate-specific antigen in monitoring prostate cancer. *Cancer Res* 41:3874–3876.
10. Vihko P, Virkkunen P, Henttu P, Roiko K, Solin T, Huhtala ML (1988) Molecular cloning and sequence analysis of cDNA encoding human prostatic acid phosphatase. *FEBS Lett* 236:275–281.
11. Lin MF, Garcia-Arenas R, Kawachi M, Lin FF (1993) Regulation of the expression of prostatic acid phosphatase in LNCaP human prostate carcinoma cells. *Cell Mol Biol Res* 39:739–750.
12. Yam LT (1974) Clinical significance of the human acid phosphatases: a review. *Am J Med* 56:604–616.
13. Vihko P (1979) Human prostatic acid phosphatases: purification of a minor enzyme and comparisons of the enzymes. *Invest Urol* 16:349–352.

14. Lin MF, Clinton GM (1987) Human prostatic acid phosphatase and its phosphotyrosyl-protein phosphatase activity. *Adv Protein Phosphatases* 4: 199–228.

15. Lin MF, Lee CL, Li SS, Chu TM (1983) Purification and characterization of a new human prostatic acid phosphatase isoenzyme. *Biochemistry* 22: 1055–1062.

16. Shaw LM, Yang N, Neat M, Croop W (1982) Immunological and clinical specificity of the immunochemical determination of prostatic acid phosphatase. *Ann NY Acad Sci* 390:73–88.

17. Ronnberg L, Vihko P, Sajanti E, Vihko R (1981) Clomiphene citrate administration to normogonadotropic subfertile men: blood hormone changes and activation of acid phosphatase in seminal fluid. *Int J Androl* 4:372–378.

18. Brillard-Bourdet M, Rehault S, Juliano L, Ferrer M, Moreau T, Gauthier F (2002) Amidolytic activity of prostatic acid phosphatase on human semenogelins and semenogelin-derived synthetic substrates. *Eur J Biochem* 269:390–395.

19. Lin MF, Clinton GM (1986) Human prostatic acid phosphatase has phosphotyrosyl protein phosphatase activity. *Biochem J* 235:351–357.

20. Nguyen L, Chapdelaine A, Chevalier S (1990) Prostatic acid phosphatase in serum of patients with prostatic cancer is a specific phosphotyrosine acid phosphatase. *Clin Chem* 36:1450–1455.

21. Li HC, Chernoff J, Chen LB, Kirschonbaum A (1984) A phosphotyrosyl-protein phosphatase activity associated with acid phosphatase from human prostate gland. *Eur J Biochem* 138:45–51.

22. Wasylewska E, Czubak J, Ostrowski WS (1983) Phosphoprotein phosphatase activity of human prostate acid phosphatase. *Acta Biochim Pol* 30:175–184.

23. Lee H, Chu TM, Lee CL (1991) Endogenous protein substrates for prostatic acid phosphatase in human prostate. *Prostate* 19:251–263.

24. Vihko P, Kurkela R, Porvari K, Herrala A, Lindfors A, Lindqvist Y, Schneider G (1993) Rat acid phosphatase: overexpression of active, secreted enzyme by recombinant baculovirus-infected insect cells, molecular properties, and crystallization. *Proc Natl Acad Sci USA* 90:799–803.

25. Lin MF, DaVolio J, Garcia-Arenas R (1992) Expression of human prostatic acid phosphatase activity and the growth of prostate carcinoma cells. *Cancer Res* 52:4600–4607.

26. Lin MF, Garcia-Arenas R, Xia XZ, Biela B, Lin FF (1994) The cellular level of prostatic acid phosphatase and the growth of human prostate carcinoma cells. *Differentiation* 57:143–149.

27. Lin MF, Meng TC, Rao PS, Chang C, Schonthal AH, Lin FF (1998) Expression of human prostatic acid phosphatase correlates with androgen-stimulated cell proliferation in prostate cancer cell lines. *J Biol Chem* 273: 5939–5947.
28. Igawa T, Lin FF, Rao P, Lin MF (2003) Suppression of LNCaP prostate cancer xenograft tumors by a prostate-specific protein tyrosine phosphatase, prostatic acid phosphatase. *Prostate* 55:247–258.
29. Lin MF, Lee MS, Zhou XW, Andressen JC, Meng TC, Johansson SL, West WW, Taylor RJ, Anderson JR, Lin FF (2001) Decreased expression of cellular prostatic acid phosphatase increases tumorigenicity of human prostate cancer cells. *J Urol* 166:1943–1950.
30. Zhang XQ, Lee MS, Zelivianski S, Lin MF (2001) Characterization of a prostate-specific tyrosine phosphatase by mutagenesis and expression in human prostate cancer cells. *J Biol Chem* 276:2544–2550.
31. Tonks NK, Neel BG (2001) Combinatorial control of the specificity of protein tyrosine phosphatases. *Curr Opin Cell Biol* 13:182–195.
32. Schneider G, Lindqvist Y, Vihko P (1993) Three-dimensional structure of rat acid phosphatase. *EMBO J* 12:2609–2615.
33. Ostanin K, Saeed A, van Etten RL (1994) Heterologous expression of human prostatic acid phosphatase and site-directed mutagenesis of the enzyme active site. *J Biol Chem* 269:8971–8978.
34. Lin MF, Clinton GM (1988) The epidermal growth factor receptor from prostate cells is dephosphorylated by a prostate-specific phosphotyrosyl phosphatase. *Mol Cell Biol* 8:5477–5485.
35. Lin MF, Meng TC (1996) Tyrosine phosphorylation of a 185 kDa phosphoprotein (pp185) inversely correlates with the cellular activity of human prostatic acid phosphatase. *Biochem Biophys Res Commun* 226:206–213.
36. Meng TC, Lin MF (1998) Tyrosine phosphorylation of c-ErbB-2 is regulated by the cellular form of prostatic acid phosphatase in human prostate cancer cells. *J Biol Chem* 273:22096–22104.
37. Lee MS, Igawa T, Lin MF (2004) Tyrosine-317 of p52[Shc] mediates androgen-stimulated proliferation signals in human prostate cancer cells. *Oncogene*, in press.
38. Lee MS, Igawa T, Yuan TC, Zhang XQ, Lin FF, Lin MF (2003) ErbB-2 signaling is involved in regulating PSA secretion in androgen-independent human prostate cancer LNCaP C-81 cells. *Oncogene* 22:781–796.
39. Reif AE, Schlesinger RM, Fish CA, Robinson CM (1973) Acid phosphatase isozymes in cancer of the prostate. *Cancer* 31:689–699.

40. Loor R, Wang MC, Valenzuela L, Chu TM (1981) Expression of prostatic acid phosphatase in human prostate cancer. *Cancer Lett* 14:63–69.
41. Hakalahti L, Vihko P, Henttu P, Autio-Harmainen H, Soini Y, Vihko R (1993) Evaluation of PAP and PSA gene expression in prostatic hyperplasia and prostatic carcinoma using northern-blot analyses, *in situ* hybridization and immunohistochemical staining with monoclonal and bispecific antibodies. *Int J Cancer* 55:590–597.
42. Lin MF, DaVolio J, Garcia-Arenas R (1992) Expression of human prostatic acid phosphatase activity and the growth of prostate carcinoma cells. *Cancer Res* 52:4600–4607.
43. Igawa T, Lin FF, Lee MS, Karan D, Batra SK, Lin MF (2002) Establishment and characterization of androgen-independent human prostate cancer LNCaP cell model. *Prostate* 50:222–235.
44. Meng TC, Lee MS, Lin MF (2000) Interaction between protein tyrosine phosphatase and protein tyrosine kinase is involved in androgen-promoted growth of human prostate cancer cells. *Oncogene* 19:2664–2677.
45. Signoretti S, Montironi R, Manola J, Altimari A, Tam C, Bubley G, Balk S, Thomas G, Kaplan I, Hlatky L, Hahnfeldt P, Kantoff P, Loda M (2000) HER-2-neu expression and progression toward androgen independence in human prostate cancer. *J Natl Cancer Inst* 92:1918–1925.
46. Yousef GM, Diamandis EP (2003) An overview of the kallikrein gene families in humans and other species: emerging candidate tumour markers. *Clin Biochem* 36:443–452.
47. Lovgren J, Valtonen-Andre C, Marsal K, Lilja H, Lundwall A (1999) Measurement of prostate-specific antigen and human glandular kallikrein 2 in different body fluids. *J Androl* 20:348–355.
48. Frazer HA, Humphrey PA, Burchette JL, Paulson DF (1992) Immunoreactive prostate-specific antigen in male periurethral glands. *J Urol* 147:246–248.
49. Clements A, Mukhtar A (1994) Glandular kallikreins and prostate specific antigen are expressed in the human endometrium. *J Clin Endocrinol Metab* 78:1536–1539.
50. Howarth DJ, Aronson IB, Diamandis EP (1997) Immunohistochemical localization of prostate-specific antigen in benign and malignant breast tissues. *Br J Cancer* 75:1646–1651.
51. Malatesta M, Mannello F, Luchetti F, Marcheggiani F, Condemi L, Papa S, Gazzanelli G (2000) Prostate-specific antigen synthesis and secretion by human placenta: a physiological kallikrein source during pregnancy. *J Clin Endocrinol Metab* 85:317–321.

52. Diamandis EP, Yu H (1995) Editorial: New biological functions of prostate-specific antigen? *J Clin Endocrinol Metab* 80:1515–1517.
53. Lilja H (2003) Biology of prostate-specific antigen. *Urology* 62:27–33.
54. Mikolajczyk SD, Millar LS, Wang TJ, Rittenhouse HG, Wolfert RL, Marks LS, Song W, Wheeler TM, Slawin KM (2000) "BPSA," a specific molecular form of free prostate-specific antigen, is found predominantly in the transition zone of patients with nodular benign prostatic hyperplasia. *Urology* 55:41–45.
55. Wang TJ, Slawin KM, Rittenhouse HG, Millar LS, Mikolajczyk SD (2000) Benign prostatic hyperplasia-associated prostate-specific antigen (BPSA) shows unique immunoreactivity with anti-PSA monoclonal antibodies. *Eur J Biochem* 267:4040–4045.
56. Robert M, Gibbs BF, Jacobson E, Gagnon C (1997) Characterization of prostate-specific antigen proteolytic activity on its major physiological substrate, the sperm motility inhibitor precursor/semenogelin I. *Biochemistry* 36:3811–3819.
57. Rehault S, Brillard-Bourdet M, Bourgeois L, Frenette G, Juliano L, Gauthier F, Moreau T (2002) Design of new and sensitive fluorogenic substrates for human kallikrein hK3 (prostate-specific antigen) derived from semenogelin sequences. *Biochim Biophys Acta* 1596:55–62.
58. Okabe E, Kajihara J, Usami Y, Hirano K (1999) The cleavage site specificity of human prostate specific antigen for insulin-like growth factor binding protein-3. *FEBS Lett* 447:87–90.
59. Cramer SD, Chen Z, Peehl DM (1996) Prostate specific antigen cleaves parathyroid hormone-related protein in the PTH-like domain: Inactivation of PTHrP-stimulated cAMP accumulation in mouse osteoblasts. *J Urol* 156 (2 Pt 1):526–531.
60. Webber MM, Waghray A, Bello D (1995) Prostate-specific antigen, a serine protease, facilitates human prostate cancer cell invasion. *Clin Cancer Res* 1:1089–1094.
61. Sutkowski DM, Goode RL, Baniel J, Teater C, Cohen P, McNulty AM, Hsiung HM, Becker GW, Neubauer BL (1999) Growth regulation of prostatic stromal cells by prostate-specific antigen. *J Natl Cancer Inst* 91:1663–1669.
62. Fortier AH, Holaday JW, Liang H, Dey C, Grella DK, Holland-Linn J, Vu H, Plum SM, Nelson BJ (2003) Recombinant prostate specific antigen inhibits angiogenesis *in vitro* and *in vivo*. *Prostate* 56:212–219.
63. Papadopoulos I, Sivridis E, Giatromanolaki A, Koukourakis MI (2001) Tumor angiogenesis is associated with MUC1 overexpression and loss of prostate-specific antigen expression in prostate cancer. *Clin Cancer Res* 7:1533–1538.

64. Horti J, Dixon SC, Logothetis CJ, Guo Y, Reed E, Figg WD (1999) Increased transcriptional activity of prostate-specific antigen in the presence of TNP-470, an angiogenesis inhibitor. *Br J Cancer* 79:1588–1593.
65. Cleutjens KB, van der Korput HA, van Eekelen CC, van Rooij HC, Faber PW, Trapman J (1997) An androgen response element in a far upstream enhancer region is essential for high, androgen-regulated activity of the prostate-specific antigen promoter. *Mol Endocrinol* 11:148–161.
66. Pilat MJ, Kamradt JM, Pienta KJ (1998–99) Hormone resistance in prostate cancer. *Cancer Metastasis Rev* 17:373–381.
67. Kuil CW, Berrevoets CA, Mulder E (1995) Ligand-induced conformational alterations of the androgen receptor analyzed by limited trypsinization. Studies on the mechanism of antiandrogen action. *J Biol Chem* 270:27569–27576.
68. Sadar MD, Hussain M, Bruchovsky N (1999) Prostate cancer: molecular biology of early progression to androgen independence. *Endocr Relat Cancer* 6:487–502.
69. Yeh S, Lin HK, Kang HY, Thin TH, Lin MF, Chang C (1999) From HER2/Neu signal cascade to androgen receptor and its coactivators: a novel pathway by induction of androgen target genes through MAP kinase in prostate cancer cells. *Proc Natl Acad Sci USA* 96:5448–5463.
70. Craft N, Shostak Y, Carey M, Sawyers CL (1999) A mechanism for hormone-independent prostate cancer through modulation of androgen receptor signaling by the HER-2/neu tyrosine kinase. *Nat Med* 5:280–285.
71. Wen Y, Hu MC, Makino K, Spohn B, Bartholomeusz G, Yan DH, Hung MC (2000) HER-2/neu promotes androgen-independent survival and growth of prostate cancer cells through the Akt pathway. *Cancer Res* 60:6841–6845.
72. Osman I, Scher HI, Drobnjak M, Verbel D, Morris M, Agus D, Ross JS, Cordon-Cardo C (2001) HER-2/neu (p185neu) protein expression in the natural or treated history of prostate cancer. *Clin Cancer Res* 7:2643–2647.
73. Price DT, Rocca GD, Guo C, Ballo MS, Schwinn DA, Luttrell LM (1999) Activation of extracellular signal-regulated kinase in human prostate cancer. *J Urol* 162:1537–1542.
74. Gioeli D, Mandell JW, Petroni GR, Frierson HF Jr, Weber MJ (1999) Activation of mitogen-activated protein kinase associated with prostate cancer progression. *Cancer Res* 59:279–284.
75. Ofelia L, Zegarra-Moro OL, Schmidt LJ, Huang H, Tindall DJ (2002) Disruption of androgen receptor function inhibits proliferation of androgen-refractory prostate cancer cells. *Cancer Res* 62:1008–1013.
76. Franco OE, Onishi T, Yamakawa K, Arima K, Yanagawa M, Sugimura Y, Kawamura J (2003) Mitogen-activated protein kinase pathway is involved in

androgen-independent PSA gene expression in LNCaP cells. *Prostate* 56:319–325.

77. Lin HK, Hu YC, Yang L, Altuwaijri S, Chen YT, Kang HY, Chang C (2003) Suppression versus induction of androgen receptor functions by the phosphatidylinositol 3-kinase/Akt pathway in prostate cancer LNCaP cells with different passage numbers. *J Biol Chem* 278:50902–50907.

78. Li J, Yen C, Liaw D, Podsypanina K, Bose S, Wang SI, Puc J, Miliaresis C, Rodgers L, McCombie R, Bigner SH, Giovanella BC, Ittmann M, Tycko B, Hibshoosh H, Wigler MH, Parsons R (1997) PTEN, a putative protein tyrosine phosphatase gene mutated in human brain, breast, and prostate cancer. *Science* 275:51943–1947.

79. Reiss K, Wang JY, Romano G, Furnari FB, Cavenee WK, Morrione A, Tu X, Baserga R (2000) IGF-I receptor signaling in a prostatic cancer cell line with a PTEN mutation. *Oncogene* 19:2687–2694.

80. Lee SO, Lou W, Hou M, Onate SA, Gao AC (2003) Interleukin-4 enhances prostate-specific antigen expression by activation of the androgen receptor and Akt pathway. *Oncogene* 22:7981–7988.

81. Furr BJ, Tucker H (1996) The preclinical development of bicalutamide: pharmacodynamics and mechanism of action. *Urology* 47(Suppl):13–45.

82. Miyake H, Nelson C, Rennie PS, Gleave ME (2000) Overexpression of insulin-like growth factor binding protein-5 helps accelerate progression to androgen-independence in the human prostate LNCaP tumor model through activation of phosphatidylinositol 3'-kinase pathway. *Endocrinol* 141:2257–2265.

83. Culig Z, Bartsch G, Hobisch A (2002) Interleukin-6 regulates androgen receptor activity and prostate cancer cell growth. *Mol Cell Endocrinol* 197: 231–238.

84. Lin DL, Whitney MC, Yao Z, Keller ET (2001) Interleukin-6 induces androgen responsiveness in prostate cancer cells through up-regulation of androgen receptor expression. *Clin Cancer Res* 7:1773–1781.

85. Qiu Y, Ravi L, Kung HJ (1998) Requirement of ErbB2 for signalling by interleukin-6 in prostate carcinoma cells. *Nature* 393:83–85.

86. Wise GJ, Marella VK, Talluri G, Shirazian D (2000) Cytokine variations in patients with hormone treated prostate cancer. *J Urol* 164:722–725.

87. Nazareth LV, Weigel NL (1996) Activation of the human androgen receptor through a protein kinase A signaling pathway. *J Biol Chem* 16:19900–19907.

88. Sadar MD, Gleave ME (2000) Ligand-independent activation of the androgen receptor by the differentiation agent butyrate in human prostate cancer cells. *Cancer Res* 15:5825–5831.

89. Chen CD, Sawyers CL (2002) NF-kappa B activates prostate-specific antigen expression and is upregulated in androgen-independent prostate cancer. *Mol Cell Biol* 22:2862–2670.

90. Kikuchi E, Horiguchi Y, Nakashima J, Kuroda K, Oya M, Ohigashi T, Takahashi N, Shima Y, Umezawa K, Murai M (2003) Suppression of hormone-refractory prostate cancer by a novel nuclear factor kappaB inhibitor in nude mice. *Cancer Res* 63:107–110.

91. Yeung F, Li X, Ellett J, Trapman J, Kao C, Chung LW (2000) Regions of prostate-specific antigen (PSA) promoter confer androgen-independent expression of PSA in prostate cancer cells. *J Biol Chem* 275:40846–40855.

92. Zelivianski S, Spellman M, Kellerman M, Kakitelashvilli V, Zhou XW, Lugo E, Lee MS, Taylor R, Davis TL, Hauke R, Lin MF (2003) ERK inhibitor PD98059 enhances docetaxel-induced apoptosis of androgen-independent human prostate cancer cells. *Int J Cancer* 107:478–485.

93. Eder JP, Kantoff PW, Roper K, Xu GX, Bubley GJ, Boyden J, Gritz L, Mazzara G, Oh WK, Arlen P, Tsang KY, Panicali D, Schlom J, Kufe DW (2000) A phase I trial of a recombinant vaccinia virus expressing prostate-specific antigen in advanced prostate cancer. *Clin Cancer Res* 6:1632–1638.

94. Heiser A, Coleman D, Dannull J, Yancey D, Maurice MA, Lallas CD, Dahm P, Niedzwiecki D, Gilboa E, Vieweg J (2002) Autologous dendritic cells transfected with prostate-specific antigen RNA stimulate CTL responses against metastatic prostate tumors. *J Clin Invest* 109:409–417.

95. Fong L, Small EJ (2003) Immunotherapy for prostate cancer. *Semin Oncol* 30:649–658.

96. Schwartz MS, Matuszewski BK (2002) Determination of a peptide-doxorubicin, prostate-specific antigen activated prodrug, and its active metabolites in human plasma using high-performance liquid chromatography with fluorescence detection. Stabilization of the peptide prodrug with EDTA. *J Chromatogr B Analyt Technol Biomed Life Sci* 780:171–182.

97. DeFeo-Jones D, Brady SF, Feng DM, Wong BK, Bolyar T, Haskell K, Kiefer DM, Leander K, McAvoy E, Lumma P, Pawluczyk JM, Wai J, Motzel SL, Keenan K, Van Zwieten M, Lin JH, Garsky VM, Freidinger R, Oliff A, Jones RE (2002) A prostate-specific antigen (PSA)-activated vinblastine prodrug selectively kills PSA-secreting cells *in vivo. Mol Cancer Ther* 1:451–459.

98. Brady SF, Pawluczyk JM, Lumma PK, Feng DM, Wai JM, Jones R, DeFeo-Jones D, Wong BK, Miller-Stein C, Lin JH, Oliff A, Freidinger RM, Garsky VM (2002) Design and synthesis of a pro-drug of vinblastine targeted at treatment of prostate cancer with enhanced efficacy and reduced systemic toxicity. *J Med Chem* 45:4706–4715.

9

EPIGENETICS IN PROSTATE CANCER

Jose A. Karam, Elie A. Benaim, Hong Chen,
Rey-Chen Pong and Jer-Tsong Hsieh

Department of Urology, UT Southwestern Medical Center
5323 Harry Hines Blvd., Dallas, TX, USA

Introduction

Prostate cancer (PCa) is the most common non-cutaneous cancer affecting males in the USA. One in six American men will be diagnosed with PCa in their lifetime. In 2004, a total of 230,110 new cases and 29,900 deaths are estimated to occur in the USA.[1] It has been well documented that alterations in genomic DNA, such as point mutations, homozygous deletions and loss of heterozygosity are linked to the pathogenesis of cancer,[2] including PCa.[3] However, the majority of studies have focused on the DNA sequence and to a lesser extent on DNA structure and its surrounding environment. Recently, investigators started looking at epigenetics as an alternative and complementary mechanism in the pathogenesis of cancer. The term "epigenetic" refers to the heritable changes in gene expression that are caused by mechanisms other than the alteration in the nucleotide sequence.[4] This concept generated tremendous new knowledge in understanding gene expression in mammalian cells.

The Role of CpG Dinucleotides in DNA Methylation

CpG dinucleotides can be either clustered as CpG islands or dispersed. In the era before completion of the human genome project, a CpG island was defined as a stretch of 200-bp of DNA with a C + G content of 50% and an observed CpG/expected CpG in excess of 0.6.[5] However, this definition included inactive and viral sequences within the human genome. When corrected for these "intrusive" sequences, a more biologically appropriate and more stringent definition of a CpG island would be a stretch of 500-bp of DNA with a C + G content of 55% and an observed CpG/expected CpG of more than 0.65.[6] Therefore, the definition of a CpG island is still arbitrary. More than half of the human genes are associated with unique CpG islands.[7] Reports from the human genome project have estimated that the human genome contains almost 30,000 CpG islands.[8]

CpG dinucleotides are present throughout the genome and are usually methylated when not associated with CpG islands. However, when the CpG dinucleotides are found in CpG islands, they are usually unmethylated, in particular if they are found in the promoter region of an active gene,[9] or methylated, when found in the 3′ end of the gene. However, CpG methylation the at 3′ end of the gene does not affect gene transcription.[10] In general, it is a rare event to find *de novo* CpG methylation in normal somatic cells. However, as cells age, especially when cultured *in vitro*, an increase in methylation has been documented.[11,12]

Cytosine methylation prevents gene expression by interfering with transcription initiation. DNA methylation has no effect on base pairing but can alter protein-DNA interaction by protruding into the major DNA groove.[13] Another explanation is that methylation results in decreased binding affinity of the transcription factors to gene promoter regions.[14]

Methyl Binding Proteins (MBP)

The first true MBP to be identified was MeCP2 (Methyl CpG-binding protein 2). It was found to specifically bind to the methyl group at position 5 of cytosine and to be active in somatic mammalian cells but not necessarily in embryonic stem cells.[15] This protein has been found most abundantly in the pericentromeric heterochromatin region[16] and its localization to this region has been shown to be dependent on the presence of methylated DNA.[17] MeCP2 specifically represses methylated promoters through a transcription repressor domain (TRD). MeCP2 can bind to DNA that contains one symmetrically methylated CpG pair and does not need chromatin disassembly in order to bind to DNA.[18] In fact, MeCP2 can displace histone H1 from

DNA and then exert its repression function, at least *in vitro*.[19] MeCP1 can also discriminate between methylated and unmethylated DNA, although needing a high amount of methylated CpG for its binding (more than 10 methylated CpGs).[20]

Four other methyl-binding domain (MBD)-containing proteins were identified by comparing the MBD domain of MeCP2 to Expressed Sequence Tags (EST) databases.[20] MBD1-mediated activity is Histone Deacetylase (HDAC)-dependent, as its actions are partially inhibited by HDAC inhibitors (HDIs). However, the identity of this HDAC is still unknown.[21] MBD1 interacts with a histone H3 methyltransferase as well as heterochromatin protein 1 (a methyl-lysine binding protein) resulting in chromatin compaction and transcription repression.[22] In the prostate, MBD1 is highly expressed in benign prostate hyperplasia and low grade PCa. However, MBD1 expression decreases in high grade PCa.[23] MBD2, which is a part of the MeCP1 complex, has transcription repression activity[24] as well as DNA demethylase activity.[25,26] MBD3 is similar in structure to MBD2, however no demethylase activity has been demonstrated.[27] MBD4 has DNA glycosylase activity, therefore effectively removing uracil or thymidine from a mismatched CpG location, at least *in vitro*. Binding experiments showed that mutations at methyl CpG sites can be reduced by the activity of MBD4.[28]

DNA Methyltransferases (DNMTs)

The conversion of cytosine (C) into 5-methylcytosine (5mC) is catalyzed by enzymes termed DNA methyl transferases (DNMTs), using S-adenosyl-methionine (SAM) as a methyl donor.[29] Three active DNMTs have been characterized. DNMT1 is responsible for methylating daughter DNA strands during the S-phase, through its interaction with Proliferating Cell Nuclear Antigen (PCNA).[30] DNMT1 is involved in maintaining the methylation status of genes and this task is possible due to its high affinity to hemi-methylated DNA.[31] When DNMT1 is absent in mice, DNA methylation is severely affected, resulting in an embryonic lethal phenotype.[32] DNMT3a and DNMT3b have some structural similarities, having the N-terminal as the regulatory subunit and the C-terminal as the catalytic subunit. In contrast to DNMT1, both DNMT3a and DNMT3b can methylate unmethylated and hemi-methylated DNA.[33]

An elegant study in *Drosophila* showed that DNMT3a, but not DNMT1, acts as a *de novo* methyltransferase.[34] Therefore, DNMT3a establishes the gene methylation pattern and then DNMT1 maintains this pattern in the future generations. When DNMT3a or DNMT3b were knocked out, the resulting mice died at 4 weeks of life or during embryonic development, respectively.[35] Increased DNMT mRNA has been documented in colon and lung cancer.[36–39] However, DNA hypermethylation is not necessarily due to overexpression of DNMT.[40]

DNMT Inhibitors

DNMT inhibitors act mainly by inhibiting methylation; however, other mechanisms are involved. After phosphorylation, these compounds incorporate into DNA or RNA.[41] After incorporating into DNA, they covalently bind DNMT resulting in its inhibition[42–44] without causing DNA demethylation *per se*.[44] Additionally, their incorporation into DNA causes structural instability resulting in DNA damage.[45]

Currently, five DNMT inhibitors have been used in preclinical/clinical trials, namely 5-azacytidine (azacytidine), 5-aza-2′-deoxycytidine (decitabine), dihydro-5-azacytidine (DHAC), arabinofuranosyl-5-azacytosine (fazarabine),[46] and most recently zebularine. Zebularine is the only DNMT inhibitor that can be given orally, while the other DNMT inhibitors are given parenterally.[47]

DNMT inhibitors have been used in preclinical studies with very good tumor control rate. However, in clinical trials, the results are not so dramatic, especially with solid tumors, where limited efficacy has been encountered.[46] Decitabine has been used in phase II trial in patients with hormone-independent metastatic prostate cancer, however, the results were not encouraging.[48] Most of the DNMT inhibitors have a relatively high cytotoxicity profile and can only demethylate genes as long as they are present in the cell surroundings, therefore limiting their potential clinical usefulness, as they cannot be administered for prolonged periods of time. However, a recent *in vitro* study showed that zebularine can suppress DNMT1 expression, demethylate p16, and restore p16 expression for up to 40 days in continuously treated T24 bladder cancer cells, without causing pronounced cytotoxicity. In addition, when zebularine is given at a lower dose following an initial dose of decitabine, a profound demethylation of p16 is observed. These results suggest the usefulness of combining an initial bolus of a parenteral DNMT inhibitor followed by a maintenance dose of the oral agent zebularine.[49] However, proof of their usefulness in a preclinical and ultimately clinical setting is yet to be established.

Recently, RNA interference (RNAi) has been used to knock out DNMT1,[50] which composes the majority of DNMT activity in cancer cells,[51] resulting in reactivation of repressed genes. Another study, however, showed that both DNMT1 and DNMT3b need to be shut down to re-express silenced genes.[52] These results imply the need to treat cancer cells with compounds that can affect more than one type of DNMT, as cancer cells might be able to overcome the deficiency in one DNMT.[53] Two phase I clinical trials using MG98, an antisense oligodeoxynucleotide against DNMT1, have been recently conducted to study the MG98 safety profile and dosage regimens in patients with cancer.[54,55]

Histones

In mammalian cells, genomic DNA is always associated with histone proteins to form chromatin structure. The basic unit of chromatin is the nucleosome, which is composed of 146 base pairs of DNA that are wrapped twice around a disk-like complex made of 8 histone proteins (2 of each of histones H2A, H2B, H3, and H4). A stable nucleosome core is assembled by H3 and H4 heterodimerization, followed by H3 dimerization resulting in a (H3-H4)$_2$ tetramer.[56] Subsequently, H2A and H2B heterodimerize and each dimer attaches to one side of the (H3-H4)$_2$ tetramer.[56] This yields an octamer of histones on which DNA can be wrapped.[57] Adjacent nucleosomes are brought together by histone H1. The N- and C-termini of histone H1 are able to bind to DNA within the nucleosome in addition to the "linker" DNA between the nucleosomes. This binding and subsequent neutralization of the acidic DNA results in the formation of higher order chromatin.[58–60] The amino acids at the N-terminal of the histone protrude out of the nucleosome, thereby allowing for specific reversible modifications and interaction with surrounding factors. This N-terminal is rich in the basic (positively charged) amino acids like lysine and serine, which allows for reversible histone modification by methylation, acetylation, phosphorylation, ubiquitination, and most recently sumoylation. When this positively charged N-terminal of the amino acid is free, it results in tight binding of histones to DNA phosphates, which are negatively charged, therefore inhibiting access of transcription factors to the gene promoter region and subsequently silencing gene expression.

Acetylation of histones is mediated by histone acetyltransferases (HATs) using acetyl CoA as the acetyl moiety donor, resulting in activation of gene transcription. HATs do not directly bind to DNA, instead, they are subunits in coactivator complexes that mediate transcriptional activity recovery. Examples of such coactivator HATs in humans are p300/CBP[61] and TAFII250,[62] which is a component of human RNA polymerase II, an enzyme involved in transcription. Steroid Receptor Coactivator-1 (SRC-1)[63] and ACTR[64] are also coactivators with HAT activity that interact with nuclear receptors in a hormone-dependent fashion. pCAF[65] has the ability to associate with p300/CBP,[66] ACTR[64] and SRC-1,[63] resulting in a multitude of HATs in the same complex. Acetylation of histones has been linked with transcriptional activation.

The second histone modification is phosphorylation of the Serine-10 of histone H3. This modification has been implicated in both activation of transcription[67] and chromosomal condensation in mitosis. This phosphorylation corresponds to the activation of early-immediate genes, such as c-Fos[68] and has been shown to occur through the Rsk-2,[69] Msk-1[70], and Snf-1 kinases.[71] Interestingly, the latter histone kinase works in concert with HAT to activate gene transcription.[71,72] Also, I kappa B kinase α (IKKα) has been reported to phosphorylate histone H3, subsequently allowing for specific H3 acetylation through CREB-binding protein (CBP), resulting in activation of nuclear factor kappa B (NF-κB) responsive genes.[73] It is not clear how histone phosphorylation activates gene transcription; however, it could be related to the fact that adding the negatively charged phosphates to histone N-termini disrupts the histone-DNA interaction, resulting in increased access of transcription factors to promoter regions.[74]

The third histone modification is due to methylation of either arginine or lysine residues. Arginine methylation at histone H3 and H4 is mediated by the histone methyltransferase (HMT) CARM1[75,76] and PRMT1,[77] respectively, through transfer of a methyl group from SAM. The end product results in gene activation. Histone lysine methylation, on the other hand, can result in either gene transcription activation or repression. Suvar3-9 has HMT activity, specifically methylating Lysine-9 of histone H3 (K9-H3),[78] subsequently attracting the heterochromatin protein HP1[79,80] resulting in heterochromatin assembly[81] and gene silencing. Human HMTs at K9-H3 include SUV39H1[82] (causing retinoblastoma (Rb)-mediated transcription repression) and EZH2 (a member of the polycomb group of transcriptional repressors).[83,84] In addition to methylation at K9-H3, EZH2 has the ability to methylate K27-H3, resulting also in transcription repression.[85] EZH2 expression was reported to be increased in metastatic prostate cancer and in localized prostate cancer. In the latter case, it indicates a poor patient prognosis and outcome.[85] Interestingly, both monomethylation[86] and trimethylation[87] at K9-H3 can control and trigger DNA methylation *per se*. Recently, it has been shown that methylation levels of K9-H3 differ depending on their location in the chromosome and that different HMTs are responsible for their methylation at each of these sites: monomethylated and dimethylated K9-H3 are localized in silenced euchromatin regions and their methylation is mediated by G9a HMT, while trimethylated K9-H3 was abundant in pericentromeric regions, with SUV39H1 and SUV39H2 responsible for their methylation.[88] In contrast, methylation at Lysine-4 of histone H3 (K4-H3) by SET7/Set9[89,90] results in transcription activation. In LNCaP prostate cancer cells, the activated androgen receptor (AR) binds to the androgen responsive element (ARE) of the prostate specific antigen (PSA) gene, resulting in decreased methylation of K4-H3 of the PSA enhancer and promoter and increased PSA transcription.[91]

The fourth covalent histone modification is ubiquitination.[92] Ubiquitin is a 76-amino acid peptide that can attach to the C-terminus of histone H2A and likely to that of H2B as well. Ubiquitination of histone H2A coincides with transcriptional activity.[93] However, ubiquitination of histone H2B results in histone H3 methylation, thereby causing transcription repression.[94]

Recently, histone sumoylation has been implicated in transcriptional repression of gene activity. SUMO (small ubiquitin-related modifier) is involved in post-translational modification of several proteins and it is mediated by the same enzymatic cascade that catalyzes ubiquitination. Sumoylation of histone H4 results in recruitment of HDAC and the heterochromatin protein HP1, therefore causing transcriptional repression.[95] Collectively, these histone modifications may constitute a "Histone code" that is able to specify patterns of gene expression.[96]

Histone Deacetylases (HDACs)

In mammals, HDACs have been grouped into 3 classes. Class I HDACs (HDAC 1, 2, 3, 8) have catalytic site homology at their C-termini and class II HDACs (HDAC 4, 5, 6, 7, 9,10) share homology at their catalytic C-termini and regulatory N-termini.[97] Class III is the conserved NAD-dependent Sir2 group of deacetylases.[97] Interestingly, class I and II, but not class III HDACs, are inhibited by Trichostatin A (TSA) and suberoylanilide hydroxamic acid (SAHA). Similar to HATs, there is evidence that HDACs do not directly bind to DNA. Instead, they are part of the transcription regulator complexes.[98] HDACs do not show complete redundancy in their functions. Class I HDACs are almost exclusively located in the nucleus. On the other hand, class II HDACs translocate between the cytoplasm and nucleus.[97,99]

Histone Deacetylase Inhibitors (HDIs)

HDIs can be classified on the basis of their different structures into hydroxamates (TSA and SAHA), cyclic tetrapeptides (apidicin depsipeptide and depudecin), carboxylates (sodium phenylbutyrate and valproic acid) and benzamides (CI-994 and MS-27-275).[100–108]

The inhibition of HDACs, as mediated by HDIs via interacting with a zinc active site in the HDAC moiety,[109] could result in induction of differentiation, growth arrest, and/or apoptosis.[110] These effects are attributed to a subset of genes whose expression has been altered, or returned back to normal upon exposure to HDIs and histone hyperacetylation,[111] as seen in single-gene,[112] as well as high-throughput studies.[113]

Several HDIs, including SAHA, phenylbutyrate, and depsipeptide have been used in Phase I and Phase II clinical trials.[114] SAHA can be administered orally or intravenously and has been shown to increase the levels of acetylated histones in peripheral blood mononuclear cells and reduce tumor activity in pretreated patients with hematologic and solid cancers.[115] SAHA was also effective in increasing the intratumor acetylated histone levels and inhibiting the growth of prostate cancer xenografts in nude mice.[116]

The Interaction Between DNA Methylation and Histone Modifications in Gene Regulation

Recently, an interaction between histone modifications and DNA methylation has been discovered and has been intensively studied. Jones and colleagues described a system where methylated cytosine attracts the methyl-binding protein MeCP2, which in turn binds a HDAC-corepressor complex, therefore resulting in transcription inhibition.[117] In addition, DNA methylation and histone methylation also interact, as MeCP2 can recruit a HMT, resulting in methylation of K9-H3.[118] More recently, it has been shown that DNMT1 and DNMT3a interact with SUV39H1 (a K9-H3 HMT) as well as HP1, providing more evidence for the close association between DNA and histone methylation.[119]

A question that has been recently addressed is whether methylation of DNA precedes histone modifications or *vice versa*.[120,121] Most of the currently available data supports the dominant role of methylation in the epigenetic control of promoter activation, as DNMT inhibitors are more important than HDAC inhibitors in initiating gene reactivation.[122] In these cases, even if HDAC inhibitors cause histone acetylation, methyl binding proteins such as MeCP2 are still bound to methylated cytosine, thereby needing a DNMT inhibitor to release the methylation and subsequently disengaging from MeCP2.[123] However, recent data showed that methylation of K9-H3 and subsequent gene silencing can occur prior to methylation of CpG in the gene promoter.[53] Both phenomena are present to some extent and the relative importance of one or the other could be dependent on specific tumor tissue, cell type, experimental conditions, and the specific gene under study.

The fact that DNA methylation and histone deacetylation cooperate to silence genes has been exploited to develop new therapeutic regimens. DNA microarray analysis[113] experiments show that the use of DNMT inhibitors and HDAC inhibitors results in a synergistic activation of specific tumor suppressor genes,[122,124,125] as well as affecting global gene expression. In addition, low doses of DNMT inhibitors and HDIs are combined in order to decrease the occurrence of side effects and cause a synergistic inhibition of tumor growth.[126] Decitabine and phenylbutyrate was found to have a synergistic effect in preventing the formation of lung tumors in mice.[127]

Epigenetics in the Pathogenesis and Diagnosis of PCa

Patra and colleagues have demonstrated that elevated DNMT and HDAC expression is associated with PCa, indicating that epigenetic regulation plays an important role in PCa pathogenesis.[128] Several genes have been described as being methylated in PCa and only to a limited extent or not at all in normal prostates. Some genes are methylated in early stages of PCa, potentially making them useful as diagnostic markers. Other genes are methylated in advanced stages of PCa and can be used as prognostic markers.

GSTP1

The most commonly studied epigenetically-controlled gene in PCa is the Glutathione-S-transferase-π1 (GSTP1) gene. GSTP1 is responsible for intracellular detoxification reactions by conjugating free radicals to glutathione.[129,130] The first evidence of GSTP1 methylation in PCa was demonstrated by Lee and colleagues,[131] when they described that GSTP1 was not expressed in several PCa cell lines due to promoter hypermethylation.

The revolution in detection of methylated DNA came in 1996 when Herman and colleagues described methylation-specific PCR (MSP), which can offer higher sensitivity and specificity in detecting minute amounts of methylated DNA.[132] Recently, Harden and colleagues employed a quantitative MSP (qMSP) assay for GSTP1 in conjunction with routine prostate biopsy histology in order to improve the PCa detection. They found that histology alone detected 39/61 tumors (64% sensitivity), while GSTP1 qMSP with histology detected 48/61 tumors (79% sensitivity) with a 100% specificity. However, when the threshold of qMSP is decreased, 4/11 samples that were labeled as normal on histology were positive on qMSP. This raises the question that such patients should be monitored more intensively, as preneoplastic lesions can harbor GSTP1 methylation. However, more controlled trials are needed to justify such a follow up.[133]

By combining laser capture microdissection and MSP, recent data demonstrated the absence of GSTP-1 methylation in patients with normal or benign hyperplastic prostates, while GSTP1 was methylated in 6.3% with prostatic proliferative inflammatory atrophy (PIA), 68.8% with high-grade prostatic intraepithelial neoplasia (HGPIN), and 90.9% with PCa. These results suggest a progressive increase in GSTP1 methylation during prostate carcinogenesis and PIA as a potential precursor of HGPIN/PCa based on the presence of GSTP1 methylation.[134]

MSP has also been used to detect GSTP1 methylation from several sources with good success, including blood, bone marrow, urine, ejaculate, lymph nodes (LNs) after pelvic LN dissection, prostate biopsies, TURP, and prostatectomy specimens (Table 1). MSP was able to detect GSTP1 methylation in all of these tissues, with a low rate of false positive results.

Table 1. GSTP1 Detection in Human Tissue/Body Fluids using MSP

Sample Origin	Patient Diagnosis	% Methylation	Reference No(s).
Prostate			
Biopsy	Cancer	89	133
Biopsy washings	Cancer	100	180
	PIN	67	
	BPH	0	
Prostate resection	Cancer	88	134
	HGPIN	69	
	PIA	6	
	BPH	0	
	Normal	0	
Pelvic lymph nodes	Cancer	90	181
	Normal	11	
Bone marrow	Cancer	40	181
Urine	Cancer	27–39	182, 183
	Normal	0–3	
Plasma	Cancer	36–72	184, 185
	Normal	0	
Ejaculate	Cancer	50	184
	Normal	0	

Detection of cancer in LN allows for a more accurate assessment of metastatic disease and better adjuvant therapy. Detection of methylated GSTP1 in blood, urine, and ejaculate potentially allows for earlier detection of PCa. In addition, its presence in blood, urine, or bone marrow could prove to be a useful prognostic marker, surrogate marker for predicting cancer volume during therapy and a means of follow up after definitive therapy.

Membrane Receptors

CD44

CD44 is an integral membrane glycoprotein involved in cell to cell adhesion and cell-extracellular matrix interaction.[135] It has been shown that CD44 promoter hypermethylation inversely correlates with the expression level of CD44 in PCa cell lines.[136] The methylation status of CD44 was examined in prostatectomy specimens, which revealed that 77.5% of PCa specimens harbored CD44 methylation, in contrast to only 10% of the matched normal controls, suggesting the possible involvement of CD44 methylation and transcriptional repression in the prostate carcinogenesis.[137] Additionally, the hypermethylation of CD44 has been found to be more common in advanced stages of PCa.[138] Recently, Woodson and colleagues reported that hypermethylation of CD44 was 1.7 times more common in black patients than in white patients with PCa.[139] Ekici and colleagues studied CD44 expression in a cohort of patients with PCa and reported that the presence of CD44 is significantly higher in non-metastatic versus metastatic groups, correlates inversely with pathologic stage and disease progression and positively with PSA-free survival.[140]

CAR

Coxsackie and adenovirus receptor (CAR), first identified as the high affinity receptor for both coxsackie and adenovirus (type 2 and 5)[141,142] is a typical immunoglobulin (Ig)-like membrane protein with two Ig domains that may have adhesion activity.[143] Like many other cell adhesion molecules, the loss of CAR is often detected in several cancer types.[144-149] In PCa, decreased expression of CAR is found in primary tumors[146] and increased expression of CAR can reduce tumor growth of

PCa *in vitro* and *in vivo*.[150] Data from our laboratory indicate that the CpG islands in the CAR promoter are unmethylated; however, the decreased expression of CAR is due to histone deacetylation at the CAR promoter.[151] In PCa, the use of HDIs increases the expression of CAR, which further enhances the adenovirus susceptibility of PCa cells.[151] Thus, combining HDIs with recombinant adenovirus could lead to a more effective treatment regimen for PCa patients.

Nuclear Receptors

AR

The AR has been shown to be down-regulated as a result of its promoter methylation.[152,153] AR is methylated in only 8% of PCas and in none of the normal prostates. The PCas with methylated AR were exclusively high stage, indicating that AR methylation is a relatively late event in prostate carcinogenesis.[154]

Estrogen Receptor (ER)

When studied in clinical specimens, ER methylation was detected in 60% of BPH, 80% of low-stage PCa and 100% of high-stage PCa specimens. The difference of ER methylation was highly significant in PCa compared to BPH.[155] Another study investigated the different subtypes of ERs in paired PCa samples and discovered that ERα-A and ERα-B gene promoters were methylated in 98% and 92% of PCa samples, respectively, while they were unmethylated in normal prostate samples. ERα-C was not methylated in any PCa samples. In addition, ERβ was methylated in 78% of PCas, with no methylation in normal prostates.[154] Such differences in ER gene methylation could imply a different role of each subtype of ER in the pathogenesis of PCa.

Retinoid Acid Receptor-β2 (RARβ2)

RARβ2 is a nuclear receptor that binds to the retinoic acid responsive element (RARE) found in retinoic acid pathway genes and other transcription factor genes.[156] The hypermethylation of RARβ2 has been reported in 53%–83% of PCas, compared to 0%–3% in normal tissues/BPH.[157–159] It has been shown that decitabine and TSA can induce RARβ2 gene expression, indicating that histone deacetylation and DNA methylation are responsible for silencing of the RARβ2 gene.[157]

Ras Effector Proteins

In PCa, enhanced expression of Ras protein correlates with increased tumor grade.[160] Several studies indicated that most metastatic tumors expressed Ras protein, while only a fifth of primary tumors did.[160–162] Surprisingly, PCa cells demonstrate an extremely low rate of mutation in the *Ras* gene.[162–164] This implies that other effectors regulating Ras activity may be involved in increasing Ras protein levels in PCa.

RASSF1A

RASSF1A, a Ras effector homologue, is a tumor suppressor gene that is down-regulated due to its promoter hypermethylation in several cancers[165,166]including PCa.[158,167] *RASSF1A* hypermethylation was found in 53%–71% of PCa specimens and it was more prevalent in patients with Gleason scores 7–10.[158,167] These results suggest that *RASSF1A* gene methylation may reflect an aggressive PCa phenotype and could potentially be used as a marker in this context.

Human Disabled-2 Interacting Protein (hDAB2IP)

hDAB2IP is a new member of Ras-GTPase activating protein family that maintains Ras inactivation status.[168] The down-regulation of hDAB2IP is often associated with many androgen-independent PCa cell lines and increased expression of hDAB2IP can suppress the growth of PCa.[168] Analysis of hDAB2IP gene promoter reveals that it is hypermethylated in PCa cell lines but not in normal epithelial cells. Both DNMT inhibitors and HDIs can induce the expression level of hDAB2IP,[169,170] indicating that the epigenetic machinery plays an important role in modulating hDAB2IP expression during PCa progression.

Nuclear Proteins

Cyclin D2

Cyclins are proteins involved in cell cycle regulation by interacting with cyclin-dependent kinases.[171] Cyclin D2 is involved in the transition from G1 to S phase during mitosis.[172] Padar and colleagues found that PCas are more commonly methylated (32%) than normal prostate tissue (6%) independent of age. In addition, methylation was significantly higher in patients with Gleason scores >7.[173] This finding suggests that loss of cyclin D2 could be involved in PCa progression.

ZNF185

ZNF185, or Zinc Finger 185 is a protein that belongs to the LIM domain protein family.[174] LIM proteins play a role in cellular growth and differentiation.[175] In a recent study, ZNF185 was found to be down-regulated in a genomic screening of PCas. After treatment of PCa cell lines with a DNMT inhibitor, ZNF185 expression was re-established. Using MSP, ZNF185 hypermethylation was detected in PCa, but not in any normal prostate samples. When stratified into different stages, ZNF185 is methylated in 36.3%, 50% and 100% of PCa samples with Gleason 6, Gleason 9 and from metastatic sites, respectively. These data indicate a role for ZNF185 promoter hypermethylation in the progression of PCa and its potential application as a tumor marker for PCa.[176]

Bone Morphogenic Protein-6 (BMP-6)

BMP-6 belongs to the transforming growth factor-β superfamily, which is involved in the formation of bone and cartilage.[177] In contrast to the above genes, where their expression has been silenced by promoter hypermethylation, BMP-6 gene methylation is decreased in PCa. This loss of BMP-6 promoter methylation and subsequent gene activation leads to overexpression of BMP-6 protein in both primary and secondary sites of PCa with advanced metastasis.[178] BMP-6 expression in PCa is associated with a decreased bone-metastasis-free survival as compared to those with no BMP-6 expression.[179] The re-expression of BMP-6 by aggressive PCa could be one way through which these cancers metastasize to bone.

Conclusion

In addition to the genetic mutations of tumor suppressor genes associated with PCa, recent data clearly indicate that epigenetic alterations are also involved in this silencing. Unlike genetic changes, epigenetic modifications are potentially reversible, which can open a new avenue of cancer therapy; several inhibitors of DNMT and HDAC are currently being studied in clinical trials for several cancers. Even so, more controlled studies on epigenetics in PCa are needed to develop new methods for early cancer detection, to predict patient prognosis and to ultimately treat patients with PCa.

References

1. Jemal A, Tiwari RC, Murray T, *et al.* (2004) Cancer statistics, 2004. *CA Cancer J Clin* 54:8–29.
2. Knudson AG, Jr (1985) Hereditary cancer, oncogenes, and antioncogenes. *Cancer Res* 45:1437–1443.
3. Ozen M, Pathak S (2000) Genetic alterations in human prostate cancer: a review of current literature. *Anticancer Res* 20:1905–1912.
4. Bird A (2002) DNA methylation patterns and epigenetic memory. *Genes Dev* 16:6–21.
5. Gardiner-Garden M, Frommer M (1987) CpG islands in vertebrate genomes. *J Mol Biol* 196:261–282.
6. Takai D, Jones PA (2002) Comprehensive analysis of CpG islands in human chromosomes 21 and 22. *Proc Natl Acad Sci USA* 99:3740–3745.
7. Antequera F, Bird A (1993) Number of CpG islands and genes in human and mouse. *Proc Natl Acad Sci USA* 90:11995–11999.
8. Lander ES, Linton LM, Birren B, *et al.* (2001) Initial sequencing and analysis of the human genome. *Nature* 409:860–921.
9. Bird AP (1986) CpG-rich islands and the function of DNA methylation. *Nature* 321:209–213.

10. Larsen F, Solheim J, Prydz H (1993) A methylated CpG island 3' in the apolipoprotein-E gene does not repress its transcription. *Hum Mol Genet* 2:775–780.

11. Jones PA, Wolkowicz MJ, Rideout WM, 3rd, *et al.* (1990) *De novo* methylation of the MyoD1 CpG island during the establishment of immortal cell lines. *Proc Natl Acad Sci USA* 87:6117–6121.

12. Antequera F, Boyes J, Bird A (1990) High levels of *de novo* methylation and altered chromatin structure at CpG islands in cell lines. *Cell* 62:503–514.

13. Razin A, Riggs AD (1980) DNA methylation and gene function. *Science* 210:604–610.

14. Clark SJ, Harrison J, Molloy PL (1997) Sp1 binding is inhibited by (m)Cp(m)CpG methylation. *Gene* 195:67–71.

15. Meehan RR, Lewis JD, Bird AP (1992) Characterization of MeCP2, a vertebrate DNA binding protein with affinity for methylated DNA. *Nucleic Acids Res* 20:5085–5092.

16. Lewis JD, Meehan RR, Henzel WJ, *et al.* (1992) Purification, sequence, and cellular localization of a novel chromosomal protein that binds to methylated DNA. *Cell* 69:905–914.

17. Nan X, Tate P, Li E, Bird A (1996) DNA methylation specifies chromosomal localization of MeCP2. *Mol Cell Biol* 16:414–421.

18. Ballestar E, Wolffe AP (2001) Methyl-CpG-binding proteins. Targeting specific gene repression. *Eur J Biochem* 268:1–6.

19. Nan X, Campoy FJ, Bird A (1997) MeCP2 is a transcriptional repressor with abundant binding sites in genomic chromatin. *Cell* 88:471–481.

20. Hendrich B, Bird A (1998) Identification and characterization of a family of mammalian methyl-CpG binding proteins. *Mol Cell Biol* 18:6538–6547.

21. Ng HH, Jeppesen P, Bird A (2000) Active repression of methylated genes by the chromosomal protein MBD1. *Mol Cell Biol* 20:1394–1406.

22. Fujita N, Watanabe S, Ichimura T, *et al.* (2003) Methyl-CpG binding domain 1 (MBD1) interacts with the Suv39h1-HP1 heterochromatic complex for DNA methylation-based transcriptional repression. *J Biol Chem* 278:24132–24138.

23. Patra SK, Patra A, Zhao H, Carroll P, Dahiya R (2003) Methyl-CpG-DNA binding proteins in human prostate cancer: expression of CXXC sequence containing MBD1 and repression of MBD2 and MeCP2. *Biochem Biophys Res Commun* 302:759–766.

24. Ng HH, Zhang Y, Hendrich B, *et al.* (1999) MBD2 is a transcriptional repressor belonging to the MeCP1 histone deacetylase complex. *Nat Genet* 23: 58–61.

25. Bhattacharya SK, Ramchandani S, Cervoni N, Szyf M (1999) A mammalian protein with specific demethylase activity for mCpG DNA. *Nature* 397:579–583.

26. Detich N, Theberge J, Szyf M (2002) Promoter-specific activation and demethylation by MBD2/demethylase. *J Biol Chem* 277:35791–35794.

27. Wade PA, Gegonne A, Jones PL, Ballestar E, Aubry F, Wolffe AP (1999) Mi-2 complex couples DNA methylation to chromatin remodelling and histone deacetylation. *Nat Genet* 23:62–66.

28. Hendrich B, Hardeland U, Ng HH, Jiricny J, Bird A (1999) The thymine glycosylase MBD4 can bind to the product of deamination at methylated CpG sites. *Nature* 401:301–304.

29. Sano H, Sager R (1980) Deoxyribonucleic acid methyltransferase from the eukaryote, *Chlamydomonas reinhardi. Eur J Biochem* 105:471–480.

30. Chuang LS, Ian HI, Koh TW, Ng HH, Xu G, Li BF (1997) Human DNA-(cytosine-5) methyltransferase-PCNA complex as a target for p21WAF1. *Science* 277:1996–2000.

31. Pradhan S, Bacolla A, Wells RD, Roberts RJ (1999) Recombinant human DNA (cytosine-5) methyltransferase. I. Expression, purification, and comparison of *de novo* and maintenance methylation. *J Biol Chem* 274: 33002–33010.

32. Li E, Bestor TH, Jaenisch R (1992) Targeted mutation of the DNA methyltransferase gene results in embryonic lethality. *Cell* 69:915–926.

33. Okano M, Xie S, Li E (1998) Cloning and characterization of a family of novel mammalian DNA (cytosine-5) methyltransferases. *Nat Genet* 19: 219–220.

34. Lyko F, Ramsahoye BH, Kashevsky H, *et al.* (1999) Mammalian (cytosine-5) methyltransferases cause genomic DNA methylation and lethality in *Drosophila. Nat Genet* 23:363–366.

35. Okano M, Bell DW, Haber DA, Li E (1999) DNA methyltransferases Dnmt3a and Dnmt3b are essential for *de novo* methylation and mammalian development. *Cell* 99:247–257.

36. Issa JP, Vertino PM, Wu J, *et al.* (1993) Increased cytosine DNA-methyltransferase activity during colon cancer progression. *J Natl Cancer Inst* 85:1235–1240.

37. Robertson KD, Uzvolgyi E, Liang G, *et al.* (1999) The human DNA methyltransferases (DNMTs) 1, 3a and 3b: coordinate mRNA expression in normal tissues and overexpression in tumors. *Nucleic Acids Res* 27: 2291–2298.

38. Belinsky SA, Nikula KJ, Baylin SB, Issa JP (1996) Increased cytosine DNA-methyltransferase activity is target-cell-specific and an early event in lung cancer. *Proc Natl Acad Sci USA* 93:4045–4050.
39. Melki JR, Warnecke P, Vincent PC, Clark SJ (1998) Increased DNA methyltransferase expression in leukaemia. *Leukemia* 12:311–316.
40. Eads CA, Danenberg KD, Kawakami K, Saltz LB, Danenberg PV, Laird PW (1999) CpG island hypermethylation in human colorectal tumors is not associated with DNA methyltransferase overexpression. *Cancer Res* 59: 2302–2306.
41. Lubbert M (2000) DNA methylation inhibitors in the treatment of leukemias, myelodysplastic syndromes and hemoglobinopathies: clinical results and possible mechanisms of action. *Curr Top Microbiol Immunol* 249:135–164.
42. Bouchard J, Momparler RL (1983) Incorporation of 5-Aza-2′-deoxycytidine-5′-triphosphate into DNA. Interactions with mammalian DNA polymerase alpha and DNA methylase. *Mol Pharmacol* 24:109–114.
43. Santi DV, Garrett CE, Barr PJ (1983) On the mechanism of inhibition of DNA-cytosine methyltransferases by cytosine analogs. *Cell* 33:9–10.
44. Juttermann R, Li E, Jaenisch R (1994) Toxicity of 5-aza-2′-deoxycytidine to mammalian cells is mediated primarily by covalent trapping of DNA methyltransferase rather than DNA demethylation. *Proc Natl Acad Sci USA* 91: 11797–11801.
45. Lin KT, Momparler RL, Rivard GE (1981) High-performance liquid chromatographic analysis of chemical stability of 5-aza-2′-deoxycytidine. *J Pharm Sci* 70:1228–1232.
46. Goffin J, Eisenhauer E (2002) DNA methyltransferase inhibitors-state of the art. *Ann Oncol* 13:1699–1716.
47. Cheng JC, Matsen CB, Gonzales FA, *et al.* (2003) Inhibition of DNA methylation and reactivation of silenced genes by zebularine. *J Natl Cancer Inst* 95:399–409.
48. Thibault A, Figg WD, Bergan RC, *et al.* (1998) A phase II study of 5-aza-2′deoxycytidine (decitabine) in hormone independent metastatic (D2) prostate cancer. *Tumori* 84:87–89.
49. Cheng JC, Weisenberger DJ, Gonzales FA, *et al.* (2004) Continuous zebularine treatment effectively sustains demethylation in human bladder cancer cells. *Mol Cell Biol* 24:1270–1278.
50. Robert MF, Morin S, Beaulieu N, *et al.* (2003) DNMT1 is required to maintain CpG methylation and aberrant gene silencing in human cancer cells. *Nat Genet* 33:61–65.

51. Rhee I, Jair KW, Yen RW, *et al.* (2000) CpG methylation is maintained in human cancer cells lacking DNMT1. *Nature* 404:1003–1007.
52. Rhee I, Bachman KE, Park BH, *et al.* (2002) DNMT1 and DNMT3b cooperate to silence genes in human cancer cells. *Nature* 416:552–556.
53. Bachman KE, Park BH, Rhee I, *et al.* (2003) Histone modifications and silencing prior to DNA methylation of a tumor suppressor gene. *Cancer Cell* 3:89–95.
54. Davis AJ, Gelmon KA, Siu LL, *et al.* (2003) Phase I and pharmacologic study of the human DNA methyltransferase antisense oligodeoxynucleotide MG98 given as a 21-day continuous infusion every 4 weeks. *Invest New Drugs* 21:85–97.
55. Stewart DJ, Donehower RC, Eisenhauer EA, *et al.* (2003) A phase I pharmacokinetic and pharmacodynamic study of the DNA methyltransferase 1 inhibitor MG98 administered twice weekly. *Ann Oncol* 14:766–774.
56. Eickbush TH, Moudrianakis EN (1978) The histone core complex: an octamer assembled by two sets of protein-protein interactions. *Biochemistry* 17:4955–4964.
57. Luger K, Mader AW, Richmond RK, Sargent DF, Richmond TJ (1997) Crystal structure of the nucleosome core particle at 2.8 A resolution. *Nature* 389:251–260.
58. Allan J, Mitchell T, Harborne N, Bohm L, Crane-Robinson C (1986) Roles of H1 domains in determining higher order chromatin structure and H1 location. *J Mol Biol* 187:591–601.
59. Carruthers LM, Bednar J, Woodcock CL, Hansen JC (1998) Linker histones stabilize the intrinsic salt-dependent folding of nucleosomal arrays: mechanistic ramifications for higher-order chromatin folding. *Biochemistry* 37:14776–14787.
60. Howe L, Iskandar M, Ausio J (1998) Folding of chromatin in the presence of heterogeneous histone H1 binding to nucleosomes. *J Biol Chem* 273: 11625–11629.
61. Ogryzko VV, Schiltz RL, Russanova V, Howard BH, Nakatani Y (1996) The transcriptional coactivators p300 and CBP are histone acetyltransferases. *Cell* 87:953–959.
62. Mizzen CA, Yang XJ, Kokubo T, *et al.* (1996) The TAF(II)250 subunit of TFIID has histone acetyltransferase activity. *Cell* 87:1261.
63. Spencer TE, Jenster G, Burcin MM, *et al.* (1997) Steroid receptor coactivator-1 is a histone acetyltransferase. *Nature* 389:194–198.
64. Chen H, Lin RJ, Schiltz RL, *et al.* (1997) Nuclear receptor coactivator ACTR is a novel histone acetyltransferase and forms a multimeric activation complex with P/CAF and CBP/p300. *Cell* 90:569–580.

65. Yang WM, Inouye C, Zeng Y, Bearss D, Seto E (1996) Transcriptional repression by YY1 is mediated by interaction with a mammalian homolog of the yeast global regulator RPD3. *Proc Natl Acad Sci USA* 93: 12845–12850.

66. Yang XJ, Ogryzko VV, Nishikawa J, Howard BH, Nakatani Y (1996) A p300/CBP-associated factor that competes with the adenoviral oncoprotein E1A. *Nature* 382:319–324.

67. Nowak SJ, Corces VG (2000) Phosphorylation of histone H3 correlates with transcriptionally active loci. *Genes Dev* 14:3003–3013.

68. Mahadevan LC, Willis AC, Barratt MJ (1991) Rapid histone H3 phosphorylation in response to growth factors, phorbol esters, okadaic acid, and protein synthesis inhibitors. *Cell* 65:775–783.

69. Sassone-Corsi P, Mizzen CA, Cheung P, *et al.* (1999) Requirement of Rsk-2 for epidermal growth factor-activated phosphorylation of histone H3. *Science* 285:886–891.

70. Thomson S, Clayton AL, Hazzalin CA, Rose S, Barratt MJ, Mahadevan LC (1999) The nucleosomal response associated with immediate-early gene induction is mediated via alternative MAP kinase cascades: MSK1 as a potential histone H3/HMG-14 kinase. *EMBO J* 18:4779–4793.

71. Lo WS, Duggan L, Tolga NC, *et al.* (2001) Snf1-a histone kinase that works in concert with the histone acetyltransferase Gcn5 to regulate transcription. *Science* 293:1142–1146.

72. Cheung P, Tanner KG, Cheung WL, Sassone-Corsi P, Denu JM, Allis CD (2000) Synergistic coupling of histone H3 phosphorylation and acetylation in response to epidermal growth factor stimulation. *Mol Cell* 5: 905–915.

73. Yamamoto Y, Verma UN, Prajapati S, Kwak YT, Gaynor RB (2003) Histone H3 phosphorylation by IKK-alpha is critical for cytokine-induced gene expression. *Nature* 423:655–659.

74. Cheung P, Allis CD, Sassone-Corsi P (2000) Signaling to chromatin through histone modifications. *Cell* 103:263–271.

75. Schurter BT, Koh SS, Chen D, *et al.* (2001) Methylation of histone H3 by coactivator-associated arginine methyltransferase 1. *Biochemistry* 40: 5747–5756.

76. Chen D, Ma H, Hong H, *et al.* (1999) Regulation of transcription by a protein methyltransferase. *Science* 284:2174–2177.

77. Wang H, Huang ZQ, Xia L, *et al.* (2001) Methylation of histone H4 at arginine 3 facilitating transcriptional activation by nuclear hormone receptor. *Science* 293:853–857.

78. Rea S, Eisenhaber F, O'Carroll D, *et al.* (2000) Regulation of chromatin structure by site-specific histone H3 methyltransferases. *Nature* 406:593–599.
79. Bannister AJ, Zegerman P, Partridge JF, *et al.* (2001) Selective recognition of methylated lysine 9 on histone H3 by the HP1 chromo domain. *Nature* 410:120–124.
80. Lachner M, O'Carroll D, Rea S, Mechtler K, Jenuwein T (2001) Methylation of histone H3 lysine 9 creates a binding site for HP1 proteins. *Nature* 410:116–120.
81. Nakayama J, Rice JC, Strahl BD, Allis CD, Grewal SI (2001) Role of histone H3 lysine 9 methylation in epigenetic control of heterochromatin assembly. *Science* 292:110–113.
82. Nielsen SJ, Schneider R, Bauer UM, *et al.* (2001) Rb targets histone H3 methylation and HP1 to promoters. *Nature* 412:561–565.
83. Kuzmichev A, Nishioka K, Erdjument-Bromage H, Tempst P, Reinberg D (2002) Histone methyltransferase activity associated with a human multiprotein complex containing the Enhancer of Zeste protein. *Genes Dev* 16: 2893–2905.
84. Czermin B, Melfi R, McCabe D, Seitz V, Imhof A, Pirrotta V (2002) *Drosophila* enhancer of Zeste/ESC complexes have a histone H3 methyltransferase activity that marks chromosomal Polycomb sites. *Cell* 111:185–196.
85. Varambally S, Dhanasekaran SM, Zhou M, *et al.* (2002) The polycomb group protein EZH2 is involved in progression of prostate cancer. *Nature* 419:624–629.
86. Tamaru H, Selker EU (2001) A histone H3 methyltransferase controls DNA methylation in *Neurospora crassa*. *Nature* 414:277–283.
87. Tamaru H, Zhang X, McMillen D, *et al.* (2003) Trimethylated lysine 9 of histone H3 is a mark for DNA methylation in *Neurospora crassa*. *Nat Genet* 34:75–79.
88. Rice JC, Briggs SD, Ueberheide B, *et al.* (2003) Histone methyltransferases direct different degrees of methylation to define distinct chromatin domains. *Mol Cell* 12:1591–1598.
89. Wang H, Cao R, Xia L, *et al.* (2001) Purification and functional characterization of a histone H3-lysine 4-specific methyltransferase. *Mol Cell* 8: 1207–1217.
90. Nishioka K, Chuikov S, Sarma K, *et al.* (2002) Set9, a novel histone H3 methyltransferase that facilitates transcription by precluding histone tail modifications required for heterochromatin formation. *Genes Dev* 16:479–489.
91. Kim J, Jia L, Tilley WD, Coetzee GA (2003) Dynamic methylation of histone H3 at lysine 4 in transcriptional regulation by the androgen receptor. *Nucleic Acids Res* 31:6741–6747.

92. Goldknopf IL, Taylor CW, Baum RM, *et al.* (1975) Isolation and characterization of protein A24, a "histone-like" non-histone chromosomal protein. *J Biol Chem* 250:7182–7187.

93. Pham AD, Sauer F (2000) Ubiquitin-activating/conjugating activity of TAFII250, a mediator of activation of gene expression in *Drosophila*. *Science* 289:2357–2360.

94. Sun ZW, Allis CD (2002) Ubiquitination of histone H2B regulates H3 methylation and gene silencing in yeast. *Nature* 418:104–108.

95. Shiio Y, Eisenman RN (2003) Histone sumoylation is associated with transcriptional repression. *Proc Natl Acad Sci USA* 100:13225–13230.

96. Turner BM (2002) Cellular memory and the histone code. *Cell* 111: 285–291.

97. Grozinger CM, Chao ED, Blackwell HE, Moazed D, Schreiber SL (2001) Identification of a class of small molecule inhibitors of the sirtuin family of NAD-dependent deacetylases by phenotypic screening. *J Biol Chem* 276: 38837–38843.

98. Khochbin S, Verdel A, Lemercier C, Seigneurin-Berny D (2001) Functional significance of histone deacetylase diversity. *Curr Opin Genet Dev* 11: 162–166.

99. de Ruijter AJ, van Gennip AH, Caron HN, Kemp S, van Kuilenburg AB (2003) Histone deacetylases (HDACs): characterization of the classical HDAC family. *Biochem J* 370:737–749.

100. Yoshida M, Kijima M, Akita M, Beppu T (1990) Potent and specific inhibition of mammalian histone deacetylase both *in vivo* and *in vitro* by trichostatin A. *J Biol Chem* 265:17174–17179.

101. Richon VM, Emiliani S, Verdin E, *et al.* (1998) A class of hybrid polar inducers of transformed cell differentiation inhibits histone deacetylases. *Proc Natl Acad Sci USA* 95:3003–3007.

102. Singh SB, Zink DL, Liesch JM, *et al.* (2002) Structure and chemistry of apicidins, a class of novel cyclic tetrapeptides without a terminal alpha-keto epoxide as inhibitors of histone deacetylase with potent antiprotozoal activities. *J Org Chem* 67:815–825.

103. Furumai R, Matsuyama A, Kobashi N, *et al.* (2002) FK228 (depsipeptide) as a natural prodrug that inhibits class I histone deacetylases. *Cancer Res* 62:4916–4921.

104. Kwon HJ, Owa T, Hassig CA, Shimada J, Schreiber SL (1998) Depudecin induces morphological reversion of transformed fibroblasts via the inhibition of histone deacetylase. *Proc Natl Acad Sci USA* 95:3356–3361.

105. Boivin AJ, Momparler LF, Hurtubise A, Momparler RL (2002) Antineoplastic action of 5-aza-2′-deoxycytidine and phenylbutyrate on human lung carcinoma cells. *Anticancer Drugs* 13:869–874.
106. Phiel CJ, Zhang F, Huang EY, Guenther MG, Lazar MA, Klein PS (2001) Histone deacetylase is a direct target of valproic acid, a potent anticonvulsant, mood stabilizer, and teratogen. *J Biol Chem* 276:36734–36741.
107. Prakash S, Foster BJ, Meyer M, *et al.* (2001) Chronic oral administration of CI-994: a phase 1 study. *Invest New Drugs* 19:1–11.
108. Saito A, Yamashita T, Mariko Y, *et al.* (1999) A synthetic inhibitor of histone deacetylase, MS-27-275, with marked *in vivo* antitumor activity against human tumors. *Proc Natl Acad Sci USA* 96:4592–4597.
109. Finnin MS, Donigian JR, Cohen A, *et al.* (1999) Structures of a histone deacetylase homologue bound to the TSA and SAHA inhibitors. *Nature* 401:188–193.
110. Marks P, Rifkind RA, Richon VM, Breslow R, Miller T, Kelly WK (2001) Histone deacetylases and cancer: causes and therapies. *Nat Rev Cancer* 1:194–202.
111. Van Lint C, Emiliani S, Verdin E (1996) The expression of a small fraction of cellular genes is changed in response to histone hyperacetylation. *Gene Expr* 5:245–253.
112. Butler LM, Zhou X, Xu WS, *et al.* (2002) The histone deacetylase inhibitor SAHA arrests cancer cell growth, up-regulates thioredoxin-binding protein-2, and down-regulates thioredoxin. *Proc Natl Acad Sci USA* 99:11700–11705.
113. Suzuki H, Gabrielson E, Chen W, *et al.* (2002) A genomic screen for genes upregulated by demethylation and histone deacetylase inhibition in human colorectal cancer. *Nat Genet* 31:141–149.
114. Marks PA, Miller T, Richon VM (2003) Histone deacetylases. *Curr Opin Pharmacol* 3:344–351.
115. Kelly WK, Richon VM, O'Connor O, *et al.* (2003) Phase I clinical trial of histone deacetylase inhibitor: suberoylanilide hydroxamic acid administered intravenously. *Clin Cancer Res* 9:3578–3588.
116. Butler LM, Agus DB, Scher HI, *et al.* (2000) Suberoylanilide hydroxamic acid, an inhibitor of histone deacetylase, suppresses the growth of prostate cancer cells *in vitro* and *in vivo*. *Cancer Res* 60:5165–5170.
117. Jones PL, Veenstra GJ, Wade PA, *et al.* (1998) Methylated DNA and MeCP2 recruit histone deacetylase to repress transcription. *Nat Genet* 19:187–191.

118. Fuks F, Hurd PJ, Wolf D, Nan X, Bird AP, Kouzarides T (2003) The methyl-CpG-binding protein MeCP2 links DNA methylation to histone methylation. *J Biol Chem* 278:4035–4040.

119. Fuks F, Hurd PJ, Deplus R, Kouzarides T (2003) The DNA methyltransferases associate with HP1 and the SUV39H1 histone methyltransferase. *Nucleic Acids Res* 31:2305–2312.

120. Jones PA, Baylin SB (2002) The fundamental role of epigenetic events in cancer. *Nat Rev Genet* 3:415–428.

121. Li E (2002) Chromatin modification and epigenetic reprogramming in mammalian development. *Nat Rev Genet* 3:662–673.

122. Cameron EE, Bachman KE, Myohanen S, Herman JG, Baylin SB (1999) Synergy of demethylation and histone deacetylase inhibition in the re-expression of genes silenced in cancer. *Nat Genet* 21:103–107.

123. El-Osta A, Kantharidis P, Zalcberg JR, Wolffe AP (2002) Precipitous release of methyl-CpG binding protein 2 and histone deacetylase 1 from the methylated human multidrug resistance gene (MDR1) on activation. *Mol Cell Biol* 22:1844–1857.

124. Shaker S, Bernstein M, Momparler LF, Momparler RL (2003) Preclinical evaluation of antineoplastic activity of inhibitors of DNA methylation (5-aza-2′-deoxycytidine) and histone deacetylation (trichostatin A, depsipeptide) in combination against myeloid leukemic cells. *Leuk Res* 27:437–444.

125. Gagnon J, Shaker S, Primeau M, Hurtubise A, Momparler RL (2003) Interaction of 5-aza-2′-deoxycytidine and depsipeptide on antineoplastic activity and activation of 14-3-3sigma, E-cadherin and tissue inhibitor of metalloproteinase 3 expression in human breast carcinoma cells. *Anticancer Drugs* 14:193–202.

126. Zhu WG, Otterson GA (2003) The interaction of histone deacetylase inhibitors and DNA methyltransferase inhibitors in the treatment of human cancer cells. *Curr Med Chem Anti-Canc Agents* 3:187–199.

127. Belinsky SA, Klinge DM, Stidley CA, et al. (2003) Inhibition of DNA methylation and histone deacetylation prevents murine lung cancer. *Cancer Res* 63:7089–7093.

128. Patra SK, Patra A, Dahiya R (2001) Histone deacetylase and DNA methyltransferase in human prostate cancer. *Biochem Biophys Res Commun* 287:705–713.

129. Coles B, Ketterer B (1990) The role of glutathione and glutathione transferases in chemical carcinogenesis. *Crit Rev Biochem Mol Biol* 25:47–70.

130. Rushmore TH, Pickett CB (1993) Glutathione S-transferases, structure, regulation, and therapeutic implications. *J Biol Chem* 268:11475–11478.
131. Lee WH, Morton RA, Epstein JI, *et al.* (1994) Cytidine methylation of regulatory sequences near the pi-class glutathione S-transferase gene accompanies human prostatic carcinogenesis. *Proc Natl Acad Sci USA* 91: 11733–11737.
132. Herman JG, Graff JR, Myohanen S, Nelkin BD, Baylin SB (1996) Methylation-specific PCR: a novel PCR assay for methylation status of CpG islands. *Proc Natl Acad Sci USA* 93:9821–9826.
133. Harden SV, Sanderson H, Goodman SN, *et al.* (2003) Quantitative GSTP1 methylation and the detection of prostate adenocarcinoma in sextant biopsies. *J Natl Cancer Inst* 95:1634–1637.
134. Nakayama M, Bennett CJ, Hicks JL, *et al.* (2003) Hypermethylation of the human glutathione S-transferase-pi gene (GSTP1) CpG island is present in a subset of proliferative inflammatory atrophy lesions but not in normal or hyperplastic epithelium of the prostate: a detailed study using laser-capture microdissection. *Am J Pathol* 163:923–933.
135. Naot D, Sionov RV, Ish-Shalom D (1997) CD44: structure, function, and association with the malignant process. *Adv Cancer Res* 71:241–319.
136. Verkaik NS, Trapman J, Romijn JC, van der Kwast TH, van Steenbrugge GJ (1999) Down-regulation of CD44 expression in human prostatic carcinoma cell lines is correlated with DNA hypermethylation. *Int J Cancer* 80:439–443.
137. Lou W, Krill D, Dhir R, *et al.* (1999) Methylation of the CD44 metastasis suppressor gene in human prostate cancer. *Cancer Res* 59:2329–2331.
138. Kito H, Suzuki H, Ichikawa T, *et al.* (2001) Hypermethylation of the CD44 gene is associated with progression and metastasis of human prostate cancer. *Prostate* 49:110–115.
139. Woodson K, Hayes R, Wideroff L, Villaruz L, Tangrea J (2003) Hypermethylation of GSTP1, CD44, and E-cadherin genes in prostate cancer among US Blacks and Whites. *Prostate* 55:199–205.
140. Ekici S, Ayhan A, Kendi S, Ozen H (2002) Determination of prognosis in patients with prostate cancer treated with radical prostatectomy: prognostic value of CD44v6 score. *J Urol* 167:2037–2041.
141. Bergelson JM, Cunningham JA, Droguett G, *et al.* (1997) Isolation of a common receptor for Coxsackie B viruses and adenoviruses 2 and 5. *Science* 275:1320–1323.
142. Tomko RP, Xu R, Philipson L (1997) HCAR and MCAR: the human and mouse cellular receptors for subgroup C adenoviruses and group B coxsackieviruses. *Proc Natl Acad Sci USA* 94:3352–3356.

143. Okegawa T, Pong RC, Li Y, Bergelson JM, Sagalowsky AI, Hsieh JT (2001) The mechanism of the growth-inhibitory effect of coxsackie and adenovirus receptor (CAR) on human bladder cancer: a functional analysis of car protein structure. *Cancer Res* 61:6592–6600.

144. Li Y, Pong RC, Bergelson JM, *et al.* (1999) Loss of adenoviral receptor expression in human bladder cancer cells: a potential impact on the efficacy of gene therapy. *Cancer Res* 59:325–330.

145. Sachs MD, Rauen KA, Ramamurthy M, *et al.* (2002) Integrin alpha(v) and coxsackie adenovirus receptor expression in clinical bladder cancer. *Urology* 60:531–536.

146. Rauen KA, Sudilovsky D, Le JL, *et al.* (2002) Expression of the coxsackie adenovirus receptor in normal prostate and in primary and metastatic prostate carcinoma: potential relevance to gene therapy. *Cancer Res* 62:3812–3818.

147. Hemmi S, Geertsen R, Mezzacasa A, Peter I, Dummer R (1998) The presence of human coxsackievirus and adenovirus receptor is associated with efficient adenovirus-mediated transgene expression in human melanoma cell cultures. *Hum Gene Ther* 9:2363–2373.

148. Miller CR, Buchsbaum DJ, Reynolds PN, *et al.* (1998) Differential susceptibility of primary and established human glioma cells to adenovirus infection: targeting via the epidermal growth factor receptor achieves fiber receptor-independent gene transfer. *Cancer Res* 58:5738–5748.

149. Okegawa T, Li Y, Pong RC, Bergelson JM, Zhou J, Hsieh JT (2000) The dual impact of coxsackie and adenovirus receptor expression on human prostate cancer gene therapy. *Cancer Res* 60:5031–5036.

150. Lucas A, Kremer EJ, Hemmi S, Luis J, Vignon F, Lazennec G (2003) Comparative transductions of breast cancer cells by three DNA viruses. *Biochem Biophys Res Commun* 309:1011–1016.

151. Pong RC, Lai YJ, Chen H, *et al.* (2003) Epigenetic regulation of coxsackie and adenovirus receptor (CAR) gene promoter in urogenital cancer cells. *Cancer Res* 63:8680–8686.

152. Jarrard DF, Kinoshita H, Shi Y, *et al.* (1998) Methylation of the androgen receptor promoter CpG island is associated with loss of androgen receptor expression in prostate cancer cells. *Cancer Res* 58:5310–5314.

153. Kinoshita H, Shi Y, Sandefur C, *et al.* (2000) Methylation of the androgen receptor minimal promoter silences transcription in human prostate cancer. *Cancer Res* 60:3623–3630.

154. Sasaki M, Tanaka Y, Perinchery G, *et al.* (2002) Methylation and inactivation of estrogen, progesterone, and androgen receptors in prostate cancer. *J Natl Cancer Inst* 94:384–390.

155. Li LC, Chui R, Nakajima K, Oh BR, Au HC, Dahiya R (2000) Frequent methylation of estrogen receptor in prostate cancer: correlation with tumor progression. *Cancer Res* 60:702–706.

156. Freemantle SJ, Spinella MJ, Dmitrovsky E (2003) Retinoids in cancer therapy and chemoprevention: promise meets resistance. *Oncogene* 22:7305–7315.

157. Nakayama T, Watanabe M, Yamanaka M, *et al.* (2001) The role of epigenetic modifications in retinoic acid receptor beta2 gene expression in human prostate cancers. *Lab Invest* 81:1049–1057.

158. Maruyama R, Toyooka S, Toyooka KO, *et al.* (2002) Aberrant promoter methylation profile of prostate cancers and its relationship to clinicopathological features. *Clin Cancer Res* 8:514–519.

159. Yamanaka M, Watanabe M, Yamada Y, *et al.* (2003) Altered methylation of multiple genes in carcinogenesis of the prostate. *Int J Cancer* 106:382–387.

160. Viola MV, Fromowitz F, Oravez S, *et al.* (1986) Expression of ras oncogene p21 in prostate cancer. *N Engl J Med* 314:133–137.

161. Sumiya H, Masai M, Akimoto S, Yatani R, Shimazaki J (1990) Histochemical examination of expression of ras p21 protein and R 1881-binding protein in human prostatic cancers. *Eur J Cancer* 26:786–789.

162. Carter BS, Epstein JI, Isaacs WB (1990) ras gene mutations in human prostate cancer. *Cancer Res* 50:6830–6832.

163. Pergolizzi RG, Kreis W, Rottach C, Susin M, Broome JD (1993) Mutational status of codons 12 and 13 of the N- and K-ras genes in tissue and cell lines derived from primary and metastatic prostate carcinomas. *Cancer Invest* 11:25–32.

164. Gumerlock PH, Poonamallee UR, Meyers FJ, deVere White RW (1991) Activated ras alleles in human carcinoma of the prostate are rare. *Cancer Res* 51:1632–1637.

165. Burbee DG, Forgacs E, Zochbauer-Muller S, *et al.* (2001) Epigenetic inactivation of RASSF1A in lung and breast cancers and malignant phenotype suppression. *J Natl Cancer Inst* 93:691–699.

166. Dammann R, Li C, Yoon JH, Chin PL, Bates S, Pfeifer GP (2000) Epigenetic inactivation of a RAS association domain family protein from the lung tumour suppressor locus 3p21.3. *Nat Genet* 25:315–319.

167. Liu L, Yoon JH, Dammann R, Pfeifer GP (2002) Frequent hypermethylation of the RASSF1A gene in prostate cancer. *Oncogene* 21:6835–6840.

168. Wang Z, Tseng CP, Pong RC, *et al.* (2002) The mechanism of growth-inhibitory effect of DOC-2/DAB2 in prostate cancer. Characterization of a novel GTPase-activating protein associated with N-terminal domain of DOC-2/DAB2. *J Biol Chem* 277:12622–12631.

169. Chen H, Pong RC, Wang Z, Hsieh JT (2002) Differential regulation of the human gene DAB2IP in normal and malignant prostatic epithelia: cloning and characterization. *Genomics* 79:573–581.

170. Chen H, Toyooka S, Gazdar AF, Hsieh JT (2003) Epigenetic regulation of a novel tumor suppressor gene (hDAB2IP) in prostate cancer cell lines. *J Biol Chem* 278:3121–3130.

171. Tsihlias J, Kapusta L, Slingerland J (1999) The prognostic significance of altered cyclin-dependent kinase inhibitors in human cancer. *Annu Rev Med* 50:401–423.

172. Zhang P (1999) The cell cycle and development: redundant roles of cell cycle regulators. *Curr Opin Cell Biol* 11:655–662.

173. Padar A, Sathyanarayana UG, Suzuki M, *et al.* (2003) Inactivation of cyclin D2 gene in prostate cancers by aberrant promoter methylation. *Clin Cancer Res* 9:4730–4734.

174. Heiss NS, Gloeckner G, Bachner D, *et al.* (1997) Genomic structure of a novel LIM domain gene (ZNF185) in Xq28 and comparisons with the orthologous murine transcript. *Genomics* 43:329–338.

175. Dawid IB, Toyama R, Taira M (1995) LIM domain proteins. *CR Acad Sci III* 318:295–306.

176. Vanaja DK, Cheville JC, Iturria SJ, Young CY (2003) Transcriptional silencing of zinc finger protein 185 identified by expression profiling is associated with prostate cancer progression. *Cancer Res* 63:3877–3882.

177. Gitelman SE, Kirk M, Ye JQ, Filvaroff EH, Kahn AJ, Derynck R (1995) Vgr-1/BMP-6 induces osteoblastic differentiation of pluripotential mesenchymal cells. *Cell Growth Differ* 6:827–836.

178. Tamada H, Kitazawa R, Gohji K, Kitazawa S (2001) Epigenetic regulation of human bone morphogenetic protein 6 gene expression in prostate cancer. *J Bone Miner Res* 16:487–496.

179. De Pinieux G, Flam T, Zerbib M, *et al.* (2001) Bone sialoprotein, bone morphogenetic protein 6 and thymidine phosphorylase expression in localized human prostatic adenocarcinoma as predictors of clinical outcome: a clinicopathological and immunohistochemical study of 43 cases. *J Urol* 166: 1924–1930.

180. Goessl C, Muller M, Heicappell R, *et al.* (2002) Methylation-specific PCR for detection of neoplastic DNA in biopsy washings. *J Pathol* 196: 331–334.

181. Kollermann J, Muller M, Goessl C, *et al.* (2003) Methylation-specific PCR for DNA-based detection of occult tumor cells in lymph nodes of prostate cancer patients. *Eur Urol* 44:533–538.

182. Cairns P, Esteller M, Herman JG, *et al.* (2001) Molecular detection of prostate cancer in urine by GSTP1 hypermethylation. *Clin Cancer Res* 7: 2727–2730.
183. Gonzalgo ML, Pavlovich CP, Lee SM, Nelson WG (2003) Prostate cancer detection by GSTP1 methylation analysis of postbiopsy urine specimens. *Clin Cancer Res* 9:2673–2677.
184. Goessl C, Krause H, Muller M, *et al.* (2000) Fluorescent methylation-specific polymerase chain reaction for DNA-based detection of prostate cancer in bodily fluids. *Cancer Res* 60:5941–5945.
185. Jeronimo C, Usadel H, Henrique R, *et al.* (2002) Quantitative GSTP1 hypermethylation in bodily fluids of patients with prostate cancer. *Urology* 60:1131–1135.

10

SIGNIFICANCE OF 5α-REDUCTASE IN PROSTATE CANCER

Jun Shimazaki

Department of Urology, Graduate School of Medicine
Chiba University, Chiba, Japan 262-8670

Introduction

Since Huggins and Hodges[1] alleviated the pain of patients with prostate cancer by androgen removal, endocrine therapy has become an important strategy for treating this disease. Of the androgens in circulation, more than 90% is testosterone secreted from the testis, and the remainder is dehydroepiandrosterone and its sulfate, and androst-4-ene-3,17-dione, from the adrenal gland. These androgens are converted to dihydrotesto-sterone (DHT, 5α-androstane-17β-ol-3-one) by 5α-reductase (EC 1.3.99.5) in the prostate, and then bound to androgen receptor, which mediates the effects of androgens. Since DHT regulates prostate growth, including the growth of malignant prostate tissues, the role of 5α-reductase in cancer development has become a focus of research.

5α-Reductase

Two types of 5α-reductase have been cloned.[2] In the human enzymes, type 1 (SRD5A1) has a deduced molecular weight of 29,000 and 259 amino acids, and type 2 (SRD5A2) has a deduced molecular weight of 28,000 and 254 amino acids. Amino acid sequence identity is approximately 50% between types 1 and 2. Sequence identity shared by human and rat isozymes is 60% for type 1 and 77% for type 2. The kinetic parameters of human enzymes are different between the two types: optimal pH and Km's for testosterone are pH 6–8.5 and 1–5 μM for type 1, and pH 5.0–5.5 and 0.075–1.0 μM for type 2.[3] Enzyme reactions of both types require NADPH as cofactor.

In the rat prostate, SRD5A1 is found in the basal cells[4] or tall secretory cells[5] of the glandular epithelium, and SRD5A2 is detected in the stromal cells. In the human prostate, early reports did not detect SRD5A1 but found SRD5A2 in the basal and stromal cells of non-malignant and cancerous prostates.[6,7] Subsequently, both types of isozymes have been shown in normal and abnormal prostates by means of immunohistochemistry,[8] RT-PCR,[9] and microarray.[10] To date, SRD5A1 and SRD5A2 have been found in many tissues such as prostate, genital and non-genital skin, and male genital organs.

Expression of SRD5A2 mRNA correlated well with the level of dihydrotestosterone estimated by 5α-reductase activity in the prostate, but no association was found between the expression of SRD5A1 mRNA and enzyme activity.[11] Using biochemical measurement, values of Km and Vmax in stroma were higher than those in epithelium from both non-malignant and cancerous tissues, indicating a higher activity of stromal 5α-reductase, although the tissue concentrations of DHT were in similar ranges between the two fractions.[12] Cancer cells reveal some 5α-reductase activity: SRD5A1 in LNCaP, PC 3 and DU145,[13–16] and SRD5A2 in LNCaP.[14,16] When cancer cells obtained from surgery were grown in culture, expression of both types of 5α-reductase could be detected, however, SRDA1 was preferentially expressed.[17] Of the cancer specimens studied, 28% showed high intensity staining for SRD5A1 in the tumor epithelium, but the hyperplastic tissues showed less intense staining in the epithelium.[18] Although some cancer cells exhibit SRD5A1, SRD5A2 seems to act as the main enzyme in the prostate, as suggested by clinical evidences. For example, the small prostate of a patient with a specific type of male pseudohermaphroditism who had normal SRD5A1 but mutated SRD5A2,[19] shrunk as the result of treatment with the SRD5A2 inhibitor, finasteride. Therefore, SRD5A2 in the stromal component may mainly act in the formation of DHT in both non-malignant and cancerous prostates, thus the SRD5A2 gene, in relation to DHT metabolism, has been widely studied in order to understand the development of prostate cancer.

Formation and Metabolism of DHT in Cancerous Prostate

In 1965, Shimazaki *et al.* first found that incubation of radiolabled testosterone with tissue extracts of rat prostate or minced tissues of normal and pathological human prostates formed radiolabled DHT and androst-4-ene-3,17-dione.[20,21] Three years later, Bruchovsky and Wilson found that DHT could be detected in isolated prostatic nuclei 2 hours after administration of ^{3}H-testosterone to rats.[22] Several months later, Anderson and Liao confirmed that nuclei of both rat ventral prostate and seminal vesicles selectively retained ^{3}H-DHT.[23] The metabolic rate of DHT formation is high in hyperplastic tissues, moderate in normal tissues, and low in cancerous tissues.[20,21] Reduced activity of 5α-reductase in the cancerous tissues was further confirmed by various procedures: incubation with minced tissues[24] and with homogenate,[25,26] RT-PCR,[11,27] and microarray.[10] Poorly differentiated cancerous tissues showed less activity than well differentiated ones. Metabolic foci in lymph nodes revealed scant activity[28] and no expression of SRD5A1 or SRD5A2 mRNA.[29] Although a few opposing findings are present,[8,9] decreased 5α-reductase activity in cancer tissues has been indicated in many other reports. In this context, hormone concentrations (pM/dry weight) in normal, benign hyperplastic, and cancerous prostate tissues were: 12.6 ± 2.3, 14.1 ± 2.4, and 39.6 ± 6.2 of testosterone; 12.9 ± 1.9, 45.5 ± 5.8, and 22.4 ± 2.4 of DHT; and no detectable level, 30.0 ± 7.6, and 42.0 ± 7.9 of androst-4-ene-3,17-dione, respectively.[30]

DHT is further metabolized to 5α-androstane-3α,17β-diol and, to a lesser extent, 5α-androstane-3β,17β-diol in the prostate. The former is converted to androsterone.[31] To assess the activity of 5α-reductase, measurements of 5α-androstane-3α,17β-diol glucuronide and androsterone glucuronide in serum are commonly used. The oxidative reaction of 5α-androstane-3α,17β-diol has been discussed, since dog prostate hyperplasia can effectively be induced with this steroid, perhaps by its conversion to DHT. However, in cases of prostate cancer, this reaction does not seem to be substantial.[32]

Percutaneous administration of dehydroepiandrosterone to healthy aged male volunteers caused an increase of androst-4-ene-3,17-dione and conjugated metabolites of DHT (glucuronides of androsterone, 5α-androstane-3α,17β-diol and 5α-androstane-3β,17β-diol) in serum, despite unchanged levels of testosterone and DHT.[33] In patients who underwent castration, the serum ratio of DHT/testosterone increased,[34] and 58% of DHT remained in the serum, in contrast to the 92% reduction of serum testosterone,[35] suggesting that adrenal androgen is a precursor of DHT. The prostate contains metabolizing enzymes for the conversion of dehydroepiandrosterone and its sulfate, and androst-4-ene-3,17-dione to DHT, including sulfatase,[36] 3β-hydroxysteroid dehydrogenase,[37] and 17β-hydroxysteroid dehydrogenase.[38,39] An estimated 30%–50% of total androgens in men are synthesized in peripheral tissues, including the prostate, from inactive adrenal precursors.[40] In a 14-year follow-up of 1008 men, the total testosterone, estrone, estradiol, and sex hormone-binding globulin levels did not correlate with the incidence of prostate cancer, but androst-4-ene-3,17-dione showed a positive dose-response gradient, suggesting an adrenal contribution.[41] Although the proportion of adrenal androgen acting as precursors of DHT is uncertain, adrenal androgen must be considered in striving for complete block of DHT formation for prostate cancer treatment. It is a clinical issue whether endocrine therapy can be achieved by suppression of the testicular hormone alone or whether elimination of influence from adrenal androgens is necessary.

Risk of DHT Formation

Men castrated at a young age and patients with male hypogonadism seldom experience prostate cancer. Ethnic differences in the incidence of clinical prostate cancer are evident, although differences in the incidence of latent cancer among the races are small. Therefore, the activity of 5α-reductase in the formation of DHT may be an etiological and/or progressive factor in clinical cancer.[42]

The levels of total and free testosterone in African-Americans were 19% and 21% higher than those in whites (both $p = 0.02$), respectively.[43] Three reports, in which testosterone, DHT, estradiol, and sex hormone-binding globulin were measured in prospective cohort studies, were reviewed by meta-analysis.[44] Men whose total testosterone level was in the highest quartile were 2.34-fold more likely to develop prostate cancer than men in the lowest quartile. Levels of DHT and estradiol did not differ significantly, but low sex hormone-binding globulin was revealed as a risk factor. Thus, levels of circulating bioavailable testosterone may be associated with prostate cancer. On the contrary, the serum testosterone level in Japanese youths was not different from that of Caucasian and African-American youths in the USA, but the latter two groups had increased serum levels of 3α,17β-androstanediol glucuronide and androsterone glucuronide, suggesting high DHT formation.[45] Racial differences in the activity of SRD5A2 continue as men age.[46] A high serum testosterone level correlates with high grade cancer[47] and increased risk of relapse.[48] Conversely, patients with high grade cancer had correlated low level of serum testosterone,[49,50] however, the initial step in the development of prostate cancer may be proceeded more by increased levels of androgen. The activity of 5α-reductase in the prostate increased by various androgens via feed-forward control.[51–53] Therefore, an increased level of testosterone, even a small increase, serves as a substrate and raises the activity of 5α-reductase, which consequently elevates the DHT level.

The gene encoding SRD5A2 contains five exons and is located on chromosome 2p23. No specific mutations or polymorphisms of 5α-reductase have been detected in the families of patients with hereditary prostate cancer.[54] Therefore, polymorphisms of SRD5A2 in a comparison between ethnic groups or in a case-control study have widely been examined. The number of dinucleotide repeats (TA)n in the 3′ untranslated region of the 5α-reductase gene was discussed in relation to the risk of prostate cancer,[55] because longer alleles may cause a modest reduction in the activity of the enzyme. Initially, differences in the number of repeats were found among the races, but no evidence revealed any correlation between the differences and the risk.[56] The (TA)n repeats were not correlated with the level of androstane-3α,17β-diol glucuronide.[57] On the contrary, in the Chinese population, which has the lowest incidence of prostate cancer, men who are heterozygous for the (TA)0/(TA)n allele had a modest risk reduction compared with men who are homozygous for the (TA)0 allele and have higher serum DHT levels.[58] Men who are homozygous for the (TA)9 or (TA)18 alleles and men who are of the (TA)9/(TA)18 genotype have a modestly reduced risk.[59] The number of (TA)n repeats was related with age at the onset of prostate cancer.[60] Of 208 patients with localized prostate cancer, 30 were (TA)n heterozygotes in peripheral lymphocytes, and this genotype was then compared with that of tumor DNA. Fifty-seven percent of the tumors showed loss of heterozygosity (LOH) or microsatellite instability in this marker. Tumors showing these somatic mutations tend to be of a high grade and stage.[61] Together with these reports, (TA)n repeat length may partly be viewed as an etiologic/progressive factor.[62]

Screening among healthy, racially/ethnically diverse male populations detected 10 missense substitutions and three double mutations that are all naturally found in human males.[63] Of the ten single amino acid substitutions, V89L (substitution of leucine for valine at codon 89) is on almost 33% of the chromosomes, followed by A49T (substitution of threonine for alanine at codon 49) on 2.0%. Other mutations are rare, at less than 2%. The Vmax of A49T is 5-fold higher than that of the wild type, and the Vmax of V89L shows 50% reduced activity.

In men with the LL genotype of V89L, the serum levels of testosterone and free testosterone were reduced by 12% and 16% respectively, and that of 5α-androstane-3α,17β-diol glucuronide was reduced by 10%.[64] The frequency of the VV genotype was the highest in African-Americans at 58.9%, lower in Caucasians at 57.1%, and the lowest in Asians at 29.4 %.[65] The VV genotype is associated with a higher serum level of 5α-androstane-3α,17β-diol glucuronide than the VL and LL genotype, thus a correlation with the higher incidence of prostate cancer in African-Americans was suggested. Men with the V allele are at a 2-fold greater risk for prostate cancer development and an additional 2-fold increase in the risk of progression when compared to men with the LL genotype.[66] Similarly, men with the VV or VL genotypes had an increased risk for prostate cancer compared with those with the LL genotype.[67] On the contrary, no correlation between the V89L genotype and prostate cancer was reported,[58–60,68] or conversely, the L allele may be of a risk but not significantly.[69–72] Finally, meta-analysis from nine studies concluded no association between SRD5A2 genotype and prostate cancer risk.[62]

An association between A49T polymorphism and prostate cancer was reported in African-Americans and Hispanic men.[73] The missense mutation in healthy men of both populations is rare, but men with AT/TT genotypes have increased risk of clinically significant cancer at 7.2-fold in African-Americans and 3.6-fold in Hispanic men. The polymorphism was correlated with extracapsular extension in Caucasians.[74] On the contrary, no association was found between this polymorphism and tumor stage, grade, or family history.[75] Men with one or two copies of the variant T allele had a 24% lower androstanediol glucuronide level than men homozygous for the wild type allele.[57] Meta-analysis, however, revealed a modest effect of T allele on cancer.[62] The T allele was not detected in the Japanese population, indicating racial differences in the polymorphism. R227Q (substitution of glutamine for arginine at codon 227) significantly reduces enzyme activity, but men with RQ phenotype are rare, and this polymorphism was not associated with prostate cancer.[58]

From these reports, it seems to be difficult to determine the risk for prostate cancer attributable to polymorphisms of SRD5A2. In each case-control study, selection of the control group could not completely exclude men with tiny foci of cancer or benign hyperplastic prostate, which is an androgen-dependent disease. The Japanese population is considered to be ethnically homogeneous, and the incidence of prostate cancer was formerly low. However, the incidence is increasing at the fastest rate of all male malignancies, therefore, the different incidences among countries can not be explained by racial differences only. Finally, reports of genetic association are influenced by study size and time of publication, thus results have been variable.[76]

The diet of Japanese men has changed to include foods with high fat and protein compositions since World War II. A diet of 25% reduced fat and the same total calories caused a 10% decrease in serum testosterone of healthy volunteers.[77] Isoflavonoids (genistein and daidzein) derived from soybean and green tea gallates (epigallocatechin-3-gallate and epicatechin-3-gallate) are favorite foods for Oriental men, and are also 5α-reductase inhibitors.[78,79] γ-Linolenic acid,[80] eicosapentaenoic acid,[81] and free fatty acids[82] are also inhibitors. Ingested foods may influence androgen metabolism, and consequently the incidence of prostate cancer.

Treatment with Inhibitors

The 5α-reductase activity in rat prostate and human skin fibroblasts was inhibited by estrogen,[83,84] progesterone, and deoxycorticosterone acetate.[85] 6-Methyleneprogesterone is also an inhibitor.[86] These inhibitors are natural steroids or their derivatives and have other hormonal effect. Subsequently, pure inhibitors have been synthesized; some specifically inhibit one type of enzyme (SRD5A1 or SRD5A2), while others inhibit both types of enzyme.[87]

4-aza-3-oxo-1-ene (finasteride, dutasteride, PNU157706), 4-aza-3-oxo-4-methyl (4MA, turosteride), 3-carboxylic steroid (SKF105657), and other androstane derivatives[88] are steroidal inhibitors, and benzoquinolinone (bexlosteride, izonsteride), ONO 3805, and FK 143 are nonsteroidal inhibitors. Bexlosteride, a SRD5A1 inhibitor, inhibits testosterone-stimulated LNCaP (possessing SRD5A1) cell growth in culture at 10 nM and 100 nM, but the compound shows no effect without testosterone.[89] In transplantable androgen-dependent tumors in animals, growth retardation was shown with the following systems; 4MA for the Noble tumor,[90] and PNU 157706 and turosteride for the Dunning R3327 tumor.[91,92] Treatment with inhibitors evokes retardation of tumor growth, but the effect is rather weak when compared with castration, suggesting that the remaining testosterone promotes tumor growth. Alternatively, weak retardation of the growth may be due to incomplete suppression of DHT formation, especially in cases where a specific SRD5A2 inhibitor is used.

Asymptomatic patients with stage D prostate cancer were treated with 10 mg of finasteride daily for up to 12 weeks, and their clinical data were compared with those from the placebo group.[93] Treatment with finasteride decreased the serum levels of PSA and DHT, but did not affect prostatic acid phosphatase, testosterone, prostate volume, or appearance of bone scan. Patients with untreated M1 cancers were treated with luteinizing hormone-releasing hormone (LHRH) analog and finasteride, flutamide, or both. After 12 weeks, PSA levels decreased in all three groups, but no differences were noticed on bone scan scores or in performance status.[94] Treatment with finasteride did not change the histological pattern of cancer.[95] Therefore, finasteride may be, if necessary, applied with other drugs to bolster the effects. Treatment with finasteride (5 mg/day) and flutamide (250 mg tid) for relapsed or metastatic cancer evoked a considerable result, accounting for 65% of the overall survival at 5 years.[96]

Prevention

The ACI/Seg rat has a 63% incidence rate of spontaneous prostate cancer by 140 weeks of age. Treatment with 20 ppm of FK 143 in the diet reduced the incidence of tumor formation to some extent, but treatment with 200 ppm of the same inhibitor showed no effect, suggesting that the lack of effect is due, at least partly, to increased testosterone in the prostate.[97] In F344 rats, treatment with dimethylaminobiphenyl causes prostate cancer. Finasteride reduced the number of visible tumors, but the total number of visible and microscopic tumors was the same as that for the control, thus finasteride may delay the development of tumors to macroscopic size.[98] Finasteride reduced prostate tumor incidence by 10% in Wistar rats treated with methylnitrosourea/testosterone propionate, and the chemopreventive activity is suspected to occur by suppression of prostatic polyamine synthesis.[99] These animal experiments suggest rather weak, if any, inhibiting effect of 5α-reductase inhibitors on the development of prostate cancer.

During treatment of benign hyperplastic prostate with a daily dose of 5 mg finasteride, occurrence of prostate cancer was surveyed. Incidence of cancer was 1% and 2% in the finasteride and placebo groups, respectively, during the 2 years of a Canadian trial.[100] In the USA, both groups showed the same cancer incidence at 5% for 4 years.[101] Fifty-two men with increased PSA but negative biopsy were divided into the finasteride and placebo groups.[102] The finasteride group showed a decrease in serum PSA by 48% and in DHT by 67%, but an increase in testosterone by 21%. The incidence of cancer was 4% (one man) in the placebo group but 30% (eight men) in the finasteride group. These results indicate that the short-term administration of finasteride cannot restrain the clinical outbreak of prostate cancer.

The Prostate Cancer Prevention Trial was started in the USA in 1993; 18,882 men 55 years of age or older with normal digital rectal examination and 3 ng/ml or less of PSA were divided into the finasteride (5 mg daily) or placebo groups.[103] After 7 years, prostate cancer was detected in 18.4% men in the finasteride group and in 24.4% of men in the placebo group, thus a 24.8% reduction in the occurrence of cancer was calculated during this period. Tumors of Gleason score 7–10 accounted for 37.0% in the finasteride group and 22.2% in the placebo group, thus the rate of malignancy increased by 1.7% with finasteride. Additionally, more sexual side effects and fewer urinary symptoms were noticed in the finasteride group. This raises the question as to whether finasteride retarded the growth of low grade cancers but could not suppress high grade cancers.

From this report, an argument on balancing diminished incidence rate and increased tumor malignancy due to finasteride has arisen. A consensus of opinion has not yet been reached (see *New Engl J Med* 2003, 349: Scardino *et al.*, p. 297, and Rubin *et al.*, p. 1569). However, chemopreventative treatments involving 5α-reductase inhibitor remain in use.

Conclusion

It is widely accepted that DHT, formed by 5α-reductase in the prostate, plays a pivotal role in the development of prostate cancer. Therefore, metabolism of DHT in the prostate is an etiologic and progressive factor. At present, the association between structural variants of 5α-reductase and prostate cancer risk might not clearly be demonstrated from the results of studies considering ethnicity as well as case-control differences. Other factors involved in androgen synthesis and metabolism may cooperate to influence the risk of prostate cancer. Application of 5α-reductase inhibitors in therapy and prevention seem to be ineffectual, thus further studies are required.

References

1. Huggins C, Hodges CV (1941) Studies of prostate cancer: I Effect of castration, estrogen and androgen injections on serum phosphatases in metastatic carcinoma of the prostate. *Cancer Res* 1:293–297.
2. Russell DW, Wilson JD (1994) Steroid 5α-reductase: Two genes/two enzymes. *Ann Rev Biochem* 63:25–61.
3. Normington K, Russell DW (1992) Tissue distribution and kinetic characteristics of rat steroid 5α-reductase isozymes. *J Biol Chem* 267: 19548–19554.
4. Berman DM, Russell DW (1993) Cell-type-specific expression of rat steroid 5α-reductase isozymes. *Proc Natl Acad Sci USA* 90:9359–9363.
5. Miyamoto T, Kagawa S, Kitagawa S, Futaki S, Yokoi H, Tsuruo Y, Ishimura K (1996) Immunocytochemical localization of 5α-reductase type I in the prostate of normal and castrated rats. *Histochem Cell Biol* 105:101–109.
6. Thigpen AE, Silver RI, Guileyardo JM, Casey ML, McConnell JD, Russell DW (1993) Tissue distribution and ontogeny of steroid 5α-reductase isozyme expression. *J Clin Invest* 92:903–910.

7. Silver RI, Wiley EL, Thigpen AE, Guileyardo JM, McConnell JD, Russell DW (1994) Cell type specific expression of 5α-reductase 2. *J Urol* 152:438–442.

8. Bonkhoff H, Stein U, Aumuller G, Remberger K (1996) Differential expression of 5α-reductase isozymes in the human prostate and prostatic carcinomas. *Prostate* 29:261–267.

9. Iehle C, Radvanyi F, de Medina SGD, Ouafik LH, Gerard H, Chopin D, Raynaud J-P, Martin P-M (1999) Differences in steroid 5α-reductase iso-enzymes expression between normal and pathological human prostate tissue. *J Steroid Biochem Mol Biol* 68:189–195.

10. Luo J, Dunn TA, Ewing CM, Walsh PC, Isaacs WB (2003) Decreased gene expression of steroid 5alpha-reductase 2 in human prostate cancer: Implications for finasteride therapy of prostate carcinoma. *Prostate* 57: 134–139.

11. Soderstrom TG, Bjelfman C, Brekkan E, Ask B, Egevad L, Norlen BJ, Rane A (2001) Messenger ribonucleic acid levels of steroid 5α-reductase 2 in human prostate predict the enzyme activity. *J Clin Endocrinol Metab* 86:855–858.

12. Bruchovsky N, Rennie P, Batzold FH, Goldenberg SL, Fletcher T, Mc Loughlin MG (1988) Kinetic parameters of 5α-reductase activity in stroma and epithelium of normal, hyperplastic, and carcinomatous human prostates. *J Clin Endocrinol Metab* 67:806–816.

13. Negri-Cesi P, Poletti A, Colciago A, Magni P, Martini P, Motta M (1998) Presence of 5alpha-reductase isozymes and aromatase in human prostate cancer cells and in benign prostate hyperplastic tissue. *Prostate* 34: 283–291.

14. Negri-Cesi P, Colciago A, Poletti A, Motta M (1999) 5alpha-reductase isozymes and aromatase are differentially expressed and active in the androgen-independent human prostate cancer cell lines DU 145 and PC-3. *Prostate* 41:224–232.

15. Delos S, Iehle C Martin P-M, Raynaud J-P (1994) Inhibition of the activity of "basic" 5α-reductase (type 1) detected in DU145 cells and expressed in insect cells. *J Steroid Biochem Mol Biol* 48:347–352.

16. Zhu YS, Cai LQ, You X, Cordero JJ, Huang Y, Imperato-McGinley J (2003) Androgen-induced prostate-specific antigen gene expression is mediated via dihydrotestosterone in LNCaP cells. *J Androl* 24:681–687.

17. Delos S, Carsol J-L, Fina F, Raynaud J-P, Martin P-M (1998) 5α-reductase and 17β-hydroxysteroid dehydrogenase expression in epithelial cells from hyperplastic and malignant human prostate. *Int J Cancer* 75:840–846.

18. Thomas LN, Douglas RC, Vessey JP, Gupta R, Fontaine D, Norman RW, Thompson IM, Troyer DA, Rittmaster RS, Lazier CB (2003) 5alpha-reductase type 1 immunostaining is enhanced in some prostate cancers compared with benign prostatic hyperplasia epithelium. *J Urol* 170: 2019–2025.

19. Thigpen AE, Davis DL, Milatovich A, Mendonca BB, Imperato-McGinley J, Griffin JE, Francke U, Wilson JD, Russell DW (1992) Molecular genetics of steroid 5alpha-reductase 2 deficiency. *J Clin Invest* 90:799–809.

20. Shimazaki J, Kurihara H, Ito Y, Shida K (1965) Testosterone metabolism in prostate: Formation of androstane-17β-ol-3-one and androst-4-ene-3,17-dione, and inhibitory effect of natural and synthetic estrogens. *Gunma J Med Sci* 14:313–325.

21. Shimazaki J, Kurihara H, Ito Y, Shida K (1965) Metabolism of testosterone in prostate (2nd report): Separation of prostatic 17β-ol-dehydrogenase and 5α-reductase. *Gunma J Med Sci* 14:326–333.

22. Bruchovsky N, Wilson JD (1968) The conversion of testosterone to 5α-androstane-17β-ol-3-one by rat prostate *in vivo* and *in vitro*. *J Biol Chem* 243:2012–2021.

23. Anderson KM, Liao S (1968) Selective retention of dihydrotestosterone by prostatic nuclei. *Nature (London)* 219:277–279.

24. Prout GR Jr, Kliman B, Daly JJ, McLaughlin RA, Griffin PP (1976) *In vitro* uptake of ^{3}H testosterone and its conversion to dihydrotestosterone by prostatic carcinoma and other tissues. *J Urol* 116:603–610.

25. Ghanadian R, Smith CB (1982) Metabolism of steroids in the prostate. In: Ghanadian R, ed. *The Endocrinology of Prostate Tumors*. MTP Press, Lancaster, pp. 113–142.

26. Brendler CB, Follansbee AL, Isaacs JT (1985) Discrimination between normal, hyperplastic, and malignant humans' prostatic tissues by enzymatic profiles. *J Urol* 133:495–501.

27. Bjelfman C, Soderstrom TG, Brekkan E, Norlen BJ, Egevad L, Unge T, Andersson S, Rane A (1997) Differential gene expression of steroid 5α-reductase 2 in core needle biopsies from malignant and benign prostatic tissue. *J Clin Endocrinol Metab* 82:2210–2214.

28. Ghanadian R, Masters JRW, Smith CB (1981) Altered androgen metabolism in carcinoma of the prostate. *Eur Urol* 7:169–170.

29. Habib FK, Ross M, Bayne CW, Bollina P, Grigor K, Chapman K (2003) The loss of 5α-reductase type I and type II mRNA expression in metastatic prostate cancer to bone and lymph node metastasis. *Clin Cancer Res* 9: 1815–1819.

30. Habib FK (1982) Factors controlling abnormal growth. In: Chisholm GD, Williams DI, eds. *Scientific Foundations of Urology*, 2nd ed. William Heineman Medical Books, London, pp. 499–505.

31. Kliman B, Prout GR, McLaughlin RA, Daly JJ, Griffin PP (1978) Altered androgen metabolism in metastatic prostate cancer. *J Urol* 119: 623–626.

32. Rizner TL, Lin HK, Peehl DM, Steckelbroeck S, Bauman DR, Penning TM (2003) Human type 3 3α-hydroxysteroid dehydrogenase (aldo-keto reductase 1C2) and androgen metabolism in prostate cells. *Endocrinology* 144: 2922–2932.

33. Labrie F, Belanger A, Cusan L, Candas B (1997) Physiological changes in dehydroepiandrosterone are not reflected by serum levels of active androgens and estrogens but of their metabolites: Intracrinology. *J Clin Endocrinol Metab* 82:2403–2409.

34. Rohl HF, Beuke H-P (1992) Effect of orchidectomy on serum concentrations of testosterone and dihydrotestosterone in patients with prostate cancer. *Scand J Urol Nephrol* 26:11–14.

35. Ying J, Yao DH, Ren XM (2003) Study of sexual hormone changes in prostate cancer patients before and after androgen deprivation therapy. *Zhonghua Nan Ke Xue* 9:191–192.

36. Farnsworth WE (1973) Human prostatic dehydroepiandrosterone sulfate sulfatase. *Steroids* 21:647–664.

37. Labrie F, Luu-The V, Lin SX, Simard J, Labrie C, El-Alfy M, Pelletier G, Belanger A (2000) Intracrinology: role of the family of 17β-hydroxysteroid dehydrogenases in human physiology and disease. *J Mol Endocrinol* 25:1–16.

38. Lin H-K, Jez JM, Schlegel BP, Peehl DM, Pachter JA, Penning TM (1997) Expression and characterization of recombinant type 2 3α-hydroxysteroid dehydrogenase (HSD) from human prostate: Demonstration of bifunctional 3α/17β-HSD activity and cellular distribution. *Mol Endocrinol* 11: 1971–1984.

39. Dufort I, Rheault P, Huang X-F, Soucy P, Luu-The V (1999) Characteristics of a highly labile human type 5 17β-hydroxysteroid dehydrogenase. *Endocrinology* 140:568–574.

40. Labrie F, Belanger A, Luu-The V, Labrie C, Simard J, Cusan L, Gomez J-L, Candas B (1998) DHEA and the intracrine formation of androgens and estrogens in peripheral target tissues: Its role during aging. *Steroids* 63: 322–328.

41. Barrett-Connor E, Garland C, McPhillips JB, Khaw K-T, Wingard DL (1990) A prospective, population-based study of androstenedione, estrogens and prostate cancer. *Cancer Res* 50:169–173.

42. Ross RK, Reichardt JKV, Ingles SA, Coetzee GA (2001) The genetic epidemiology of prostate cancer. In: Chung LWK, Isaacs WB, Simons JW, eds. *Prostate Cancer.* Humana Press, Totowa, NJ, pp. 111–121.

43. Ross R, Bernstein L, Judd H, Hanisch R, Pike M, Henderson B (1986) Serum testosterone levels in healthy young black and white men. *J Natl Cancer Inst* 76:45–48.

44. Shaneyfelt T, Husein R, Bubley G, Mantzoros CS (2000) Hormonal predictors of prostate cancer: A meta-analysis. *J Clin Oncol* 18:847–853.

45. Ross RK, Bernstein L, Lobo RA, Shimizu H, Stanczyk FZ, Pike MC, Henderson BE (1992) 5-alpha-reductase activity and risk of prostate cancer among Japanese and US white and black males. *Lancet* 339:887–889.

46. Wu AH, Whittemore AS, Kolonel LN, Stanczyk FZ, John EM, Gallagher RP, West DW (2001) Lifestyle determinants of 5α-reductase metabolites in older African-American, White, and Asian-American men. *Cancer Epidemiol Biomarkers Prev* 10:533–538.

47. Gustafsson O, Norming U, Gustafsson S, Eneroth P, Astrom G, Nyman CR (1996) Dihydrotestosterone and testosterone levels in men screened for prostate cancer: a study of a randomized population. *Br J Urol* 77:433–440.

48. Zagars GK, Pollack A, von Eschenbach AC (1997) Serum testosterone — a significant determinant of metastatic relapse for irradiated localized prostate cancer. *Urology* 49:327–334.

49. Schatzl G, Madersbacher S, Thurridl T, Waldmuller J, Kramer G, Haitel A, Marberger M (2001) High-grade prostate cancer is associated with low serum testosterone levels. *Prostate* 47:52–58.

50. Zhang PL, Rosen S, Veeramachaneni R, Kao J, De Wolf WC, Bubley G (2002) Association between prostate cancer and serum testosterone levels. *Prostate* 53:179–182.

51. Shimazaki J, Ohki Y, Matsushita M, Tanaka M, Shida K (1972) Further studies on testosterone 5α-reduction in rat ventral prostate. *Endocrinol Japan* 19:69–75.

52. Wilson JD (1975) Metabolism of testicular androgens, In: Hamilton DW, Greep RO, eds. *Handbook of Physiology, Section 7, Endocrinology, Vol 7.* American Physiological Society, Washington, pp. 491–508.

53. Torres JM, Ruiz E, Ortega E (2003) Development of a quantitative RT-PCR method to study 5α-reductase mRNA isozymes in rat prostate in different androgen status. *Prostate* 56:74–79.

54. Chang BL, Zheng SL, Isaacs CD, Turner AR, Bleecker ER, Walsh PC, Meyers DA, Isaacs WB, Xu J (2003) Evaluation of SDR5A2 sequence variants in susceptibility to hereditary and sporadic prostate cancer. *Prostate* 56:37–44.

55. Kantoff P, Febbo P, Giovannuci E, Krithivas K, Dahl D, Chang G, Hennekens C, Brown M, Stampfer M (1997) A polymorphism of the 5α-reductase gene and its association with prostate cancer: A case-control analysis. *Cancer Epidemiol Biomarkers Prev* 6:189–192.

56. Ross RK, Pike MC, Coetzee GA, Reichardt JKV, Yu MC, Feigelson H, Stanczyk FZ, Kolonel LN, Henderson BE (1998) Androgen metabolism and prostate cancer: Establishing a model of genetic susceptibility. *Cancer Res* 58:4497–4504.

57. Allen NE, Reichardt JK, Nguyen H, Key TJ (2003) Association between two polymorphisms in the SRD5A2 gene and serum androgen concentrations in British men. *Cancer Epidemiol Biomarkers Prev* 12:578–581.

58. Hsing AW, Chen C, Chokkalingam AP, Gao YT, Dightman DA, Nguyen HT, Deng J, Cheng J, Sesterhenn IA, Mostofi FK, Stanczyk FZ, Reichardt JK (2001) Polymorphic markers in the SRD5A2 gene and prostate cancer risk: a population-based case-control study. *Cancer Epidemiol Biomarkers Prev* 10:1077–1082.

59. Lamharzi N, Johnson MM, Goodman G, Etzioni R, Weiss NS, Dightman DA, Barnett M, Di Tommaso D, Chen C (2003) Polymorphic markers in the 5alpha-reductase type II gene and the incidence of prostate cancer. *Int J Cancer* 105:480–483.

60. Latil AG, Azzouzi R, Cancel GS, Guillaume EC, Cochan-Priollet B, Berthon PL, Cussenot O (2001) Prostate carcinoma risk and allelic variants of genes involved in androgen biosynthesis and metabolism pathways. *Cancer* 92:1130–1137.

61. Akalu A, Elmajian DA, Highshaw RA, Nicholls PW, Reichardt JK (1999) Somatic mutations at the SRD5A2 locus encoding prostatic steroid 5alpha-reductase during prostate cancer progression. *J Urol* 161:1355–1358.

62. Ntais C, Polycarpou A, Ioannidis JP (2003) SRD5A2 gene polymorphisms and the risk of prostate cancer: a meta-analysis. *Cancer Epidemiol Biomarkers Prev* 12:618–624.

63. Makridakis NM, di Salle E, Reichardt JK (2000) Biochemical and pharmacogenetic dissection of human steroid 5alpha-reductase type II. *Pharmacogenetics* 10:407–413.

64. Allen NE, Forrest MS, Key TJ (2001) The association between polymorphisms in the CYP 17 and 5α-reductase (SRD5A2) genes and serum androgen concentrations in men. *Cancer Epidemiol Biomarkers Prev* 10: 185–189.

65. Makridakis N, Ross RK, Pike MC, Chang L, Stanczyk FZ, Kolonel LN, Shi CY, Yu MC, Henderson BE, Reichardt JK (1997) A prevalent missense

substitution that modulates activity of prostatic steroid 5alpha-reductase. *Cancer Res* 57:1020–1022.

66. Nam RK, Toi A, Vesprini D, Ho M, Chu W, Harvie S, Sweet J, Trachtenberg J, Jewett MAS, Narod SA (2001) V89L polymorphism of type-2, 5-alpha reductase enzyme gene predicts prostate cancer presence and progression. *Urology* 57:199–205.

67. Li Z, Habuchi T, Mitsumori K, Kamoto T, Kinoshitu H, Segawa T, Ogawa O, Kato T (2003) Association of V89L SRD5A2 polymorphism with prostate cancer development in a Japanese population. *J Urol* 169: 2378–2381.

68. Febbo PG, Kantoff PW, Platz EA, Casey D, Batter S, Giovannucci E, Hennekens CH, Stampfer MJ (1999) The V89L polymorphism in the 5α-reductase type 2 gene and risk of prostate cancer. *Cancer Res* 59: 5878–5881.

69. Lunn RM, Bell DA, Mohler JL, Taylor JA (1999) Prostate cancer risk and polymorphism in 17 hydroxylase (CYP 17) and steroid reductase (SRD5A2). *Carcinogenesis* 20:1727–1731.

70. Yamada Y, Watanabe M, Murata M, Yamanaka M, Kubota Y, Ito H, Kato T, Kawamura J, Yatani R, Shiraishi T (2001) Impact of genetic polymorphisms of 17-hydroxylase cytochrome P-450 (CYP 17) and steroid 5α-reductase type II (SRD5A2) genes on prostate-cancer risk among the Japanese population. *Int J Cancer* 92:683–686.

71. Soderstrom T, Wadelius M, Andersson SO, Johansson JE, Johansson S, Granath F, Rane A (2002) 5alpha-reductase 2 polymorphisms as risk factors in prostate cancer. *Phamacogenetics* 12:307–312.

72. Shibata A, Gurcia MI, Cheng I, Stamey TA, McNeal JE, Brooks JD, Henderson S, Yemoto CE, Peehl DM (2002) Polymorphisms in the androgen receptor and type II 5α-reductase genes and prostate cancer prognosis. *Prostate* 52:269–278.

73. Makridakis NM, Ross RK, Pike MC, Crocitto LE, Kolonel LN, Pearce CL, Henderson BE, Reichardt JK (1999) Association of missense substitution in SRD5A2 gene with prostate cancer in African-American and Hispanic men in Los Angeles, USA. *Lancet* 354:975–978.

74. Jaffe JM, Malkowicz SB, Walker AH, MacBride S, Peschel R, Tomaszewski J, van Arsdalen K, Wein AJ, Rebbeck TR (2000) Association of SRD5A2 genotype and pathological characteristics of prostate tumors. *Cancer Res* 60:1626–1630.

75. Mononen N, Ikonen T, Syrijakoski K, Matikainen M, Schleutker J, Tammela TL, Koivisto PA, Kallioniemi OP (2001) A missense substitution

A49T in the steroid 5-α-reductase gene (SRD5A2) is not associated with prostate cancer in Finland. *Br J Cancer* 84:1344–1347.

76. Loannidis JPA, Trikalinos TA, Ntzani EE, Contopoulos-Ioannidis DG (2003) Genetic associations in large versus small studies: an empirical assessment. *Lancet* 361:567–571.

77. Hamalainen E, Adlercreutz H, Puska P, Pietinen P (1984) Diet and serum sex hormones in healthy men. *J Steroid Biochem* 20:459–464.

78. Evans BAJ, Griffiths K, Morton M (1995) Inhibition of 5alpha-reductase in genital skin fibroblasts and prostate tissue by dietary ligands and isoflavonoids. *J Endocrinol* 147:295–302.

79. Liao S, Hiipakka RA (1995) Selective inhibition of steroid 5α-reductase isozymes by tea epicatechin-3-gallate and epigallocatechin-3-gallate. *Biochem Biophys Res Commun* 214:833–838.

80. Kokontis JM, Liao S (1999) Molecular action of androgen in the normal and neoplastic prostate. *Vitamin Hormone* 55:219–307.

81. Pham H, Ziboh VA (2002) 5alpha-reductase-catalyzed conversion of testosterone to dihydrotestosterone is increased in prostatic adenocarcinoma cells: suppression by 15-lipoxygenase metabolites of gamma-linolenic and eicosapentaenoic acids. *J Steroid Biochem Mol Biol* 82:393–400.

82. Raynaud JP, Cousse H, Martin PM (2002) Inhibition of type 1 and type 2 5alpha reductase activity by free fatty acids, active ingredients of permixon. *J Steroid Biochem Mol Biol* 82:233–239.

83. Shimazaki J, Ohki Y, Koya A, Shida K (1972) Inhibition of nuclear testosterone 5α-reductase in rat ventral prostate by estrogens and anti-androgens. *Endocrinol Japan* 19:585–588.

84. Lee DKH, Young JC, Tamura Y, Patterson DC, Bird CE, Clark AF (1973) *In vitro* effects of estrogens on the Δ^4–reduction of testosterone by rat prostate and liver preparations. *Can J Biochem* 51:735–740.

85. Voigt W, Fernandez EP, Hsia S (1970) Transformation of testosterone into 17β-hydroxy-5α-androstan-3-one by microsomal preparations of human skin. *J Biol Chem* 245:5594–5499.

86. Petrow V, Wang Y-S, Lack L, Sandberg A, Kadohama N, Kendle K (1983) Prostate cancer II. Inhibitors of rat prostatic 4-ene-3-ketosteroid 5α-reductase derived from 6-methylene-4-androsten-3-ones. *J Steroid Biochem* 19: 1491–1502.

87. Shimazaki J (2002) The role of 5α-reductase in prostate disease and male pattern baldness. In: Chang C, ed. *Androgens and Androgen Receptor.* Kluwer Academic Pub, pp. 155–196.

88. Nnane IP, Kato K, Liu Y, Lu Q, Wang X, Ling Y-Z, Brodie A (1998) Effects of some novel inhibitors of $C_{17,20}$-lyase and 5α-reductase *in vitro* and *in vivo* and their potential role in the treatment of prostate cancer. *Cancer Res* 58:3826–3832.

89. Sutkowski DM, Audia JE, Goodie RL, Hsiao KC, Leibovitch IY, McNulty AM and Neubauer BL (1996) Responses of LNCaP prostatic adenocarcinoma cell cultures to LY 300502, a benzoquinolinone human type 1 5α-reductase inhibitor. *Prostate* 6(Suppl):62–66.

90. Kadohama N, Wakisaka M, Kim U, Karr JP, Murphy GP, Sandberg AA (1985) Retardation of prostate tumor progression in the Noble rat by 4-methyl-4-aza-steroidal inhibitors of 5α-reductase. *J Natl Cancer Inst* 74:475–486.

91. Di Salle E, Giudici D, Racice A, Zaccheo T, Ornati G, Nesi M, Panzeri A, Delos S, Martin PM (1998) PNU 157706, a novel dual type I and II 5α-reductase inhibitor. *J Steroid Biochem Mol Biol* 64:179–186.

92. Zaccheo T, Giudici D, di Salle E (1998) Effect of early treatment of prostate cancer with the 5α-reductase inhibitor turosteride in Dunning R3327 prostatic carcinoma in rats. *Prostate* 35:237–242.

93. Presti JC Jr, Fair WR, Andriole G, Sogami PC, Seidmon EJ, Ferguson D, Ng J, Gormley GJ (1992) Multicenter, randomized, double-blind, placebo controlled study to investigate the effect of finasteride (MK-906) on stage D prostate cancer. *J Urol* 148:1201–1204.

94. Kirby R, Robertson C, Turkes A, Griffiths K, Denis LJ, Boyle P, Altwein J, Schroeder F (1999) Finasteride in association with either flutamide or goserelin as combination hormonal therapy in patients with stage M1 carcinoma of the prostate gland. *Prostate* 40:105–114.

95. Yang XJ, Lecksell K, Short K, Gottesman J, Peterson L, Bannow J, Schellhammer PF, Fitch WP, Hodge GB, Perra R, Rouse S, Waldsteicher J, Epstein JI (1999) PLESS study group. Does long-term finasteride therapy affect the histologic features of benign prostatic tissue and prostate cancer on needle biopsy? *Urology* 53:696–700.

96. Oh WK, Manola J, Bittmann L, Brufsky A, Kaplan ID, Smith MR, Kaufman DS, Kantoff PW (2003) Finasteride and flutamide therapy in patients with advanced prostate cancer: response to subsequent castration and long-term follow-up. *Urology* 62:99–104.

97. Homma Y, Kaneko M, Kondo Y, Kawabe K, Kakizoe T (1997) Inhibition of rat prostate carcinogenesis by a 5alpha-reductase inhibitor, FK 143. *J Natl Cancer Inst* 89:803–807.

98. Tsukamoto S, Akaza H, Onozawa M, Shirai T, Ideyama Y (1998) A five-alpha reductase inhibitor or antiandrogen prevents the progression of microscopic prostate carcinoma to macroscopic carcinoma in rats. *Cancer* 82: 531–537.

99. Esmat AY, Refaie FM, Shaheen MH, Said MM (2002) Chemoprevention of prostate carcinogenesis by DFMO and/or finasteride treatment in male Wistar rats. *Tumori* 88:513–521.

100. Nickel JC, Fradet Y, Boake RC, Pommerville PJ, Perreault J-P, Afridi SK, Elhilali MM (1996) Prospect Study Group 1996. Efficacy and safety of finasteride therapy for benign prostatic hyperplasia: results of a 2-year randomized controlled trial (the PROSPECT Study). *Can Med Assoc J* 155:1251–1259.

101. McConnell JD, Bruskewitz R, Walsh P, Andriole G, Lieber M, Holtgrewe HL, Albertsen P, Roehrborn CG, Nickel JC, Wang DZ, Taylor AM, Waldstreicher J (1998) The effect of finasteride on the risk of acute urinary retention and the need for surgical treatment among men with benign prostatic hyperplasia. *New Engl J Med* 338:557–563.

102. Cote RJ, Skinner EC, Salem CE, Mertes SJ, Stanczyk FZ, Henderson BE, Pike MC, Ross RK (1998) The effect of finasteride on the prostate gland in men with elevated serum prostate-specific antigen levels. *Br J Cancer* 78:413–418.

103. Thompson IM, Goodman PJ, Tangen CM, Lucia MS, Miller GJ, Ford LG, Lieber MM, Cespedes RD, Atkins JN, Lippman SM, Carlin SM, Ryan A, Szczepanek CM, Crowley JJ, Coltman Jr CA (2003) The influence of finasteride on the development of prostate cancer. *New Engl J Med* 349: 215–224.

11

ROLES OF VITAMIN E IN PROSTATE AND PROSTATE CANCER

Shuyuan Yeh, Jing Ni, Eugene Chang, Yi Yin and Ming Chen

Departments of Urology and Pathology
University of Rochester Medical Center, Rochester, New York

Introduction

In the United States, prostate cancer is the second leading cause of new cancer cases, accounting for approximately 33% of all new cases in males and is the second leading cause of cancer-related death of men, behind lung cancer.[1] Factors such as diet, exercise, and environment are all aspects related in the subsequent development of cancers. For example, statistics from the American Cancer Society show that the death rates of prostate cancer are greater in the United States compared to China.[1]

Epidemiological studies have indicated the protective roles of certain vitamins and minerals in prostate cancer.[2-4] Among these vitamins and minerals, vitamin E has been identified by researchers as a potent anticancer agent in the delay or prevention of prostate cancer. There is a variety of factors that affect the performance and effectiveness of vitamin E in the body. The method by which vitamin E is taken into the body is an area of concern. Another consideration is the efficacy of different isoforms of vitamin E including four tocopherols and four tocotrienols.[5] There are also numerous synthetic vitamin E analogs that have been proven to be effective *in vivo*, such as α-vitamin E succinate (VES).

In vivo animal and clinical studies support *in vitro* data on the effectiveness of vitamin E in curbing the growth of cancers through a variety of mechanisms including cell cycle inhibition, apoptosis, gene regulation, and antioxidation. This review discusses anticancer mechanisms of vitamin E other than its antioxidant activity, and supporting animal and clinical data. Upcoming clinical trials and a look at future study directions are also included.

Vitamin E and Its Analogs

Vitamin E refers to a family of compounds called tocopherols and tocotrienols. Both groups are further divided into four isoforms: α, β, γ, and δ. α-Tocopherol is the most commonly found natural form of vitamin E as it accounts for about 90% of all tocopherols in most mammalian tissues.[5] It has several esterified analogs including α-tocopheryl acetate (α-vitamin E acetate, VEA), α-tocopheryl nicotinate (α-vitamin E nicotinate, VEN), and α-tocopheryl succinate (α-vitamin E succinate, VES). Of all these forms, VES (vitamin E succinate) is the most effective in terms of its anticancer properties. Both *in vitro* and *in vivo* studies have shown that VES is capable of inducing apoptosis and inhibiting cell proliferation in cancer cells without affecting the proliferation of most normal cells.[6] VES can be hydrolyzed by esterase in the gastrointestinal tract and may thus lose some of its potency. *In vivo* animal studies have shown that an intraperitoneal injection is an effective delivery strategy of the VES.[7] A non-hydrolyzable ether forms, α-tocopheryl oxybutyric acid and ether acetic acid analogs, have been created as a solution for this loss of potency.[8–10]

In addition, Birringer *et al.* have shown that the modification of different functional moieties of the vitamin E molecule can enhance its proapoptotic properties. Analogs of VES with a lower number of methyl substitutions on the aromatic ring were less active than VES itself. Replacement of the succinyl group with a maleyl group greatly enhanced the activity. However, methylation of the free succinyl carboxyl group on VES completely abolished the apoptogenic activity of these compounds.[11]

Vitamin E Absorption and Transport

Major dietary sources of vitamin E include vegetable oils, margarine, nuts, seeds, whole grains, soybeans, eggs, and avocados. The recommended dietary allowance of vitamin E is 15 mg/day (15 mg = 22.5 IU),[12] however, common doses range from 100 to 800 IU/day with no significant adverse side effects, and have not been associated with mutagenic or teratogenic properties.[13]

Vitamin E is absorbed in the intestine and circulates through the lymphatic system. It is absorbed together with lipids, packed into chylomicrons, and transported to the liver. This process is similar for the various forms of vitamin E. After transport to the liver, α-tocopherol will be absorbed and released to the plasma. Most other ingested β-, γ-, and δ-tocopherols and tocotrienols are secreted into bile, or not absorbed and excreted in the feces.[5]

In the American diet the level of consumption of γ-tocopherol ranges from two to four times higher than the level of α-tocopherol. Both forms are equally well absorbed by the intestines, bound with chylomicron lipoprotein, and transported to liver, yet the plasma level of α-tocopherol is five to ten times higher than plasma levels of γ-tocopherol. This is attributed to α-tocopherol's higher affinity to a liver cytosolic tocopherol transfer protein (TTP) compared to γ-tocopherol. Therefore, TTP is a major determinant of plasma tocopherol levels. There have been studies that show that dietary supplementation with α-tocopherol will actually decrease levels of γ-tocopherol in the blood and adipose tissue[14,15] due to the limited binding capacity of the hepatic TTP.

Furthermore, Bonina's study indicates that α-tocopherol and VES (α-tocopheryl succinate) are incorporated into erythrocyte membranes with the help of specific transport proteins. The study suggested that other vitamin E transfer or binding proteins could exist and differences in membrane incorporation of α-tocopherol and VES might contribute to their variant cytoprotective properties.[16] Indeed, other vitamin E binding proteins, the tocopherol associated protein and tocopherol binding protein, were identified, but their functions were not fully characterized.[17–19]

Functional Mechanisms of Vitamin E in Prostate Cancer

Currently, a new clinical trial, SELECT,[20,21] has been initiated in the US, and an earlier epidemiological study also indicated that daily supplements of Vitamin E could reduce the incidence and mortality of prostate cancer.[2] However, the functional mechanisms remain largely unclear. We summarize the functional mechanisms of vitamin E as follows.

Vitamin E and Its Analogs Induce Proapoptotic Properties in Prostate Cancer Cells

α-Vitamin E (α-tocopherol) has been shown by researchers to have proapoptotic properties in human prostate cancer LNCaP cells. Their data showed that vitamin E administration resulted in reduced DNA synthesis and enhanced DNA fragmentation, as well as a general inhibition of cell proliferation.[22]

Another study by Gunawardena and colleagues, showed that α-tocopherol stimulated apoptosis in three different human prostate cancer cell lines: DU-145 (androgen-unresponsive), LNCaP (androgen-responsive), and ALVA-101 (moderately androgen-responsive). The group cited nucleosome fragmentation as evidence of apoptosis following α-tocopherol treatment in these different prostate cancer cell lines.[23]

Furthermore, results from other researchers indicated that the apoptosis-triggering properties of VES may be due to its modulation of Fas signaling. Fas belongs to the tumor necrosis factor receptor and nerve growth factor receptor superfamily, and contains a cytoplasmic death domain that can initiate an apoptotic cascade. Using two prostate cancer cell lines (LNCaP and PC-3) and the normal prostate epithelial cells (PrEC) the investigators showed that VES induced apoptosis only in cancer cells. They also showed that VES administration enhanced Fas ligand expression and increased Fas levels in the membrane, both of which are important events in Fas-induced apoptosis.[24]

Vitamin E and Its Analogs Inhibit Cell Cycle Progression

VES has been shown to inhibit the proliferation of prostate cancer cell lines through the inhibition of cell cycle. Our group has found that VES effectively inhibits prostate cancer LNCaP cell growth by causing cell cycle arrest in the G1 phase with a reduction of cells in S phase. VES decreases the expression of several cell cycle regulatory proteins such as cyclin D1, D3, E, cdk2, and cdk4, but not cdk6.[25] In addition, Ni et al. also found that VES can inhibit the phosphorylation of retinoblastoma (Rb), and consequently inhibit the E2F activity.[25] Another group, Venkasteswaran et al., has observed similar inhibitory effects of VES. Their data shows VES-induced

G1 arrest in LNCaP and G2/M arrest in PC-3 prostate cancer cells. Their data also showed a G1 phase arrest, and the mechanism credited for the increased amounts of p27 by VES.[26]

In addition to α-tocopherol, γ-tocopherol is another isoform of vitamin E that has demonstrated anticancer properties. A study by Gysin and colleagues showed that γ-tocopherol inhibits cell proliferation more significantly than α-tocopherol in DU-145 and LNCaP cells. They also showed that the mechanisms of γ-tocopherol are through inhibition of DNA synthesis, defects of cell cycle with decreased S-phase cell population, and down-regulation of cyclin D1 and cyclin E levels. Based on their results, γ-tocopherol is more potent than α-tocopherol in those two cell lines.[27] However, the absorption efficiency of γ-tocopherol is lower than that of α-tocopherol in human.[14]

VES Inhibits the Expressions of PSA and the Androgen Receptor (AR)

A functional AR is essential for the development and progression of prostate cancer.[28–30] In prostate, AR can bind to the promoter of and regulate the expression of prostate-specific antigen (PSA), the most popular detection marker for prostate cancer. Results from our earlier report suggested that VES, at a non-toxic concentration and *in vivo* achievable level, could selectively inhibit the expression of both AR and PSA, but not retinoid X receptor α (RXRα) and peroxisome proliferators-activated receptor α (PPARα), in prostate cancer LNCaP cells. Results from further investigation indicated that VES can affect the translational efficiency of AR. Overall, the results suggested that VES-mediated inhibition of prostate cancer cell growth can be partly due to the inhibition of AR function.[31]

VES Inhibits Activity of MMP9 Secreted From Prostate Cancer Cells

Most of the tumors of prostate cancer patients become incurable once their cancers progress to metastatic stage. Metastasis of cancer cells employs complicated processes including degradation of extracellular matrix, migration, homing and angiogenesis. Our group has found that

VES can affect the invasiveness of prostate cancer PC-3 and DU-145 cells. Results from mechanism investigation suggested that VES could affect the matrix metalloproteinase-9 (MMP-9) activity, but not the tissue inhibitor of metalloproteinases (TIMPs). The inhibition of MMP-9 activity and cancer metastasis through matrigel could be observed with 24 h treatment of VES. This time frame is shorter then the event of VES mediated disturbance of the cell cycle distribution and cell growth, which takes action upon longer VES treatment. Thus, the inhibition of MMP-9 activity could be an event independent of VES-mediated cell growth inhibition and cell cycle progression of prostate cancer cells.[32]

In vivo Animal Study of Vitamin E's Role in Prostate and Prostate Cancer

One study has investigated the effects of vitamin E deficiency on pubertal growth and maturation of the rat prostate. The rats were placed on a vitamin E deficient diet at four weeks of age and were followed for 15–26 weeks. The study showed that vitamin E deficiency in the body led to a less significant increase in weight, DNA, and protein in the lateral lobe of prostate compared with control rats. The group also concluded that vitamin E deficiency may contribute to the delay of prostate differentiation.[33]

In spite of the constructive role of vitamin E in the development of prostate, the role of vitamin E in the incidence and progression of prostate cancer are controversial in animal models. In 3,2′-dimethyl-4-aminobiphenyl (DMBA)-initiated rat prostate carcinogenesis, the modifying effects of six naturally occurring antioxidants, including α-tocopherol, were investigated. Atypical hyperplasias and carcinomas of the prostate were observed in the ventral lobe in all groups treated with DMAB. However, the incidence of these lesions was not significantly different between carcinogen control and antioxidant-treated groups. There were also no significant increases or decreases in the incidence of tumors in any other organs.[34]

Fleshner *et al.* also investigated the effects between vitamin E and a high-fat diet on prostate cancer development. Tumors were induced by subcutaneous injection of LNCaP cells in nude mice and they were treated with dl-α-tocopherol at 11.4 mg/kg body weight/day while divided into four different groups (regular diet, high-fat diet, regular diet with supplemental vitamin E, high-fat diet with supplemental vitamin E). They concluded that the mechanism for fat induced growth of prostate cancer cells is mediated by oxidative stress, thus making vitamin E an effective solution.[35]

Vitamin E has been shown to enhance the growth-inhibitory effects of adriamycin on human prostatic carcinoma cells *in vitro*. Vitamin E used in combination with adriamycin was evaluated in the treatment of Nb rat prostate adenocarcinoma. The adriamycin-vitamin E treatment groups had the lowest average final tumor volume, but the mortality rate increased. These results suggest that vitamin E may play a role in enhancing the cytotoxic effects of adriamycin.[36] Recently, the antineoplastic effects of VES, selenium, and lycopene were tested on Lady mouse prostate cancer model. The results suggested that oral feeding of VES, selenium, and lycopene will elicit a better antineoplastic effects.[37] Overall the antineoplastic effects of vitamin E and its analogs need further evaluation in animals.

Clinical Study of Vitamin E in Prostate Cancer

There have been numerous studies focusing on the effect of vitamin E supplement and its correlation to cancer occurrence. Results from a finished Alpha-Tocopherol, Beta-Carotene (ATBC) Cancer Prevention Study (n = 29,133) of male smokers suggested that the daily supplement of α-tocopherol could reduce the incidence and mortality of prostate cancer.[2]

In addition, the association between prostate cancer and baseline vitamin E and selenium was evaluated in the trial-based cohort of the ATBC study. During nine years of follow-up, 317 men developed incident prostate cancer. The report found that there were no significant associations between baseline serum α-tocopherol, regular dietary vitamin E, or selenium and prostate cancer.[38] Overall, their results indicated a protective effect for total vitamin E among those who received the α-tocopherol intervention.[38] In another study, the investigators examined the associations between prediagnostic blood levels of micronutrients and prostate cancer risk in two nested case-control studies of 9,804 and 10,456 male residents of Washington County, Maryland, who donated blood in 1974 (CLUE I) and 1989 (CLUE II), respectively. They found serum α-tocopherol might be weakly associated with prostate cancer risk.[39] Furthermore, a study was done on 10,456 male residents from Washington County, Maryland using donated blood samples. The results showed that the risk of prostate cancer declined with increasing concentrations of γ-tocopherol although not linearly. Men having γ-tocopherol levels in the top fifth had a five-fold reduced risk compared to the bottom fifth. In this study, statistically significant protective effects are associated with high levels of selenium and α-tocopherol are observed only when γ-tocopherol concentrations are high.[3,40]

An additional population-based, case-control study in King County, Washington examined supplement dietary use in 697 incident prostate cancer cases (ages 40–64). The results suggested that individual supplements of zinc, vitamin C, and vitamin E may be protective.[3] However, the suggested supplemental vitamin E may not have a beneficial effect on the risk of prostate cancer in non-smokers.[41]

Furthermore, the relation of baseline levels of serum α-tocopherol and serum sex hormones in older men was studied.[36] Their results suggested that serum α-tocopherol was significantly inversely associated with serum androstenedione, testosterone, sex hormone-binding globulin, and estrogen levels. These results indicated that α-tocopherol may affect concentrations of several sex hormones in older men and may have implications for the protective effect of vitamin E in relation to prostate cancer in the ATBC Study.[42] Moreover, another group analyzed whether long-term supplementation with α-tocopherol affected VEGF levels, a cytokine integrally involved in endothelial cell proliferation, vascular permeability, and regulation of angiogenesis. Two hundred Finnish men were randomly assigned to placebo and α-tocopherol pills (50 mg) daily. There was an 11% reduction in VEGF levels in the α-tocopherol group compared to a 10% increase for the control group. The result suggests that α-tocopherol may suppress prostate cancer angiogenesis through reducing VEGF levels.[3,43]

Due to controversial data from various studies, whether the supplement of α-tocopherol and its analogs could lower the risk of prostate cancer remains to be elucidated. Currently, there is a big clinical trial, Selenium and Vitamin E Clinical Trial (SELECT) in the US. The SELECT trial is a randomized, prospective, double-blind study that intends to determine whether selenium and vitamin E, singly or in combination, can reduce the risk of prostate cancer in healthy men. The study will provide 200 μg

L-selenomethionine and 400 mg racemic α-tocopheryl acetate. The trial began in 2001 and final results are expected in 2013.[21] The outcomes of this clinical trial will provide a comprehensive investigation of the association between the prostate cancer risk and the supplement of vitamin E and/or selenium.

Summary

Although some controversial data exists, the epidemiological and clinical studies suggested that the incidence and mortality of prostate cancer may be reduced with daily supplement of α-tocopherol analogs. We and other researchers have devoted efforts on exploring these underlying mechanisms. Currently, the identified mechanisms include inhibition of DNA synthesis,[22] inducing apoptosis and FAS ligand activity,[24] affecting the expression and function of AR and PSA,[31] targeting on cell cycle molecules,[25,26] and inhibiting the invasiveness of prostate cancer cells.[32] There are still several fields have not been addressed. First, it is of great interest to know whether α-tocopherol and its analogs can affect the growth factor and kinase signals, oncogene function, bone metastasis, and angiogenesis in prostate cancer cells. Second, as most of the published results rely on the *in vitro* cell line studies, it is important to use animal models to test the anticancer effects of α-tocopherol and its analogs. The application of animal models, including cancer cell xenografts on nude mice, transgenic mice such as TRAMP model,[44] LADY prostate cancer model,[45,46] knockout mice models such as NKX3.1knockout mice,[47] pTENknockout mice[48] and others, could advance our insights of how α-tocopherol affects the development of prostate cancer *in vivo*. Third, there is a need to identify the α-tocopheryl derivatives with better efficacy and stability than the parental chemical version. Fourth, the exploration of the roles of tocopherol-associated protein (TAP) and tocopherol transfer protein (TTP) are also important. Till now, TTP is the only protein that has been linked to the absorption of tocopherol into liver and then subsequently into circulating systems.[49,50] However, the roles of another tocopherol binding protein, TAP, have not been well-explored. Fifth, among these fat-soluble vitamins, A, D, E, and K, the receptors of vitamin A and vitamin D have been identified. It is interesting to investigate whether vitamin E has a specific receptor, which can bind and propagate the function and signal of vitamin E. Overall, the anticancer effects of vitamin E and its analogs have been observed, yet the underlying mechanisms need more intensive investigations. Although there have been many advances in radiotherapy, chemotherapy, and surgery, the use of complementary therapies for cancer remains of key interest. Understanding the functional mechanisms of vitamin E are important, as they will provide a base for the combinational therapy with other compounds. In the long run, cancer patients could benefit from a cocktail therapy via combining different treatments with complementary or synergistic effects.

References

1. Jemal A, Tiwari RC, Murray T, Ghafoor A, Samuels A, Ward E, Feuer EJ, Thun MJ (2004) Cancer statistics, 2004. *CA Cancer J Clin* 54:8–29.
2. The Alpha-Tocopherol, Beta Carotene Cancer Prevention Study Group (1994) The effect of vitamin E and beta carotene on the incidence of lung cancer and other cancers in male smokers. *N Engl J Med* 330:1029–1035.
3. Kristal AR, Stanford JL, Cohen JH, Wicklund K, Patterson RE (1999) Vitamin and mineral supplement use is associated with reduced risk of prostate cancer. *Cancer Epidemiol Biomarkers Prev* 8:887–892.
4. Chiu BC, Ji BT, Dai Q, Gridley G, McLaughlin JK, Gao YT, Fraumeni JF, Jr, Chow WH (2003) Dietary factors and risk of colon cancer in Shanghai, China. *Cancer Epidemiol Biomarkers Prev* 12:201–208.
5. Brigelius-Flohe R, Traber MG (1999) Vitamin E: function and metabolism. *FASEB J* 13:1145–1155.
6. Prasad KN, Kumar B, Yan XD, Hanson AJ, Cole WC (2003) Alpha-tocopheryl succinate, the most effective form of vitamin E for adjuvant cancer treatment: a review. *J Am Coll Nutr* 22:108–117.
7. Malafa MP, Neitzel LT (2000) Vitamin E succinate promotes breast cancer tumor dormancy. *J Surg Res* 93:163–170.
8. Fariss MW, Fortuna MB, Everett CK, Smith JD, Trent DF, Djuric Z (1994) The selective antiproliferative effects of alpha-tocopheryl hemisuccinate and cholesteryl hemisuccinate on murine leukemia cells result from the action of the intact compounds. *Cancer Res* 54:3346–3351.
9. Lawson KA, Anderson K, Menchaca M, Atkinson J, Sun L, Knight V, Gilbert BE, Conti C, Sanders BG, Kline K (2003) Novel vitamin E analogue decreases syngeneic mouse mammary tumor burden and reduces lung metastasis. *Mol Cancer Ther* 2:437–444.

10. Anderson K, Simmons-Menchaca M, Lawson KA, Atkinson J, Sanders BG, Kline K (2004) Differential response of human ovarian cancer cells to induction of apoptosis by vitamin E succinate and vitamin E analogue, alpha-TEA. *Cancer Res* 64:4263–4269.

11. Birringer M, EyTina JH, Salvatore BA, Neuzil J (2003) Vitamin E analogues as inducers of apoptosis: structure-function relation. *Br J Cancer* 88: 1948–1955.

12. Institute of Medicine (2000) *Dietary Reference Intakes for Vitamin C, Vitamin E, Selenium, and Carotenoids.* National Academies Press, Washington, DC.

13. Fleshner NE (2002) Vitamin E and prostate cancer. *Urol Clin North Am* 29:107–113, ix.

14. Huang HY, Appel LJ (2003) Supplementation of diets with alpha-tocopherol reduces serum concentrations of gamma- and delta-tocopherol in humans. *J Nutr* 133:3137–3140.

15. Baker H, Handelman GJ, Short S, Machlin LJ, Bhagavan HN, Dratz EA, Frank O (1986) Comparison of plasma alpha and gamma tocopherol levels following chronic oral administration of either all-rac-alpha-tocopheryl acetate or RRR-alpha-tocopheryl acetate in normal adult male subjects. *Am J Clin Nutr* 43:382–387.

16. Bonina F, Lanza M, Montenegro L, Salerno L, Smeriglio P, Trombetta D, Saija A (1996) Transport of alpha-tocopherol and its derivatives through erythrocyte membranes. *Pharm Res* 13:1343–1347.

17. Zimmer S, Stocker A, Sarbolouki MN, Spycher SE, Sassoon J, Azzi A (2000) A novel human tocopherol-associated protein: cloning, *in vitro* expression, and characterization. *J Biol Chem* 275:25672–25680.

18. Dutta-Roy AK, Gordon MJ, Leishman DJ, Paterson BJ, Duthie GG, James WP (1993) Purification and partial characterisation of an alpha-tocopherol-binding protein from rabbit heart cytosol. *Mol Cell Biochem* 123:139–144.

19. Gordon MJ, Campbell FM, Duthie GG, Dutta-Roy AK (1995) Characterization of a novel alpha-tocopherol-binding protein from bovine heart cytosol. *Arch Biochem Biophys* 318:140–146.

20. Klein EA, Thompson IM, Lippman SM, Goodman PJ, Albanes D, Taylor PR, Coltman C (2001) SELECT: the next prostate cancer prevention trial. Selenum and Vitamin E Cancer Prevention Trial. *J Urol* 166:1311–1315.

21. Klein EA, Lippman SM, Thompson IM, Goodman PJ, Albanes D, Taylor PR, Coltman C (2003) The selenium and vitamin E cancer prevention trial. *World J Urol* 21:21–27.

22. Sigounas G, Anagnostou A, Steiner M (1997) dl-alpha-tocopherol induces apoptosis in erythroleukemia, prostate, and breast cancer cells. *Nutr Cancer* 28:30–35.

23. Gunawardena K, Murray DK, Meikle AW (2000) Vitamin E and other anti-oxidants inhibit human prostate cancer cells through apoptosis. *Prostate* 44:287–295.

24. Israel K, Yu W, Sanders BG, Kline K (2000) Vitamin E succinate induces apoptosis in human prostate cancer cells: role for Fas in vitamin E succinate-triggered apoptosis. *Nutr Cancer* 36:90–100.

25. Ni J, Chen M, Zhang Y, Li R, Huang J, Yeh S (2003) Vitamin E succinate inhibits human prostate cancer cell growth via modulating cell cycle regulatory machinery. *Biochem Biophys Res Commun* 300:357–363.

26. Venkateswaran V, Fleshner NE, Klotz LH (2002) Modulation of cell proliferation and cell cycle regulators by vitamin E in human prostate carcinoma cell lines. *J Urol* 168:1578–1582.

27. Gysin R, Azzi A, Visarius T (2002) Gamma-tocopherol inhibits human cancer cell cycle progression and cell proliferation by down-regulation of cyclins. *FASEB J* 16:1952–1954.

28. Heinlein CA, Chang C (2002) Androgen receptor (AR) coregulators: an overview. *Endocr Rev* 23:175–200.

29. Yeh S, Kang HY, Miyamoto H, Nishimura K, Chang HC, Ting HJ, Rahman M, Lin HK, Fujimoto N, Hu YC, Mizokami A, Huang KE, Chang C (1999) Differential induction of androgen receptor transactivation by different androgen receptor coactivators in human prostate cancer DU145 cells. *Endocrine* 11:195–202.

30. Yeh S, Lin HK, Kang HY, Thin TH, Lin MF, Chang C (1999) From HER2/Neu signal cascade to androgen receptor and its coactivators: a novel pathway by induction of androgen target genes through MAP kinase in prostate cancer cells. *Proc Natl Acad Sci USA* 96:5458–5463.

31. Zhang Y, Ni J, Messing EM, Chang E, Yang CR, Yeh S (2002) Vitamin E succinate inhibits the function of androgen receptor and the expression of prostate-specific antigen in prostate cancer cells. *Proc Natl Acad Sci USA* 99:7408–7413.

32. Zhang M, Altuwaijri S, Yeh S (2004) RRR-alpha-tocopheryl succinate inhibits human prostate cancer cell invasiveness. *Oncogene* 23:3080–3088.

33. Wilson MJ, Kaye D, Smith WE, Quach HT, Sinha AA, Vatassery GT (2003) Effect of vitamin E deficiency on the growth and secretory function of the rat prostatic complex. *Exp Mol Pathol* 74:267–275.

34. Nakamura A, Shirai T, Takahashi S, Ogawa K, Hirose M, Ito N (1991) Lack of modification by naturally occurring antioxidants of 3,2′-dimethyl-4-aminobiphenyl-initiated rat prostate carcinogenesis. *Cancer Lett* 58:241–246.

35. Fleshner N, Fair WR, Huryk R, Heston WD (1999) Vitamin E inhibits the high-fat diet promoted growth of established human prostate LNCaP tumors in nude mice. *J Urol* 161:1651–1654.

36. Nesbitt JA, Smith J, McDowell G, Drago JR (1988) Adriamycin-vitamin E combination therapy for treatment of prostate adenocarcinoma in the Nb rat model. *J Surg Oncol* 38:283–284.

37. Venkateswaran V, Fleshner NE, Sugar LM, Klotz LH (2004) Antioxidants block prostate cancer in lady transgenic mice. *Cancer Res* 64:5891–5896.

38. Hartman TJ, Albanes D, Pietinen P, Hartman AM, Rautalahti M, Tangrea JA, Taylor PR (1998) The association between baseline vitamin E, selenium, and prostate cancer in the alpha-tocopherol, beta-carotene cancer prevention study. *Cancer Epidemiol Biomarkers Prev* 7:335–340.

39. Huang HY, Alberg AJ, Norkus EP, Hoffman SC, Comstock GW, Helzlsouer KJ (2003) Prospective study of antioxidant micronutrients in the blood and the risk of developing prostate cancer. *Am J Epidemiol* 157:335–344.

40. Helzlsouer KJ, Huang HY, Alberg AJ, Hoffman S, Burke A, Norkus EP, Morris JS, Comstock GW (2000) Association between alpha-tocopherol, gamma-tocopherol, selenium, and subsequent prostate cancer. *J Natl Cancer Inst* 92:2018–2023.

41. Chan JM, Stampfer MJ, Ma J, Rimm EB, Willett WC, Giovannucci EL (1999) Supplemental vitamin E intake and prostate cancer risk in a large cohort of men in the United States. *Cancer Epidemiol Biomarkers Prev* 8:893–899.

42. Hartman TJ, Dorgan JF, Virtamo J, Tangrea JA, Taylor PR, Albanes D (1999) Association between serum alpha-tocopherol and serum androgens and estrogens in older men. *Nutr Cancer* 35:10–15.

43. Woodson K, Triantos S, Hartman T, Taylor PR, Virtamo J, Albanes D (2002) Long-term alpha-tocopherol supplementation is associated with lower serum vascular endothelial growth factor levels. *Anticancer Res* 22:375–378.

44. Greenberg NM, DeMayo FJ, Sheppard PC, Barrios R, Lebovitz R, Finegold M, Angelopoulou R, Dodd JG, Duckworth ML, Rosen JM, *et al.* (1994) The rat probasin gene promoter directs hormonally and developmentally regulated expression of a heterologous gene specifically to the prostate in transgenic mice. *Mol Endocrinol* 8:230–239.

45. Kasper S, Sheppard PC, Yan Y, Pettigrew N, Borowsky AD, Prins GS, Dodd JG, Duckworth ML, Matusik RJ (1998) Development, progression, and androgen-dependence of prostate tumors in probasin-large T antigen transgenic mice: a model for prostate cancer. *Lab Invest* 78:319–333.

46. Masumori N, Thomas TZ, Chaurand P, Case T, Paul M, Kasper S, Caprioli RM, Tsukamoto T, Shappell SB, Matusik RJ (2001) A probasin-large T antigen transgenic mouse line develops prostate adenocarcinoma and neuroendocrine carcinoma with metastatic potential. *Cancer Res* 61:2239–2249.

47. Bhatia-Gaur R, Donjacour AA, Sciavolino PJ, Kim M, Desai N, Young P, Norton CR, Gridley T, Cardiff RD, Cunha GR, Abate-Shen C, Shen MM (1999) Roles for Nkx3.1 in prostate development and cancer. *Genes Dev* 13:966–977.

48. Kim MJ, Cardiff RD, Desai N, Banach-Petrosky WA, Parsons R, Shen MM, Abate-Shen C (2002) Cooperativity of Nkx3.1 and Pten loss of function in a mouse model of prostate carcinogenesis. *Proc Natl Acad Sci USA* 99:2884–2889.

49. Leonard SW, Terasawa Y, Farese RV, Jr, Traber MG (2002) Incorporation of deuterated RRR- or all-rac-alpha-tocopherol in plasma and tissues of alpha-tocopherol transfer protein–null mice. *Am J Clin Nutr* 75:555–560.

50. Ouahchi K, Arita M, Kayden H, Hentati F, Ben Hamida M, Sokol R, Arai H, Inoue K, Mandel JL, Koenig M (1995) Ataxia with isolated vitamin E deficiency is caused by mutations in the alpha-tocopherol transfer protein. *Nat Genet* 9:141–145.

12

VITAMIN D AND PROSTATE CANCER

Yi-Fen Lee, Huei-Ju Ting and Bo-Ying Bao

Departments of Pathology & Laboratory Medicine and Urology
University of Rochester Medical Center
Rochester, New York, USA

Introduction

Nutritional factors have been hypothesized to be critical in the development of numerous cancers, and this holds true for prostate cancer. On the basis of geographic patterns of ultraviolet radiation throughout the contiguous United States, and on epidemiological data on prostate cancer incidence, the hypothesis was raised by Schwartz and colleagues that vitamin D deficiency may be a prostate cancer risk factor, and that increased exposure to sunlight may protect against clinical prostate cancer.[1] *In vitro* studies have shown that treatment with $1\alpha, 25(OH)_2D_3$ (1,25-VD), a active form of vitamin D, decreases proliferation and increases differentiation of prostate cancer cells. Prostate cancer cells contain a specific receptor for 1,25-VD (the vitamin D receptor, VDR) that is known to mediate inhibition of proliferation, tumor invasiveness, the induction of apoptosis, and differentiation of prostate cancer cells. In this chapter, we will summarize recent progress in the study of vitamin D in prostate cancer, including epidemiological analyses, the vitamin D anti-tumor mechanisms, and vitamin D-based treatment in clinical trials. Understanding how vitamin D acts in the prostate is of great importance for the continued advancement of prostate cancer therapy and prevention.

Epidemiology Study

On the basis of geographic patterns of ultraviolet radiation throughout the United States and epidemiological data on prostate cancer incidence, a hypothesis was raised by Schwartz and colleagues that vitamin D deficiency might be a risk factor and that increased sunlight exposure may protect against prostate cancer.[1] It was initially found that prostate cancer mortality rates were higher in northern latitudes. Because casual exposure to sunlight results in the production of vitamin D, it was postulated that vitamin D promotes differentiation of prostate cells and that inadequate levels of vitamin D may permit the growth of prostate cancer. Later, it was reported that prostate cancer mortality rates by county within the United States were inversely correlated with the availability of UV radiation, lending further support to the vitamin D hypothesis.[2] Men with prostate cancer have been found to have lower serum levels of 1,25-VD before diagnosis of the disease.[3] This is further supported by the Ahonen group study comprised of a 13-year follow-up of about 19,000 middle-aged men who were free of clinically verified prostate cancer. They found that among those who developed prostate cancer, more than half had vitamin D deficiency (serum level of vitamin D3 [1,25-VD$_3$] below 50 nmol/l). Low 1,25-VD$_3$ concentrations in the younger men were associated with more aggressive prostate cancer, and high 1,25-VD$_3$ levels delayed the appearance of clinically verified prostate cancer by 1.8 years. Therefore, Vitamin D deficiency may increase the risk of initiation and progression of prostate cancer.[4]

One of the most recent studies of 200,000 samples from Nordic men, including men from Norway, Finland, and Sweden, found that the normal average serum concentration of 25(OH)-vitamin D (40–60 nmol/l) was associated with the lowest risk of prostate cancer, and that both low ($\leq$19 nmol/l) and high ($\geq$80 nmol/l) 25(OH)-vitamin D serum concentrations were associated with higher prostate cancer risk. High vitamin D levels might enhance expression of 24-hydroxylase, the enzyme that inactivates 1,25-VD. Therefore, the U-shaped risk of prostate cancer might be due to the availability of 1,25-VD within the prostate.[5]

Vitamin D Action

1,25-VD, the bioactive form of vitamin D, was identified as a nutrient a century ago, and is the major regulator of calcium and phosphate homeostasis, responsible for maintenance of bone integrity, and also plays an important role in hair follicle cycling and mammary gland development. The biological effects of 1,25-VD are mainly mediated through the VDR, a member of the nuclear receptor superfamily, which heterodimerizes with the retinoid X receptor (RXR) and binds to response elements located in the promoters of target genes in various tissues, such as bone (osteocalcin, osteopontin, and beta 3 integrin), kidney (24-hydroxylase), and intestine (calbindin).[6,7] Like other nuclear receptors, VDR contains an amino-terminal activation function 1 (AF-1) domain, a DNA binding domain (DBD), composed of two hexameric half-sites organized as direct repeats that recognize specific DNA response elements, and a ligand binding domain (LBD) that contains a ligand-regulated transcriptional activation function 2 (AF-2) region.[8] Ligand-induced conformational changes in the LBD of VDR create an interface for protein-protein interaction between receptors and a group of intermediate proteins, termed coregulators, that may connect liganded receptors to basal transcription machinery, or that remodel the chromatin structure to facilitate transcription initiation.[9]

Several coregulators that modulate VDR activity have been identified. Included are positive coregulators such as SRC-1, TIF2/GRIP-1, SRC-3/RAC3/AIB-1, HMG-1/2, TAF(II)55, Smad3, and TRAP220, as well as negative coregulators such as NCoRs, Smad7, and Stat1.[10–18] The VDR-interacting protein (DRIP) complex, identified by affinity column assay, consists of several components, promotes transactivation of VDR *in vitro*, and demonstrates chromatin remodeling activity.[19] Large numbers of coregulators have been identified, and it is believed that they may form several multiprotein complexes to serve particular functions in modulating receptor transactivation. For example, the SWI/SNF complex possesses ATP-dependent chromatin remodeling activity, the CBP and p/CAF complexes possess histone acetyltransferase activity, and the DRIP complex functions to recruit basal transcription factors.[20]

The phosphorylation status of VDR is also important for modulation of receptor function. For example, phosphorylation of VDR by casein kinase-II promotes its transactivation activity, while phosphorylation of VDR by PKC is thought to negatively regulate its activity. In addition, the tyrosine-phosphorylated VDR exerts increasing affinity for DRIP205, a component of a coregulator complex that acts as a bridge between the basal transcription machinery and VDR.[21] A recent report showed that the p38 and JNK-triggered c-Jun/AP-1 pathways transactivate VDR and sensitize breast cancer to vitamin D-induced growth inhibition.[22] These lines of evidence indicate that cross-talk between growth factors and VDR-mediated vitamin D action may be involved in modulating vitamin D-mediated growth arrest in cancer cells.

Mechanism of Anti-tumor Action in Prostate Cancer by Vitamin D

A key feature of cancer cells is their increased rate of growth relative to normal cells, and this can be attributed to increased cell proliferation, decreased cell death, or a combination of the two. 1,25-VD has been demonstrated to regulate cellular differentiation and proliferation in a number of normal and malignant cells, including prostate cancer cells, however the response to 1,25-VD in cancer cells appears to be cell type-specific. The majority of the 1,25-VD-mediated signals function through the VDR. The sensitivity and responsiveness of cells to vitamin D are therefore partly dependent on the activation of VDR. Miller *et al.* first demonstrated the presence of VDR in the LNCaP human prostate cancer cell line.[23] VDRs have since been found in other prostate cancer cell lines, as well as in normal prostate epithelial and stromal cells grown in culture.[24] Several studies have demonstrated that 1,25-VD and its analogs inhibit the growth of prostate cancer cell lines as well as primary prostate cancer cells in culture.[23–26] The 1,25-VD responsiveness is variable among cell lines tested, however the context of VDR and the 1,25-VD-mediated VDR transcriptional activity did not fully explain the different vitamin D anti-proliferative responses among cell lines. Our data and that of other investigators show that the cross-talk between vitamin D and androgen/AR signaling contributes to some degree of growth inhibition. The vitamin D anti-proliferation effect is greater in AR-expressing prostate cancer cells, such as LNCaP and CWR22R, than in AR-negative prostate cancer cells, such as DU145 and PC-3. Treatment with vitamin D enhances the AR expression, and inhibition of AR expression by antiandrogen-treatment, AR RNAi, or AR targeted disruption resulted in diminished vitamin D growth inhibition effects.[27–29] Therefore, androgen/AR signaling plays important roles in the anti-proliferative action of vitamin D in prostate cancer cell lines as summarized in Fig. 1.

Different mechanisms have been proposed for the inhibition of cell growth by vitamin D. The most common feature of response to 1,25-VD in cancer cells is the induction of G1/G0 cell cycle arrest, however, the 1,25-VD-induced G1/G0 arrest pathways are likely multi-factorial. In LNCaP cells, vitamin D treatment decreases retinoblastoma protein phosphorylation, represses E2F transcriptional activity, slightly increases levels of cyclin-dependent kinase (CDK) inhibitor p21, and decreases CDK activity, finally resulting in G0/G1 accumulation.[29,30] In other cancer models, such as U937 myelomonocytes, p21 appears to be the most highly up-regulated

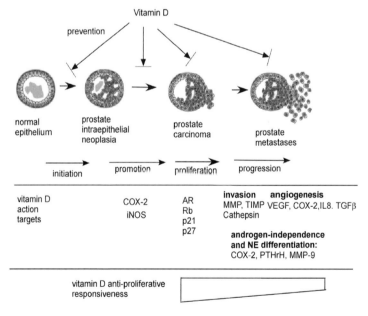

Fig. 1. Illustration of vitamin D anti-tumor effects and of putative vitamin D responsive genes.

gene, yet, in head and neck squamous cell carcinoma (SCC), p21 is not increased, but p27 is up-regulated. Identification of a vitamin D response element (VDRE) in the p21 promoter regions suggested direct regulation of p21 activity by vitamin D/VDR, and the cell context is likely to be another determining factor. In addition to G1/G0 arrest, induction of apoptosis and differentiation of the prostate cancer cells may also contribute to the antiproliferative activity of vitamin D in some prostate cancer cells.[31] Studies in breast cancer cells suggest that the vitamin D/VDR pathway seems to be involved in stimulating the mitochondria to release cytochrome C rather than a pathway relying on upstream caspases.[32] The mechanisms by which 1,25-VD induces apoptosis remain to be further investigated.

In addition to its antiproliferative effect, 1,25-VD can inhibit prostate cancer cell invasion, adhesion, and migration through modulation of select cell surface adhesion molecules, such as integrins (alpha 4 and beta 4),[33] and by inhibition of metallo-proteases (MMP-2 and MMP-9).[34] These data suggest that 1,25-VD can not only inhibit the growth of the tumor cells, but can also stop tumor cell migration, penetration, and metastasis. Such data stimulated clinical trials of vitamin D as therapeutic agents for treatment of prostate cancer.[35,36] In one of our most recent studies, we found that vitamin D prevents the prostate cancer cell invasion via modulation of selective proteinase activity. In our current study using the zymographic assay, we found that 1,25-VD inhibited MMP-9 activity and enhanced tissue inhibitors of metalloproteinase-1 (TIMP-1) activity, but had less of an effect on plasminogen activators and Cathepsin.[37] Real-time PCR analysis demonstrated that 1,25-VD inhibited MMP-9 and induced TIMP-1 transcript expression in a time dependent manner. The vitamin D effects on the TIMP-1 promoter activity further suggested a potential cross-talk between AP-1 and vitamin D/VDR signalings, which might contribute to the suppression of TIMP-1. In contrast, the regulation of MMP-9 by vitamin D did not seem to be regulated at the transcriptional level, suggesting some post-transcriptional modifications, or RNA stability might contribute to the suppression of MMP-9 activity by vitamin D.[37] From our study, we concluded that vitamin D modulates the activity of selective proteinases, such as MMP-9 and TIMP-1, to inhibit the prostate cancer cell invasion, and thus provides proof of the concept for treating advanced stage prostate cancer patients with vitamin D to stop disease progression.

Development of New Vitamin D Analogs and Their Use in Combination Therapy for Prostate Cancer

The beneficial effects of 1,25-VD against cancer cell proliferation have been supported by many *in vitro* studies, yet the therapeutic window of 1,25-VD usefulness is extremely narrow and effective doses cannot be administered without inducing hypercalcemia. The increase in calcium is achieved both by enhanced intestinal absorption and by liberation of calcium from the bone, eventually leading to decreased bone mass at higher doses. Therefore, much effort has been directed toward the identification of new analogs, which retain the favorable activities of 1,25-VD while avoiding the side effects. Several synthetic vitamin D analogs have been reported to exert promising anti-cancer effects with reduced hypercalcemia. Skowronski *et al.* showed that selected vitamin D analogs displayed reduced calcemic effects and that potency was even greater than 1,25-VD.[38] Among those vitamin D analogs, one of the most promising synthetic analogs is Seocalcitol (EB1089, Leo Pharmaceutical Products). A considerable number of *in vitro* studies have been carried out with EB1089 and show that the analog is more potent than 1,25-VD with respect to regulation of cancer cell growth and differentiation, and the effect of EB1089 on calcium metabolism *in vivo* is approximately 50% less than that of 1,25-VD. The anti-cancer effects of EB1089 without induction of hypercalcemia were also demonstrated *in vivo* in a rat model of mammary gland carcinoma. Similar effects were seen in an *in vivo* prostate cancer study where EB1089 inhibited prostate cancer cell proliferation and reduced tumorigenesis as well as tumor metastases. Several other vitamin D analogs or structural VDR activators, such as Maxacalcitol (OCT) (Chugai Pharmaceutical Co. Ltd), 16-ene analogs (Hoffmann LaRoche, Inc.), 19-nor analogs (Hoffmann LaRoche, Inc.), 1α-hydroxyvitamin D5.[39] LG190119 (Ligand Pharmaceuticals Inc.), and 1α-hydroxyvitamin D2 have been developed and tested in clinical trials in the advanced prostate cancer patients.[40,41] These compounds may have promise as therapeutic agents for cancer and other diseases, with fewer side effects than 1,25-VD.

Another strategy to preserve vitamin D anti-tumor effects while avoiding the side effects is vitamin D-based combination therapy in which other agents that either promote vitamin D responsiveness or reduce the hyper-calcemia are used. The regimens used for vitamin D combination therapy include the chemotherapy drug (Paclitaxel, Taxotere),[42,43] anti-mitotic agents (Genistein),[44] differentiation agents (retinoic acid),[45,46] and the agents that modulate vitamin D/VDR action (Dexamethasone).[47] All reg-imens were shown to potentiate the anti-tumor effects of vitamin D and reduce vitamin-D associated hypercalcemia in prostate cancer cells and animal models, yet detailed mechanisms are not yet known and more clinical trials need to be done.

Vitamin D-Based Clinical Trials

Evidence accumulated from both experimental and epidemiological stud-ies supports the idea that vitamin D could be used as a therapeutic drug to control prostate cancer, and several vitamin D-based clinical trials have been conducted, mainly enlisting patients with advanced androgen-independent prostate cancer (AIPC). Pilot studies from small numbers of patients that took daily orally doses of calcitriol found that the PSA levels in those patients were significantly lower before calcitriol therapy. However, there is incidence of hypercalciuria or hypercalcemia, and the development of renal stones in some patients, which limits its clinical usefulness.[35] One Phase I clinical trial was conducted by injection of calcitriol subcutaneously every other day in the advanced malignancy patients and tested the tolerable toxicity via this route.[48] Then, different calcitriol-based clinical trials, with either modifications in the schedules and route of administration, or combinations with dexamethasone, pacli-taxel have been developed.[49] In addition to the calcitriol, its analogs such as 1α-hydroxyvitamin D_2 have been tested in clinical trial Phase I and II in the AIPC patients.[40,41] The results from all these clinical trials suggest further clinical investigation of this disease with vitamin D, its analogs, or in combination with other agents, such as chemotherapy, should be further pursued.

In the past, chemotherapy was considered ineffective, however, newer chemotherapeutic drugs and drug combinations are now demonstrating improved response rates. Among those chemotherapy drugs, taxotere, a semisynthetic taxane, is commonly used as a chemotherapeutic agent by itself and in combination regimens in the treatment of hormone refractory prostate cancer (HRPC). 1,25-VD has been shown to sensitize prostate cancer cells to cytotoxic drugs, such as paclitaxel, platinum compounds, and Taxotere. The Phase II clinical trial of Taxotere® plus calcitriol has shown approximately twice the PSA decline response rate compared with taxotere alone,[43] which provide very promising strategies for treatment of AIPC. Quality of life (QOL) and pain relief were also checked during the calcitriol and taxotere combination therapy. Significant analgesic activity was demonstrated, yet worsening in several QOL parameters was also observed in patients experiencing relatively low pain intensity.[50]

Loss of Vitamin D Anti-proliferative Responsiveness in Prostate Cancer

While current efforts focus on developing strategies to use vitamin D analogs to control prostate cancer, it is possible that prostate cancer cells could become resistant to the tumor suppressive effects of vitamin D. Some prostate cancer cells are already known to be resistant to growth inhibition by vitamin D. Analyses of experimental model systems reveal that prostate cancer cells become less sensitive to vitamin D through loss of vitamin D receptors, loss of signaling molecules that modulate vitamin D action, or through changes in metabolic enzymes, such as 1α-hydroxylase and 24-hydroxylase, that sensitize or degrade vitamin D compounds.[51] Such changes have been found in experimental models, yet whether these alterations occur in human prostate cancer tissues *in vivo*, and the associated frequencies of occurrences still need to be determined. One study suggested that VDR levels were decreased in the prostate after age 60, which might be linked with increased incidence of prostate cancer with age,[52] and development of vitamin D resistance during the disease progression.

In one of our current studies, we identified a prostate cancer cell subline, CWR22R-2, which displays more aggressive behavior in the tumor invasiveness than its parental CWR22R cells. This aggressive CWR22R-2 line displays reduced vitamin D anti-proliferative effects compared to CWR22R cells, which provides evidence that prostate cancer cells might develop resistance to vitamin D during disease progression. Further characterization of these two cell lines found reduced vitamin D transcriptional activity in CWR22R-2 cells, which might correlate with higher expression of VDR co-repressors such as SMRT and NCoR, and eventually result in reduced vitamin D responsiveness.[53] More evidence from other prostate cancer cell lines with different vitamin D responses and from prostate cancer patient samples is needed to confirm our findings.

Future Perspectives

With increasing numbers of people being diagnosed with prostate cancer each year, there is great interest in developing better strategies to treat, and even to prevent, prostate cancer. Vitamin D has been proven to inhibit prostate cancer growth, progression, and metastases in both *in vitro* and *in vivo* animal models. However, the therapeutic use of vitamin D is limited. Development of vitamin D-based treatment with improved therapeutic indices, so that desired activity can be maximized while the tendency toward hypercalcemia can be minimized, is necessary.

The Figure summarizes our studies and those of others regarding vitamin D action in prostate cancer. Vitamin D may work through multiple pathways to prevent prostate cancer growth and progression via direct or indirect modulation of intracellular signals or secreted proteins, which are involved in the tumor growth, invasion, and angiogenesis. Whether the vitamin D-mediated changes of gene profiles occur *in vivo* as they occur *in vitro*, remain to be answered. Development of the prostate cancer patient tissue array technique by combination of classical histochemical analyses with advanced molecular techniques might provide powerful tools to study prostate cancer progression and its correlation with the clinical features at the molecular level. Through analysis of the expression of those vitamin D responsive genes identified from *in vitro* studies using prostate cancer tissue array samples, we might be able to generate a vitamin D-response human database in prostate cancer and thus directly translate *in vitro* study results into clinical application. These will certainly help to predict outcomes of vitamin D-based treatment and enhance the treatment efficacy based on individual patients' biochemical and molecular profiles.

References

1. Schwartz GG, Hulka BS (1990) Is vitamin D deficiency a risk factor for prostate cancer? (Hypothesis). *Anticancer Res* 10:1307–1311.
2. Hanchette CL, Schwartz GG (1992) Geographic patterns of prostate cancer mortality. Evidence for a protective effect of ultraviolet radiation. *Cancer* 70:2861–2869.
3. Corder EH, Guess HA, Hulka BS, et al. (1993) Vitamin D and prostate cancer: a prediagnostic study with stored sera. *Cancer Epidemiol Biomarkers Prev* 2:467–472.
4. Ahonen MH, Tenkanen L, Teppo L, Hakama M, Tuohimaa P (2000) Prostate cancer risk and prediagnostic serum 25-hydroxyvitamin D levels (Finland). *Cancer Causes Control* 11:847–852.
5. Tuohimaa P, Tenkanen L, Ahonen M, et al. (2004) Both high and low levels of blood vitamin D are associated with a higher prostate cancer risk: a longitudinal, nested case-control study in the Nordic countries. *Int J Cancer* 108:104–108.
6. Glass CK (1994) Differential recognition of target genes by nuclear receptor monomers, dimers, and heterodimers. *Endocr Rev* 15:391–407.
7. Kato S (2000) The function of vitamin D receptor in vitamin D action. *J Biochem (Tokyo)* 127:717–722.
8. Haussler MR, Haussler CA, Jurutka PW, et al. (1997) The vitamin D hormone and its nuclear receptor: molecular actions and disease states. *J Endocrinol* 154(Suppl):S57–73.
9. Freedman LP (1999) Multimeric coactivator complexes for steroid/nuclear receptors. *Trends Endocrinol Metab* 10:403–407.
10. Boonyaratanakornkit V, Melvin V, Prendergast P, et al. (1998) High-mobility group chromatin proteins 1 and 2 functionally interact with steroid hormone receptors to enhance their DNA binding *in vitro* and transcriptional activity in mammalian cells. *Mol Cell Biol* 18:4471–4487.
11. Leo C, Li H, Chen JD (2000) Differential mechanisms of nuclear receptor regulation by receptor-associated coactivator 3. *J Biol Chem* 275:5976–5982.
12. Liu YY, Nguyen C, Peleg S (2000) Regulation of ligand-induced heterodimerization and coactivator interaction by the activation function-2 domain of the vitamin D receptor. *Mol Endocrinol* 14:1776–1787.
13. May M, Mengus G, Lavigne AC, Chambon P, Davidson I (1996) Human TAF(II28) promotes transcriptional stimulation by activation function 2 of the retinoid X receptors. *EMBO J* 15:3093–3104.

14. Subramaniam N, Leong GM, Cock TA, *et al.* (2001) Cross-talk between 1,25-dihydroxyvitamin D3 and transforming growth factor-beta signaling requires binding of VDR and Smad3 proteins to their cognate DNA recognition elements. *J Biol Chem* 276:15741–15746.

15. Tagami T, Lutz WH, Kumar R, Jameson JL (1998) The interaction of the vitamin D receptor with nuclear receptor corepressors and coactivators. *Biochem Biophys Res Commun* 253:358–363.

16. Takeshita A, Ozawa Y, Chin WW (2000) Nuclear receptor coactivators facilitate vitamin D receptor homodimer action on direct repeat hormone response elements. *Endocrinology* 141:1281–1284.

17. Vidal M, Ramana CV, Dusso AS (2002) Stat1-vitamin D receptor interactions antagonize 1,25-dihydroxyvitamin D transcriptional activity and enhance stat1-mediated transcription. *Mol Cell Biol* 22:2777–2787.

18. Takeyama K, Masuhiro Y, Fuse H, *et al.* (1999) Selective interaction of vitamin D receptor with transcriptional coactivators by a vitamin D analog. *Mol Cell Biol* 19:1049–1055.

19. Rachez C, Suldan Z, Ward J, *et al.* (1998) A novel protein complex that interacts with the vitamin D3 receptor in a ligand-dependent manner and enhances VDR transactivation in a cell-free system. *Genes Dev* 12: 1787–1800.

20. Rosenfeld MG, Glass CK (2001) Coregulator codes of transcriptional regulation by nuclear receptors. *J Biol Chem* 276:36865–36868.

21. Barletta F, Freedman LP, Christakos S (2002) Enhancement of VDR-mediated transcription by phosphorylation: correlation with increased interaction between the VDR and DRIP205, a subunit of the VDR-interacting protein coactivator complex. *Mol Endocrinol* 16:301–314.

22. Qi X, Pramanik R, Wang J, *et al.* (2002) The p38 and JNK pathways cooperate to trans-activate vitamin D receptor via c-Jun/AP-1 and sensitize human breast cancer cells to vitamin D(3)-induced growth inhibition. *J Biol Chem* 277:25884–25892.

23. Miller GJ, Stapleton GE, Ferrara JA, *et al.* (1992) The human prostatic carcinoma cell line LNCaP expresses biologically active, specific receptors for 1 alpha,25-dihydroxyvitamin D3. *Cancer Res* 52:515–520.

24. Peehl DM, Skowronski RJ, Leung GK, Wong ST, Stamey TA, Feldman D (1994) Antiproliferative effects of 1,25-dihydroxyvitamin D3 on primary cultures of human prostatic cells. *Cancer Res* 54:805–810.

25. Skowronski RJ, Peehl DM, Feldman D (1993) Vitamin D and prostate cancer: 1,25 dihydroxyvitamin D3 receptors and actions in human prostate cancer cell lines. *Endocrinology* 132:1952–1960.

26. Schwartz GG, Oeler TA, Uskokovic MR, Bahnson RR (1994) Human prostate cancer cells: inhibition of proliferation by vitamin D analogs. *Anticancer Res* 14:1077–1078.

27. Hsieh TY, Ng CY, Mallouh C, Tazaki H, Wu JM (1996) Regulation of growth, PSA/PAP and androgen receptor expression by 1 alpha,25-dihydroxyvitamin D3 in the androgen-dependent LNCaP cells. *Biochem Biophys Res Commun* 223:141–146.

28. Hsieh T, Wu JM (1997) Induction of apoptosis and altered nuclear/cytoplasmic distribution of the androgen receptor and prostate-specific antigen by 1alpha,25-dihydroxyvitamin D3 in androgen-responsive LNCaP cells. *Biochem Biophys Res Commun* 235:539–544.

29. Bao BY, Ting HJ, Hu YC, Lee YF (2004) Androgen signaling is required in vitamin D mediated growth inhibition in prostate cancer cells. *Oncogene* (in press).

30. Zhuang SH, Burnstein KL (1998) Antiproliferative effect of 1alpha,25-dihydroxyvitamin D3 in human prostate cancer cell line LNCaP involves reduction of cyclin-dependent kinase 2 activity and persistent G1 accumulation. *Endocrinology* 139:1197–1207.

31. Blutt SE, McDonnell TJ, Polek TC, Weigel NL (2000) Calcitriol-induced apoptosis in LNCaP cells is blocked by overexpression of Bcl-2. *Endocrinology* 141:10–17.

32. Weitsman GE, Ravid A, Liberman UA, Koren R (2003) Vitamin D enhances caspase-dependent and -independent TNFalpha-induced breast cancer cell death: The role of reactive oxygen species and mitochondria. *Int J Cancer* 106:178–186.

33. Sung V, Feldman D (2000) 1,25-Dihydroxyvitamin D3 decreases human prostate cancer cell adhesion and migration. *Mol Cell Endocrinol* 164: 133–143.

34. Schwartz GG, Wang MH, Zang M, Singh RK, Siegal GP (1997) 1 alpha,25-Dihydroxyvitamin D (calcitriol) inhibits the invasiveness of human prostate cancer cells. *Cancer Epidemiol Biomarkers Prev* 6:727–732.

35. Gross C, Stamey T, Hancock S, Feldman D (1998) Treatment of early recurrent prostate cancer with 1,25-dihydroxyvitamin D3 (calcitriol). *J Urol* 159:2035–2039; discussion pp. 2039–2040.

36. Trump D, Lau YK (2003) Chemotherapy of prostate cancer: present and future. *Curr Urol Rep* 4:229–232.

37. Bao BY, Lee YF (2004) 1,25-vitamin D3 inhibits prostate cancer cell invasion by modulation MMPs, TIPs, and cystein protease activities. *Oncogene* (submitted).

38. Skowronski RJ, Peehl DM, Feldman D (1995) Actions of vitamin D3, analogs on human prostate cancer cell lines: comparison with 1,25-dihydroxyvitamin D3. *Endocrinology* 136:20–26.
39. Mehta RG, Mehta RR (2002) Vitamin D and cancer. *J Nutr Biochem* 13:252–264.
40. Liu G, Oettel K, Ripple G, *et al.* (2002) Phase I trial of 1alpha-hydroxyvitamin D(2) in patients with hormone refractory prostate cancer. *Clin Cancer Res* 8:2820–2827.
41. Liu G, Wilding G, Staab MJ, *et al.* (2003) Phase II study of 1alpha-hydroxyvitamin D(2) in the treatment of advanced androgen-independent prostate cancer. *Clin Cancer Res* 9:4077–4083.
42. Hershberger PA, Yu WD, Modzelewski RA, Rueger RM, Johnson CS, Trump DL (2001) Calcitriol (1,25-dihydroxycholecalciferol) enhances paclitaxel antitumor activity *in vitro* and *in vivo* and accelerates paclitaxel-induced apoptosis. *Clin Cancer Res* 7:1043–1051.
43. Beer TM, Eilers KM, Garzotto M, Egorin MJ, Lowe BA, Henner WD (2003) Weekly high-dose calcitriol and docetaxel in metastatic androgen-independent prostate cancer. *J Clin Oncol* 21:123–128.
44. Rao A, Woodruff RD, Wade WN, Kute TE, Cramer SD (2002) Genistein and vitamin D synergistically inhibit human prostatic epithelial cell growth. *J Nutr* 132:3191–3194.
45. Zhao XY, Ly LH, Peehl DM, Feldman D (1999) Induction of androgen receptor by 1alpha,25-dihydroxyvitamin D3 and 9-cis retinoic acid in LNCaP human prostate cancer cells. *Endocrinology* 140:1205–1212.
46. Ikeda N, Uemura H, Ishiguro H, *et al.* (2003) Combination treatment with 1alpha,25-dihydroxyvitamin D3 and 9-cis-retinoic acid directly inhibits human telomerase reverse transcriptase transcription in prostate cancer cells. *Mol Cancer Ther* 2:739–746.
47. Johnson CS, Hershberger PA, Bernardi RJ, McGuire TF, Trump DL (2002) Vitamin D receptor: a potential target for intervention. *Urology* 60:123–130; discussion pp. 130–131.
48. Smith DC, Johnson CS, Freeman CC, Muindi J, Wilson JW, Trump DL (1999) A Phase I trial of calcitriol (1,25-dihydroxycholecalciferol) in patients with advanced malignancy. *Clin Cancer Res* 5:1339–1345.
49. Blutt SE, Weigel NL (1999) Vitamin D and prostate cancer. *Proc Soc Exp Biol Med* 221:89–98.
50. Beer TM, Eilers KM, Garzotto M, Hsieh YC, Mori M (2004) Quality of life and pain relief during treatment with calcitriol and docetaxel in symptomatic metastatic androgen-independent prostate carcinoma. *Cancer* 100:758–763.

51. Peehl DM, Feldman D (2003) The role of vitamin D and retinoids in controlling prostate cancer progression. *Endocr Relat Cancer* 10:131–140.
52. Krill D, DeFlavia P, Dhir R, *et al.* (2001) Expression patterns of vitamin D receptor in human prostate. *J Cell Biochem* 82:566–572.
53. Ting HJ, Bao BY, Lee YF (2004) Loss of 1,25-dihydroxyvitamin D3 responsiveness in aggressive androgen-independent prostate cancer cells. *Mol Biol Cell* (submitted).

13

FUNCTIONS OF ESTROGEN RECEPTOR IN PROSTATE AND PROSTATE CANCER

Shuyuan Yeh, Ming Chen, Jing Ni, Yi Yin, Eugene Chang, Min Zhang and Xingqing Wen

Departments of Urology and Pathology
University of Rochester Medical Center, Rochester, New York

Introduction

It has long been known that the functions of estrogen and estrogen receptor (ER) are important for the female reproductive system, mammary gland development, and cancer progression.[1] Accumulated evidence from various studies indicated that ER is expressed and functions in the male reproductive system, including prostate. Earlier studies only identified one traditional ER, ERalpha (ERα), which was thought to be responsible for all the estrogen-mediated responses in prostate. Recently, ERbeta (ERβ) was identified and shown to express in prostate epithelia.[2] Results from PCR, immunohistochemical staining and receptor knockout (KO) mice suggested that estrogens, ERα and ERβ play significant roles in prostate development and the initiation and progression of prostate cancer. In this chapter, we will focus on the distribution of ERα and ERβ, potential target genes, ER association proteins, their potential roles in the development of prostate, and the progression of prostate cancer based on the results from prostate tissues, cancer cell lines, and animal models, including αERKO, βERKO, αβERKO, and hypogonadal (hpg) mice.

Distribution of ERα and ERβ in Prostate Tissues, Cancer Specimens and Cancer Cell Lines

Estrogen has been used for the treatment of prostate cancer since the early 1940s.[3] It is generally believed this action is indirectly mediated at the hypothalamic level to suppress the circulating androgens.[4] However, in the early 1960s, a direct action of estrogen via their own receptors in the prostate was proposed by Mangan *et al.*[5] Recently, the evidences that ER expressed in normal prostate, benign prostatic hyperplasia (BPH), prostate cancer specimens, and different prostate cancer cell lines, along with the demonstration of the stimulatory or inhibitory effects of estrogen on prostate cancer cells growth suggested estrogen may exert direct effects on prostate via their own receptors.[6-11] The following sections will discuss the distribution of ERα and ERβ in prostate tissues, cancer specimens, and cancer cell lines.

Both ERα and ERβ express in the human prostate tissue.[2,12] In normal prostate tissue ERα is mostly expressed in stromal cells with occasional expression in the basal epithelial cells,[8,11,13-15] whereas ERβ is abundantly present in basal epithelial cells.[8,11,13] The complementary location of both ERα and ERβ might explain why some early studies reported ERα in both the stroma and epithelium of the normal prostate, which may be caused by cross reaction against both ER subtypes.[16]

In BPH, ERα immunostaining could not be detected in several studies.[15,16] Using enzyme immunoassay, Mobbs *et al.* (1990) found high positivity of ERα in BPH.[17] The latter immunostaining studies found ERα was stronger in BPH than in normal prostates and localized in both epithelial and stromal cells.[8] Immunoexpression of ERβ in BPH was also higher than in normal prostates and localized only in the epithelium.[8]

In prostate cancer specimens, the expressions of both ERα and ERβ have been studied for years,[6,8,13,18] however, the relative expression levels and location of ERs in prostate cancer are still controversial. Using methods of immunohistochemistry staining, loss or down-regulation of ERα in prostate cancer has been reported.[19,20] It appears ERα gene is transcriptionally inactivated by DNA methylation in most prostate cancer cells lines and specimens.[11,21] Conversely, several groups reported the higher ERα expression in the prostate cancer specimens than in BPH and normal prostate tissue, which is consistent with other reports that abundance of ERα is positively correlated with the malignancy of prostate cancer.[7,17]

In terms of ERβ expression, Royuela *et al*. (2001) reported the ERβ has increasing epithelial staining in both BPH and prostate cancer, and some stromal cells acquire ERβ in prostate cancer specimens, not in normal prostate and BPH. These findings suggest the involvement of ERβ in prostate cancer. However, recent reports showed a frequent loss of ERβ expression in prostate cancer samples relative to normal prostate tissue.[13,18,22] In the primary prostate tumor sites, ERβ was strongly expressed in low grade prostate carcinoma and was markedly diminished in higher grade tumor.[18,22,23] These results suggested ERβ may protect against abnormal prostate cell growth.[11,13,22] Loss of ERβ may cause prostate epithelial cells to escape the control of proliferation by ERβ in prostate cancer. Further studies indiated ERβ protein expression was significantly elevated in metastatic prostate tumor.[13] Currently it is unclear why the ERβ expression will be decreased in the higher grade prostate cancer and re-elevated in metastases. One hypothesis is that the failure to lose ERβ may allow the cancer cells to gain the metastatic potential, and another could be the local environment in the distal metastatic sites may induce ERβ expression. Although the controversy of ERs expression exists, the accumulating evidence shows the abnormality of ER signaling may contribute to the pathogenesis of prostate cancer.

The expression patterns of both ERs in different prostate cancer cell lines has been studied recently. The earlier studies on the effect of estrogens on prostate cancer cells growth showed the direct role of estrogen via their own receptors, but the specific ER has not been defined. Using RT-PCR, Lau *et al*. (1999) showed ERβ, but not ERα, was found in normal prostate epithelia cells, along with pS2 and PR mRNA expression. Only ERβ is detectable in LNCaP and DU145 cell lines, whereas PC-3 and BPH-1 expressed both ERα and ERβ.[11] Currently, there are two ERβ isoforms, ERβ1 and ERβ2. Only ERβ1 was detectable in PC-3, DU145, and LNCaP cell lines, whereas ERβ2 was absent.[24] Together, these studies suggested ERβ could be the key player of estrogen-mediated effects in prostate cancer cell lines.

In rodents, it was found that ERα mRNA was the major type of ER expressed in two-week-old rat prostate and that as the rat aged ERβ became the dominant expression.[25] In agreement with the results from human prostate, it was found that ERα protein is predominantly located in the stroma cells of ventral prostate of adult rodents, with over 90% of the epithelial cells stained positive for ERβ.[26]

Estrogen Regulated Genes in Prostate Cancer

Estrogens and ER have been shown to play important roles in prostate carcinogenesis.[27] The detailed mechanisms however, are not well known. Currently, some estrogen target genes have been identified, which may contribute to the diversified estrogen effect on prostate cancer. Those genes include telomerase,[27] endothelin-1,[28] eNOS,[29] E-cadherin,[30] metallothionein II,[31] CGA gene,[32] androgen receptor,[26] and glutathione-peroxidase.[33]

In addition, PS2 and progesterone receptor (PR), have an estrogen responsive element (ERE) in the promoter regions, and are also expressed in the prostate, suggesting they can be regulated by estrogen in human prostate.[11] In mouse prostate, diethylstilbestrol (DES) treatment induces PR synthesis in secretory epithelial cells, which is usually low in the untreated prostate. Although a functional role for progesterone in regulating prostate growth is unknown, PR synthesis is an effective marker of estrogen action in the prostate. It was found that the acute DES exposure of WT male mice, the prostatic responses were similar, including induction of squamous metaplasia (SQM), and up-regulation of PR.[34] Table 1 lists the identified estrogen target genes in the prostate. In comparison, many other estrogen target genes have been identified in the breast or other estrogen target organs. For better understanding of the estrogen signal in prostate, ERα and ERβ target genes and their roles in prostate need to be identified and characterized.

Table 1. Estrogen Regulated Genes in Prostate

Function	Genes	Up- or Down-regulation	Estrogen Response Element (ERE)
Carcinogenesis	Telomerase	↑	+
Angiogenesis	eNOS	↑	N/A
Metastasis	E-cadherin	↑	N/A
Metastasis	Endothelin-1	↓	N/A
Homeostasis	Metallothionein II	↑	N/A
Hormones	CGA gene	↑	N/A (link with ERα)
Oxidant enzyme	Glutathione-peroxidase	↑	N/A
Transcription factor	Androgen receptor	↓	N/A
Transcription factor	Progesterone receptor	↑	+
Unknown	PS2	↑	+

ER Coregulators in Prostate

ERs are ligand-dependent transcription factors which bind to the ERE to regulate the transcription of target genes. The transcription initiation is a complex process which involves the cooperative interaction between ERs and multiple factors at the promoter region of target genes. The occurrence of transcriptional interference between nuclear receptors in early transient receptor/reporter co-transfection assays suggested the existence of common rate limiting cofactors, other than general transcription factors (GTFs), required for ERs activation function.[35,36] In this regard, coregulators were identified, and defined as coactivators or corepressors required for transcriptional regulation.[37] In this chapter, we will mainly focus on the expression pattern of some identified ER coactivators in the prostate tissue and prostate cancer cell lines.

To date, there are numerous ER coregulators that have been identified and the most well characterized ER coactivators belong to the p160 family, including SRC-1, SRC-2 (TIF2/GRIP1) and SRC-3 (AIB1/RAC3).[37] Among these identified ER coactivators, SRC-3/RAC3/AIB1 is the most well studied in prostate cancer cell lines. Using Western blotting, Gnanapragasam *et al.* showed that SRC3/RAC3/AIB1 protein has the highest expression in LNCaP cells, moderate expression in PC-3 cells, and low-level expression in DU145 cells.[38] In the human prostate tissue, the levels of SRC-3/RAC3/AIB1 expression is significantly correlated with tumor grade and stage of disease, but not with serum PSA levels.[38] SRC-1 is expressed as a major RNA transcript of 7.5 kb in many tissues, including prostate. The expression levels of SRC-1 were found to be elevated in the cancer specimens with a higher grade or poor response to endocrine therapy, than in those with a lower grade or good response to endocrine therapy.[39] In addition to SRC-1 and SRC-3, other ER co-regulators, CBP/p300, SMRT, and N-CoR, are also expressed in prostate.[40]

Overall, most of ER co-regulators identified to date are not specific to ER, and can interact with other nuclear receptors, including AR.[41] Therefore, how these co-regulators regulate ER function in prostate development and neoplastic transformation remains to be elucidated. In addition, whether any ER specific associated proteins exist in prostate needs further investigation.

Histological Changes in Prostates of αERKO and βERKO Mice

To understand the roles of estrogen, ERα and ERβ in the development of prostate glands, the gene knockout strategy has been used. The adult male αERKO mouse prostate shows normal development and histology, specifically in the ventral prostate (VP)[42,43] and anterior prostate (AP).[44] With aging, the weights of αERKO seminal vehicle (SV) and AP increased,[45] although they remain histologically indistinguishable from that of WT littermates.[42,44]

The initial description of targeted disruption of the gene encoding ERβ reported some evidence of epithelial hyperplasia in βERKO prostates.[46] Weihua et al.[26] further reported that βERKO mice had multiple hyperplastic foci in the peripheral and central zones of the VP at five months; by one year of age, eight of ten βERKO VPs had multiple hyperplastic lesions, and most epithelial cells stained positively for the proliferation antigen Ki-67. However, other studies of the prostate phenotype in ERβ-deficient mice,[42,43,47] failed to corroborate the initial report of Krege et al.,[46] and no hyperplasia was seen in prostate lobes of βERKO line at 12–20 months.[42,43,47] The reason for discrepant results from mice with the same apparent genotype is unclear, yet other factors might affect the mice, such as diet or infection. In general, there is no significant histological changes in prostates of αERKO mice, and with controversial observation in prostate of βERKO Mice.

Estrogen Imprinting Effect on the Development of Prostate

Although estrogen levels are low or undetectable in adult male mice, administration of exogenous estrogens during development[48] dramatically affects prostate growth and function.[49–54] The effects of estrogens vary according to timing and duration of exposure, in addition to the type and dose of estrogen administered. Furthermore, the individual lobes of the prostate exhibit varied degrees of response to estrogens and androgens.

The neonatal period after birth is very fundamental for the rodent prostate development in which the prostate involves branching morphogenesis followed by functional differentiation. In this period, brief exposure of male rats or mice to high-level estrogens will cause irreversible alterations in development and function of the prostate gland and a reduced responsiveness to androgens during adulthood.[50,55–57] The estrogen imprinting effect is associated with an aging-related prostatic lesion, which includes the hyperplasia of prostatic epithelial cells or severe dysplasia similar to high grade prostatic intra-epithelial neoplasia (PIN) and extensive immune cell infiltrate.[51,58–61]

As early as 1978, Rajfer and Coffey reported that if high dose of 17β-estradiol at 500 μg per day, or estradiol benzoate at 250 μg per day, or estradiol dipropionate at 100 μg per day, is administered to intact male rats for 2 days during the 1st week after birth, the prostate, at adulthood, is diminutive in size and is inert to the action of exogenous androgens. If immature rodents are exposed to exogenous estrogen before puberty, the aging animals develop prostatic epithelial hyperplasia[50] or even dysplasia if androgen is given together with estrogen.[61] A series of studies by McLachlan *et al.* demonstrated that perinatal exposure to the synthetic estrogen, DES, results in an assortment of apparently direct defects in the murine male reproductive tract, including undescended testes, epididymal cysts, aberrant expression of estrogen inducible genes, adenocarcinoma, and sterility.[61–65]

In addition to morphological and histological changes, several groups characterized the other hallmarks of neonatal estrogen imprinting in the rat model as well as in different mouse strains. These included transient up-regulation of ERα, down-regulation of androgen receptor (AR), decreased ERβ levels in adult prostate epithelium, lack of dorsal lateral prostate (DLP) secretory protein, up-regulated proto-oncogene c-fos, reduced TGFβ type I receptor levels in the prostate epithelium, but not in stroma, whereas there was no effect on TGFβ type II receptor. p21 (cip-1/waf-1) is a cyclin-dependent kinase inhibitor, and is known to be inducible by TGFβ1 in the prostate. Neonatal estrogenization prevented this transient expression of p21 (cip-1/waf-1) in the prostate epithelium cells. Those changes in molecular levels suggested they could be good markers for estrogenization in the prostate.[66–72]

Estrogen Treatment of αERKO, βERKO, and Hypogonadal (*hpg*) Mouse Models

Intact adult αERKO mice treated with DES showed no change in organ weight, no induction of SQM, or synthesis of CK10 or PR in any prostate lobe.[44] In contrast, the intact adult βERKO mouse treated with DES showed a full response, similar to that of WT mice.[44] In spite of normal ERβ levels in the αERKO prostate, these animals showed no morphological or molecular effects of estrogen in the prostate. These data suggest that these actions or effects of exogenous estrogen on the adult mouse prostate are predominantly mediated through ERα. ERα is thus the predominant receptor mediating mitogenic estrogen action in the prostate, and a role for ERβ remains to be identified.

Because classic estrogen responses (SQM and up-regulation of PR) were seen in the βERKO but not in the αERKO mice, it is assumed that ERα mediates these responses in the adult prostate. A recent report involving tissue recombination examined the role of ERα in mediating estrogenic responses in prostate, using combinations of WT and αERKO prostate epithelial and stromal cells.[44] The recombinant tissues were grafted under the kidney capsule of immunologically deprived nude mice exposed to DES treatment for 21 days. ERα is required for the induction of SQM, but not for the up-regulation of PR synthesis, which occurred in all recombinants, even though this response was absent after the *in vivo* DES treatment of αERKO mice.[44] The functional significance of the separation of these two end points (SQM and PR synthesis) suggests that additional mechanisms are involved in mediating estrogen responses.

Exposure to estrogens during the neonatal period causes both acute and long-term effects on the prostate gland. Neonatally estrogenized WT animals show inhibited prostate growth during development and subsequently display evidence of dysplasia and an attenuated response to androgens.[50,52–54,67] When estrogenized animals are castrated and then treated with androgen (testosterone) implants, the observed effects are not completely blocked, suggesting that much of the phenotype is the result of permanent alterations within the prostate tissue caused by direct estrogen action.[67] The neonatal studies described above were all conducted in a rat model system with high doses of DES. By contrast, a single report showed increased prostate size following low-dose maternal estrogen administration to male mouse fetuses.[49,73] The discrepancies between rat and mouse models, and high- and low-dose estrogen, emphasize the compounding influences of timing, duration, and dose of estrogen in similar studies. Recently, Prins *et al.*[42] utilized αERKO and βERKO mice to demonstrate that both acute and chronic effects of neonatal DES treatment are predominantly mediated by ERα in mouse prostate.

Investigation of intact male mice with prostatic response to estrogen treatment requires analysis of both indirect and direct effects. Indirect actions occur via regulation of the hypothalamic-pituitary-gonadal (HPG) axis. They alter androgen production and the endocrine status of the mice. Direct responses to estrogen by the prostate differ and occur in response to local or intraprostatic changes in estrogen synthesis via aromatase enzyme activity or modulation of the ERs. More recently, the direct actions of estrogens *in vivo* were evaluated using the hypogonadal (*hpg*) mouse model[74] that is deficient in pituitary gonadotropin and sex steroid production. Mature male *hpg* mice were exposed to estradiol for 6 weeks, and proliferative changes were recorded in the prostate with specific effects observed in the stroma and epithelium; estradiol administration stimulated growth and expansion of the stromal, epithelial and luminal compartments of the mouse prostate lobes.[75] The epithelial cells became multi-layered and squamous, showing immunoexpression of high molecular weight cytokeratins and cytokeratin 10 (CK10) that is characteristic of the pathology known as squamous metaplasia (SQM).[44,76] The stromal response was characterized by an increase in fibroblastic stroma that penetrated the smooth muscle layer, accompanied by a reduction and disorganization in α-actin-positive smooth muscle cells surrounding the glandular ducts. Additionally, neutrophils were identified in the stroma and were shown to migrate through the epithelium to the lumen. Although secretory activity of prostate epithelial cells was significantly reduced by estradiol exposure, the lumen was distended as a result of accumulated cellular debris comprising epithelial cells, inflammatory cells, and anuclear keratinised deposits.[75]

Overall, results from these genomic-manipulated mice suggested that ERα is the dominant ER form mediating the developmental estrogenization of the prostate gland. Estrogens induced direct proliferative changes in the prostate of male *hpg mice*, which do not have physiological levels of androgen.

Estrogen Effect on Initiation, Growth, and Progression of Prostate Cancer

While androgens play essential roles in the development and growth of prostate and pathogenesis of prostate cancer, extensive *in vivo* and *in vitro* studies suggested that estrogens are required for carcinogenesis of prostate cancer. It was demonstrated that treatment with both estrogen and testosterone will induce 100% dorsolaterol prostate carcinoma in rats.[77] In human, direct estrogen effects and the balance of androgens and estrogens may contribute to these estrogen activities. Men synthesize both estrogens and androgens and as men age, the plasma levels of androgen decreases while estrogen remains constant. However, the expression pattern and activity of aromatase, the enzyme that turns testosterone into estrogen, suggests that local synthesized estrogen may have significant consequences in tumorigenesis of prostate.[78,79] Here we will focus on estrogens effects on prostate cancer cells from *in vitro* and *in vivo* approaches. While this approach provides some insights to explain the *in vivo* observation from clinical and mouse study, many unclear and controversial data remain.

In prostate, estrogen induced cancerous transformation may be partially due to their genotoxic metabolites, including 2-hydroxy-estrogens, 4-hydroxy-estrogens, quinone, and semiquinone intermediates. These metabolites may directly induce genomic damage or function via formation of reactive oxygen species (ROS).[80,81] In addition, the enzymes responsible for the formation or inactivation of these estrogen metabolites may also play critical roles in the estrogen mediated transformation in prostate. These enzymes include (1) cytochrome p4501A1, which can convert estrogen into 2-hydroxy-estrogens, (2) cytochrome p4501B1, which can concert estrogens to 4-hydroxy-estrogens, (3) cathecol-O-methyl-transferase, which can inactivate 2- and 4-hydroxy-estrogens, and (4) glutathione-S-transferases that detoxify ROS.[81–83] Although these may be important factors for estrogen mediated effects in prostate, few of them have been investigated for their contribution in prostate cancer.

As the aromatase can convert androgens into estrogens, thus it could be one of the risk factor of prostate cancer.[84,85] However, the aromatase transgenic mice and knockout mice have numerous endocrine defects,[34,86] thus these mice cannot be used as good models to study the relationship between estrogen formation and prostate cancer risk. The studies will be advanced by producing mice with prostate specific expression or knock-out of aromatase in the future.

In adult WT mice, administration of high-dose DES, a potent synthetic estrogen, causes regression of the prostate and induces SQM in the epithelium. The reduced organ size is associated with declining androgen levels, whereas SQM is considered to be a direct, ERα mediated response to estrogen.[44] Prostatic SQM is characterized by proliferation of basal cells, leading to formation of stratified squamous epithelium and altered CK10 synthesis. In mouse prostate, DES treatment induces PR synthesis in secretory epithelial cells, which is usually low in the untreated prostate.

Although studies suggested that estrogens are required for carcinogenesis of prostate cancer, yet extensive *evidences also* suggest that estrogens can suppress prostate cancer growth. It has been found that estrogen inhibits the cell growth of PC-3, an androgen independent prostate cancer cell line,[9] while it can stimulate the growth of LNCaP, an androgen responsive prostate cancer cell line.[10] This difference may be due to different ER forms and ER levels in these two cell lines[85,86] and other mechanisms. Although estrogen stimulates both ERα and ERβ, it is generally believed that ERα stimulates cell proliferation whereas ERβ counteracts ERα activity. In the prostate, ERα is exclusively expressed in stroma, while ERβ is largely expressed in epithelial cells. In tumors, ERα is expressed in both stroma and epithelial. Many studies support the expression pattern of ERα and ERβ, and the interaction between stroma and epithelial of prostate largely contributes to the different estrogen effects on the prostate cancer cells growth *in vivo* and *in vitro*.[11,87–89] However, the expression pattern of ERα and ERβ in normal and tumor prostate tissue, and prostate cancer cell lines are different. More studies need to be elucidated.

The effect of estrogen regulation of prostate cancer cell growth was also tested with the estrogen metabolite, 2-methoxyestradiol (2-ME), which can arrest the cell cycle and induce apoptosis.[90,91] However, the 10 μM dose of 2-ME used in the study is much higher than physiological concentration. Cellular component concentrations are another important factor for the cellular growth or signal. Homeostatic changes might also contribute to malignant growth. Estrogen can increase intracellular Ca (2+) in PC-3 cells.[92] Estrogen also reduces the uptake of rubidium chloride, suggesting an estrogen effect on ion transport and change of cellular membrane permeability.[93]

Although estrogen effects on prostate cancer cell growth are somewhat controversial, the fact that estrogen is required for prostate carcinogenesis is consistent. It was reported that a low ratio of androgen to estrogen results in a higher risk for the prostate cancer. *In vivo* animal studies also supported that estrogen, in a milieu of decreasing androgen, contributes significantly to the prostate hyperplasia, prostate dysplasia, and prostate cancer. βERKO mice cannot be induced by estrogen treatment to grow prostate cancer.[76,94] Therefore, estrogens and ERs, together with androgen, are required for the pathogenesis of prostate cancer. Recently, telomerase, whose activity increased during tumorigenesis, has been shown to be stimulated by estrogen in primary cultured cells from BPH and normal prostate tissue. Telomerase contains ERE in its promoter, thus could be a target gene of ER.[27] This may be one of the mechanisms by which estrogens stimulate carcinogenesis. Antiestrogen treatment therefore may prevent prostate cancer.

It is very significant that in the transgenic adenocarcinoma mouse prostate (TRAMP) mouse model of adenocarcinoma of the ventral prostate,[95] the selective estrogen receptor modulator (SERM), toremifene,[96] and the phytoestrogen genistein,[97] prevent the development of cancer. Although it has been suggested that this protection results from inhibition of ERα in the prostate stroma, an equally acceptable explanation is that these agents, acting as ERβ agonists, prevent proliferation of the prostate epithelium. Such a mechanism is likely in view of the role of ERβ in preventing proliferation of the ventral prostate epithelium in the mouse and strongly suggests a role for ERβ agonists in the treatment and/or prevention of prostate cancer.

Implantation of prostate cancer xenografts (LuCaP 35, LuCaP 49, LuCaP 58, LuCaP 73, PC-3, and LNCaP) into intact and ovariectomized female mice was done by Corey *et al.* to characterize growth and uptake rates in the absence of androgens.[98] Significant inhibition of prostate cancer growth in intact *vs.* ovariectomized female animals was observed in five of six prostate cancer xenograft lines (except for PC-3). E2 supplements given to ovariectomized female mice led to inhibition of tumor establishment and diminished growth of LuCaP 35, similar to that observed in intact female mice. RT-PCR showed that these xenografts express the ERβ message. Two hypothetical mechanisms may be suggested to explain how E2 can affect prostate cancer tumor growth in female mice in the absence of androgens: (1) E2 exerts direct inhibitory effects via ER expressed on prostate cancer cells or via other, as yet unidentified, mechanisms; and (2) E2 exerts effects on other cells, which then secrete signaling molecules that inhibit prostate cancer growth.

Together, these *in vivo* and *in vitro* studies suggested that estrogens may have dual roles: (1) estrogens are required for tumorigenecity of prostate cancer; and (2) Estrogens may suppress growth of prostate cancer.

Conclusion

To date, results from various studies clearly demonstrated that estrogens and ERs play important roles in prostate development and tumorigenesis. However, the roles are still not completely elucidated. Results from αERKO male mice suggest that ERα plays roles in the initiation of BPH and SQM.[86] Results from βERKO male mice indicated that when mice aged they may develop hypertrophy[26] suggesting that ERβ plays a negative role or is a factor controlling prostatic cell growth. However, results from other groups are not entirely consistent with that conclusion.[99] It is currently unclear whether nutritional and environmental factors contribute to the discrepancy. Furthermore, the number and function of different isoforms of ERβ that exist in the prostate have not been conclusively determined.

References

1. Russo IH, Russo J (1998) Role of hormones in mammary cancer initiation and progression. *J Mammary Gland Biol Neoplasia* 3:49–61.
2. Mosselman S, Polman J, Dijkema R (1996) ER beta: identification and characterization of a novel human estrogen receptor. *FEBS Lett* 392:49–53.
3. Huggins C, Hodges CV (1941) Studies on prostatic cancer. I. The effect of castration, of estrogen and androgen injection on serum phosphatases in metastatic carcinoma of the prostate. *Cancer Res* 1:293–297.

4. Huggins C, Hodges CV (1972) Studies on prostatic cancer. I. The effect of castration, of estrogen and androgen injection on serum phosphatases in metastatic carcinoma of the prostate. *CA Cancer J Clin* 22:232–240.

5. Mangan FR, Neal GE, Williams DC (1967) The effects of diethylstilboestrol and castration on the nucleic acid and protein metabolism of rat prostate gland. *Biochem J* 104:1075–1081.

6. Brolin J, Skoog L, Ekman P (1992) Immunohistochemistry and biochemistry in detection of androgen, progesterone and estrogen receptors in benign and malignant human prostatic tissue. *Prostate* 20:281–295.

7. Bonkhoff H, Fixemer T, Hunsicker I, Remberger K (1999) Estrogen receptor expression in prostate cancer and premalignant prostatic lesions. *Am J Pathol* 155:641–647.

8. Royuela M, de Miguel MP, Bethencourt FR, Sanchez-Chapado M, Fraile B, Arenas MI, Paniagua R (2001) Estrogen receptors alpha and beta in the normal, hyperplastic and carcinomatous human prostate. *J Endocrinol* 168:447–54.

9. Carruba G, Pfeffer U, Fecarotta E, Coviello DA, D'Amato E, Lo Castro M, Vidali G, Castagnetta L (1994) Estradiol inhibits growth of hormone-nonresponsive PC3 human prostate cancer cells. *Cancer Res* 54:1190–1193.

10. Castagnetta LA, Carruba G (1995) Human prostate cancer: a direct role for oestrogens. *Ciba Found Symp* 191:269–286; discussion 286–289.

11. Lau KM, LaSpina M, Long J, Ho SM (2000) Expression of estrogen receptor (ER)-alpha and ER-beta in normal and malignant prostatic epithelial cells: regulation by methylation and involvement in growth regulation. *Cancer Res* 60:3175–3182.

12. Kuiper GG, Carlsson B, Grandien K, Enmark E, Haggblad J, Nilsson S, Gustafsson JA (1997) Comparison of the ligand binding specificity and transcript tissue distribution of estrogen receptors alpha and beta. *Endocrinology* 138:863–870.

13. Leav I, Lau KM, Adams JY, McNeal JE, Taplin ME, Wang J, Singh H, Ho SM (2001) Comparative studies of the estrogen receptors beta and alpha and the androgen receptor in normal human prostate glands, dysplasia, and in primary and metastatic carcinoma. *Am J Pathol* 159:79–92.

14. Chaisiri N, Pierrepoint CG (1980) Examination of the distribution of oestrogen receptor between the stromal and epithelial compartments of the canine prostate. *Prostate* 1:357–366.

15. Ehara H, Koji T, Deguchi T, Yoshii A, Nakano M, Nakane PK, Kawada Y (1995) Expression of estrogen receptor in diseased human prostate assessed by non-radioactive *in situ* hybridization and immunohistochemistry. *Prostate* 27:304–313.

16. Schulze H, Claus S (1990) Histological localization of estrogen receptors in normal and diseased human prostates by immunocytochemistry. *Prostate* 16:331–343.
17. Mobbs BG, Johnson IE, Liu Y (1990) Quantitation of cytosolic and nuclear estrogen and progesterone receptor in benign, untreated and treated malignant human prostatic tissue by radioligand binding and enzyme-immunoassays. *Prostate* 16:235–244.
18. Latil A, Bieche I, Vidaud D, Lidereau R, Berthon P, Cussenot O, Vidaud M (2001) Evaluation of androgen, estrogen (ER alpha and ER beta), and progesterone receptor expression in human prostate cancer by real-time quantitative reverse transcription-polymerase chain reaction assays. *Cancer Res* 61:1919–1926.
19. Konishi N, Nakaoka S, Hiasa Y, Kitahori Y, Ohshima M, Samma S, Okajima E (1993) Immunohistochemical evaluation of estrogen receptor status in benign prostatic hypertrophy and in prostate carcinoma and the relationship to efficacy of endocrine therapy. *Oncology* 50:259–263.
20. Hobisch A, Hittmair A, Daxenbichler G, Wille S, Radmayr C, Hobisch-Hagen P, Bartsch G, Klocker H, Culig Z (1997) Metastatic lesions from prostate cancer do not express oestrogen and progesterone receptors. *J Pathol* 182:356–361.
21. Li LC, Chui R, Nakajima K, Oh BR, Au HC, Dahiya R (2000) Frequent methylation of estrogen receptor in prostate cancer: correlation with tumor progression. *Cancer Res* 60:702–706.
22. Horvath LG, Henshall SM, Lee CS, Head DR, Quinn DI, Makela S, Delprado W, Golovsky D, Brenner PC, O'Neill G, Kooner R, Stricker PD, Grygiel JJ, Gustafsson JA, Sutherland RL (2001) Frequent loss of estrogen receptor-beta expression in prostate cancer. *Cancer Res* 61:5331–5335.
23. Tsurusaki T, Aoki D, Kanetake H, Inoue S, Muramatsu M, Hishikawa Y, Koji T (2003) Zone-dependent expression of estrogen receptors alpha and beta in human benign prostatic hyperplasia. *J Clin Endocrinol Metab* 88:1333–1340.
24. Hanstein B, Liu H, Yancisin MC, Brown M (1999) Functional analysis of a novel estrogen receptor-beta isoform. *Mol Endocrinol* 13:129–137.
25. Asano K, Maruyama S, Usui T, Fujimoto N (2003) Regulation of estrogen receptor alpha and beta expression by testosterone in the rat prostate gland. *Endocr J* 50:281–287.
26. Weihua Z, Makela S, Andersson LC, Salmi S, Saji S, Webster JI, Jensen EV, Nilsson S, Warner M, Gustafsson JA (2001) A role for estrogen receptor beta in the regulation of growth of the ventral prostate. *Proc Natl Acad Sci USA* 98:6330–6335.

27. Nanni S, Narducci M, Della Pietra L, Moretti F, Grasselli A, De Carli P, Sacchi A, Pontecorvi A, Farsetti A (2002) Signaling through estrogen receptors modulates telomerase activity in human prostate cancer. *J Clin Invest* 110:219–227.

28. Grande M, Carlstrom K, Stege R, Pousette A, Faxen M (2002) Estrogens affect endothelin-1 mRNA expression in LNCaP human prostate carcinoma cells. *Eur Urol* 41:568–572; discussion 573–574.

29. Grande M, Carlstrom K, Stege R, Pousette A, Faxen M (2000) Estrogens increase the endothelial nitric oxide synthase (ecNOS) mRNA level in LNCaP human prostate carcinoma cells. *Prostate* 45:232–237.

30. Carruba G, Miceli D, D'Amico D, Farruggio R, Comito L, Montesanti A, Polito L, Castagnetta LA (1995) Sex steroids up-regulate E-cadherin expression in hormone-responsive LNCaP human prostate cancer cells. *Biochem Biophys Res Commun* 212:624–631.

31. Harris H, Henderson R, Bhat R, Komm B (2001) Regulation of metallothionein II messenger ribonucleic acid measures exogenous estrogen receptor-beta activity in SAOS-2 and LNCaPLN3 cells. *Endocrinology* 142:645–652.

32. Bieche I, Latil A, Parfait B, Vidaud D, Laurendeau I, Lidereau R, Cussenot O, Vidaud M (2002) CGA gene (coding for the alpha subunit of glycoprotein hormones) overexpression in ER alpha-positive prostate tumors. *Eur Urol* 41:335–341.

33. Weihua Z, Warner M, Gustafsson JA (2002) Estrogen receptor beta in the prostate. *Mol Cell Endocrinol* 193:1–5.

34. McPherson SJ, Wang H, Jones ME, Pedersen J, Iismaa TP, Wreford N, Simpson ER, Risbridger GP (2001) Elevated androgens and prolactin in aromatase-deficient mice cause enlargement, but not malignancy, of the prostate gland. *Endocrinology* 142:2458–2467.

35. Meyer ME, Gronemeyer H, Turcotte B, Bocquel MT, Tasset D, Chambon P (1989) Steroid hormone receptors compete for factors that mediate their enhancer function. *Cell* 57:433–442.

36. Tora L, White J, Brou C, Tasset D, Webster N, Scheer E, Chambon P (1989) The human estrogen receptor has two independent nonacidic transcriptional activation functions. *Cell* 59:477–487.

37. McKenna NJ, Lanz RB, O'Malley BW (1999) Nuclear receptor coregulators: cellular and molecular biology. *Endocr Rev* 20:321–344.

38. Gnanapragasam VJ, Leung HY, Pulimood AS, Neal DE, Robson CN (2001) Expression of RAC 3, a steroid hormone receptor co-activator in prostate cancer. *Br J Cancer* 85:1928–1936.

39. Fujimoto N, Mizokami A, Harada S, Matsumoto T (2001) Different expression of androgen receptor coactivators in human prostate. *Urology* 58:289–294.

40. Misiti S, Schomburg L, Yen PM, Chin WW (1998) Expression and hormonal regulation of coactivator and corepressor genes. *Endocrinology* 139:2493–2500.
41. McKenna NJ, O'Malley BW (2002) Minireview: nuclear receptor coactivators — an update. *Endocrinology* 143:2461–2465.
42. Prins GS, Birch L, Couse JF, Choi I, Katzenellenbogen B, Korach KS (2001) Estrogen imprinting of the developing prostate gland is mediated through stromal estrogen receptor alpha: studies with alphaERKO and betaERKO mice. *Cancer Res* 61:6089–6097.
43. Couse JF, Curtis Hewitt S, Korach KS (2000) Receptor null mice reveal contrasting roles for estrogen receptor alpha and beta in reproductive tissues. *J Steroid Biochem Mol Biol* 74:287–296.
44. Risbridger G, Wang H, Young P, Kurita T, Wang YZ, Lubahn D, Gustafsson JA, Cunha G, Wong YZ (2001) Evidence that epithelial and mesenchymal estrogen receptor-alpha mediates effects of estrogen on prostatic epithelium. *Dev Biol* 229:432–442.
45. Couse JF, Korach KS (1999) Estrogen receptor null mice: what have we learned and where will they lead us? *Endocr Rev* 20:358–417.
46. Krege JH, Hodgin JB, Couse JF, Enmark E, Warner M, Mahler JF, Sar M, Korach KS, Gustafsson JA, Smithies O (1998) Generation and reproductive phenotypes of mice lacking estrogen receptor beta. *Proc Natl Acad Sci USA* 95:15677–15682.
47. Dupont S, Krust A, Gansmuller A, Dierich A, Chambon P, Mark M (2000) Effect of single and compound knockouts of estrogen receptors alpha (ERalpha) and beta (ERbeta) on mouse reproductive phenotypes. *Development* 127:4277–4291.
48. Jarred RA, Cancilla B, Prins GS, Thayer KA, Cunha GR, Risbridger GP (2000) Evidence that estrogens directly alter androgen-regulated prostate development. *Endocrinology* 141:3471–3477.
49. vom Saal FS, Timms BG, Montano MM, Palanza P, Thayer KA, Nagel SC, Dhar MD, Ganjam VK, Parmigiani S, Welshons WV (1997) Prostate enlargement in mice due to fetal exposure to low doses of estradiol or diethylstilbestrol and opposite effects at high doses. *Proc Natl Acad Sci USA* 94:2056–2061.
50. Prins GS (1992) Neonatal estrogen exposure induces lobe-specific alterations in adult rat prostate androgen receptor expression. *Endocrinology* 130:3703–3714.
51. Prins GS (1997) Developmental estrogenization of the prostate gland. In: Naz RK, ed. *Prostate: Basic and Clinical Aspects*, pp. 247–265.

52. Prins GS, Birch L (1995) The developmental pattern of androgen receptor expression in rat prostate lobes is altered after neonatal exposure to estrogen. *Endocrinology* 136:1303–1314.

53. Prins GS (1989) Differential regulation of androgen receptors in the separate rat prostate lobes: androgen independent expression in the lateral lobe. *J Steroid Biochem* 33:319–326.

54. Prins GS, Jung MH, Vellanoweth RL, Chatterjee B, Roy AK (1996) Age-dependent expression of the androgen receptor gene in the prostate and its implication in glandular differentiation and hyperplasia. *Dev Genet* 18:99–106.

55. Rajfer J, Coffey DS (1979) Effects of neonatal steroids on male sex tissues. *Invest Urol* 17:3–8.

56. Rajfer J, Coffey DS (1978) Sex steroid imprinting of the immature prostate. Long-term effects. *Invest Urol* 16:186–190.

57. Naslund MJ, Coffey DS (1986) The differential effects of neonatal androgen, estrogen and progesterone on adult rat prostate growth. *J Urol* 136:1136–1140.

58. Prins GS, Woodham C, Lepinske M, Birch L (1993) Effects of neonatal estrogen exposure on prostatic secretory genes and their correlation with androgen receptor expression in the separate prostate lobes of the adult rat. *Endocrinology* 132:2387–2398.

59. Pylkkanen L, Makela S, Valve E, Harkonen P, Toikkanen S, Santti R (1993) Prostatic dysplasia associated with increased expression of c-myc in neonatally estrogenized mice. *J Urol* 149:1593–1601.

60. Arai Y, Chen CY, Nishizuka Y (1978) Cancer development in male reproductive tract in rats given diethylstilbestrol at neonatal age. *Gann* 69:861–862.

61. Santti R, Newbold RR, Makela S, Pylkkanen L, McLachlan JA (1994) Developmental estrogenization and prostatic neoplasia. *Prostate* 24:67–78.

62. McLachlan JA, Newbold RR, Bullock B (1975) Reproductive tract lesions in male mice exposed prenatally to diethylstilbestrol. *Science* 190:991–992.

63. Newbold RR, Bullock BC, McLachlan JA (1986) Adenocarcinoma of the rete testis. Diethylstilbestrol-induced lesions of the mouse rete testis. *Am J Pathol* 125:625–628.

64. Newbold RR, Bullock BC, McLachlan JA (1985) Lesions of the rete testis in mice exposed prenatally to diethylstilbestrol. *Cancer Res* 45:5145–5150.

65. Beckman WC, Jr, Newbold RR, Teng CT, McLachlan JA (1994) Molecular feminization of mouse seminal vesicle by prenatal exposure to diethylstilbestrol: altered expression of messenger RNA. *J Urol* 151:1370–1378.

66. Driscoll SG, Taylor SH (1980) Effects of prenatal maternal estrogen on the male urogenital system. *Obstet Gynecol* 56:537–542.

67. Prins GS, Birch L (1997) Neonatal estrogen exposure up-regulates estrogen receptor expression in the developing and adult rat prostate lobes. *Endocrinology* 138:1801–1809.

68. Prins GS, Marmer M, Woodham C, Chang W, Kuiper G, Gustafsson JA, Birch L (1998) Estrogen receptor-beta messenger ribonucleic acid ontogeny in the prostate of normal and neonatally estrogenized rats. *Endocrinology* 139:874–883.

69. Chang WY, Wilson MJ, Birch L, Prins GS (1999) Neonatal estrogen stimulates proliferation of periductal fibroblasts and alters the extracellular matrix composition in the rat prostate. *Endocrinology* 140:405–415.

70. Chang WY, Birch L, Woodham C, Gold LI, Prins GS (1999) Neonatal estrogen exposure alters the transforming growth factor-beta signaling system in the developing rat prostate and blocks the transient p21(cip1/waf1) expression associated with epithelial differentiation. *Endocrinology* 140:2801–2813.

71. Sabharwal V, Putz O, Prins GS (2000) Neonatal estrogen exposure induces progesterone receptor expression in the developing prostate gland. In: *95th Annual Meeting of the American Urologic Association*, p. 97.

72. Habermann H, Chang WY, Birch L, Mehta P, Prins GS (2001) Developmental exposure to estrogens alters epithelial cell adhesion and gap junction proteins in the adult rat prostate. *Endocrinology* 142:359–369.

73. Putz O, Schwartz CB, Kim S, LeBlanc GA, Cooper RL, Prins GS (2001) Neonatal low- and high-dose exposure to estradiol benzoate in the male rat: I. Effects on the prostate gland. *Biol Reprod* 65:1496–1505.

74. Cattanach BM, Iddon CA, Charlton HM, Chiappa SA, Fink G (1977) Gonadotrophin-releasing hormone deficiency in a mutant mouse with hypogonadism. *Nature* 269:338–340.

75. Bianco JJ, Handelsman DJ, Pedersen JS, Risbridger GP (2002) Direct response of the murine prostate gland and seminal vesicles to estradiol. *Endocrinology* 143:4922–4933.

76. Cunha GR, Wang YZ, Hayward SW, Risbridger GP (2001) Estrogenic effects on prostatic differentiation and carcinogenesis. *Reprod Fertil Dev* 13:285–296.

77. Han X, Liehr JG, Bosland MC (1995) Induction of a DNA adduct detectable by 32P-postlabeling in the dorsolateral prostate of NBL/Cr rats treated with estradiol-17 beta and testosterone. *Carcinogenesis* 16:951–954.

78. Cunha GR, Hayward SW, Wang YZ, Ricke WA (2003) Role of the stromal microenvironment in carcinogenesis of the prostate. *Int J Cancer* 107:1–10.

79. Risbridger GP, Bianco JJ, Ellem SJ, McPherson SJ (2003) Oestrogens and prostate cancer. *Endocr Relat Cancer* 10:187–191.
80. Cavalieri E, Frenkel K, Liehr JG, Rogan E, Roy D (2000) Estrogens as endogenous genotoxic agents — DNA adducts and mutations. *J Natl Cancer Inst Monogr* 75–93.
81. Yager JD (2000) Endogenous estrogens as carcinogens through metabolic activation. *J Natl Cancer Inst Monogr* 67–73.
82. Yager JD, Liehr JG (1996) Molecular mechanisms of estrogen carcinogenesis. *Annu Rev Pharmacol Toxicol* 36:203–232.
83. Tanaka Y, Sasaki M, Kaneuchi M, Shiina H, Igawa M, Dahiya R (2002) Polymorphisms of the CYP1B1 gene have higher risk for prostate cancer. *Biochem Biophys Res Commun* 296:820–826.
84. Di Salle E, Briatico G, Giudici D, Ornati G, Panzeri A (1994) Endocrine properties of the testosterone 5-alpha-reductase inhibitor turosteride (FCE 26073). *J Steroid Biochem Mol Biol* 48:241–248.
85. Hiramatsu M, Maehara I, Ozaki M, Harada N, Orikasa S, Sasano H (1997) Aromatase in hyperplasia and carcinoma of the human prostate. *Prostate* 31:118–124.
86. Li X, Nokkala E, Yan W, Streng T, Saarinen N, Warri A, Huhtaniemi I, Santti R, Makela S, Poutanen M (2001) Altered structure and function of reproductive organs in transgenic male mice overexpressing human aromatase. *Endocrinology* 142:2435–2442.
87. Ito T, Tachibana M, Yamamoto S, Nakashima J, Murai M (2001) Expression of estrogen receptor (ER-alpha and ER-beta) mRNA in human prostate cancer. *Eur Urol* 40:557–563.
88. Linja MJ, Savinainen KJ, Tammela TL, Isola JJ, Visakorpi T (2003) Expression of ERalpha and ERbeta in prostate cancer. *Prostate* 55:180–186.
89. Maruyama S, Fujimoto N, Asano K, Ito A, Usui T (2000) Expression of estrogen receptor alpha and beta mRNAs in prostate cancers treated with leuprorelin acetate. *Eur Urol* 38:635–639.
90. Bu S, Blaukat A, Fu X, Heldin NE, Landstrom M (2002) Mechanisms for 2-methoxyestradiol-induced apoptosis of prostate cancer cells. *FEBS Lett* 531:141–151.
91. Qadan LR, Perez-Stable CM, Anderson C, D'Ippolito G, Herron A, Howard GA, Roos BA (2001) 2-Methoxyestradiol induces G2/M arrest and apoptosis in prostate cancer. *Biochem Biophys Res Commun* 285:1259–1266.
92. Huang JK, Jan CR (2001) Mechanism of estrogens-induced increases in intracellular Ca(2+) in PC3 human prostate cancer cells. *Prostate* 47: 141–148.

93. Widmark A, Grankvist K, Bergh A, Henriksson R, Damber JE (1995) Effects of estrogens and progestogens on the membrane permeability and growth of human prostatic carcinoma cells (PC-3) *in vitro. Prostate* 26:5–11.

94. Jarred RA, McPherson SJ, Bianco JJ, Couse JF, Korach KS, Risbridger GP (2002) Prostate phenotypes in estrogen-modulated transgenic mice. *Trends Endocrinol Metab* 13:163–168.

95. Gingrich JR, Barrios RJ, Morton RA, Boyce BF, DeMayo FJ, Finegold MJ, Angelopoulou R, Rosen JM, Greenberg NM (1996) Metastatic prostate cancer in a transgenic mouse. *Cancer Res* 56:4096–4102.

96. Raghow S, Hooshdaran MZ, Katiyar S, Steiner MS (2002) Toremifene prevents prostate cancer in the transgenic adenocarcinoma of mouse prostate model. *Cancer Res* 62:1370–1376.

97. Mentor-Marcel R, Lamartiniere CA, Eltoum IE, Greenberg NM, Elgavish A (2001) Genistein in the diet reduces the incidence of poorly differentiated prostatic adenocarcinoma in transgenic mice (TRAMP). *Cancer Res* 61: 6777–6782.

98. Corey E, Quinn JE, Emond MJ, Buhler KR, Brown LG, Vessella RL (2002) Inhibition of androgen-independent growth of prostate cancer xenografts by 17beta-estradiol. *Clin Cancer Res* 8:1003–1007.

99. Couse JE, Mahato D, Eddy EM, Korach KS (2001) Molecular mechanism of estrogen action in the male: insights from the estrogen receptor null mice. *Reprod Fertil Dev* 13:211–219.

14

EPIDEMIOLOGY OF PROSTATE CANCER

Ann W. Hsing

Division of Cancer Epidemiology and Genetics
National Cancer Institute,
Bethesda, Maryland 20852-7234, USA

Anand P. Chokkalingam

Celera Diagnostics, LLC
Alameda, California 94502, USA

Introduction

Prostate cancer is the most common non-skin cancer in most western populations, and although worldwide incidence rates were on the rise through the 1990s,[1] they now appear to be declining slightly.[2] In western countries, the rise in incidence in the late 1970s and early 1980s was due, in part, to the increased use of transurethral resection of the prostate for benign prostatic hyperplasia (BPH).[3] However, the increase in incidence between 1986 and 1992 was largely due to the increasing use of prostate specific antigen (PSA) testing for early detection of prostate cancer.[4] Although incidence rates in Asian countries are low, their recent relative increases are larger than those of western countries and have been attributed to increased westernization.[1]

Despite prostate cancer's high morbidity, its etiology remains obscure. The only established risk factors are age, race and a family history of prostate cancer. Many putative factors, such as hormones, diet, obesity, physical inactivity, occupation, vasectomy, smoking, sexual factors, and genetic susceptibility, have been implicated, but the epidemiologic evidence is inconclusive. An overview of these factors is presented below.

Table 1. Summary of Epidemiologic Risk Factors for Prostate Cancer

	Observation	Evidence	Implications
Established Factors			
Age	Incidence rises with age	Consistent	Latency is long and progression is slow
Race	African-Americans have the highest reported rates in the world, while Chinese men living in China have the lowest reported rates.	Consistent	Suggests both environmental and genetic factors may have a role in prostate cancer
	Migrants have much higher risk than their counterparts in ancestral countries	Consistent	Suggests a role of environmental factors Suggests westernization may be related to an increased risk
Family history of prostate cancer	Familial aggregation	Consistent	Suggests a role of genetic predisposition
Probable Factors			
Diet	Animal fat and red meat intake is associated with an increased risk	Somewhat consistent	Suggests fat or other constituents in meat may contribute to prostate carcinogenesis
	Selenium and vitamin E are associated with a reduced risk	Somewhat consistent	Suggests anti-carcinogenic effect of these compounds Chemoprevention trials are underway to evaluate these effects
	Consumption of tomato products is associated with a decreased risk	Somewhat consistent	Lycopene may protect against prostate cancer

Table 1 (*Continued*)

	Intake of cruciferous vegetables may be associated with decreased risk	Suggestive	Suggests intake of broccoli, cauliflower, Brussels sprouts and other cruciferous vegetables may protect against prostate cancer
	Allium vegetable intake may be associated with decreased risk	Needs confirmation	
	Intake of fish and marine fats may be associated with a decreased risk	Needs confirmation	
	Calcium may be associated with increased risk	Inconsistent	
	Intake of total vegetables may be associated with decreased risk	Inconsistent	
IGFs	Higher serum/plasma levels of IGF-I and lower levels of IGFBP-3 may be related to an increased risk	Somewhat consistent	Suggests IGFs may be related to the progression of prostate cancer Clinical utility of IGFs is under evaluation
Occupation	Farmers have ~10% excess risk	Consistent	Suggests exposures to herbicides or pesticides or lifestyles among farmers may be related to prostate cancer risk
	Workers in heavy metal and rubber industries may have an increased risk	Suggestive	Suggests exposures to certain chemicals may increase prostate cancer risk
Androgens	Higher serum levels of androgens may be associated with an increased risk	Suggestive	Suggests androgenic action is involved in prostate carcinogenesis
Obesity	Abdominal obesity may be related to an increased risk	Suggestive	Suggests that alteration of hormone synthesis or metabolism may have a role in prostate cancer etiology

Table 1 (*Continued*)

	Observation	Evidence	Implications
Chronic inflammation	Inflammation is found in prostate biopsies and resected prostate tissue, and pro-inflammatory markers are associated with increased risk	Suggestive	Suggests that factors contributing to inflammatory states may have a role in prostate cancer initiation or promotion
Vitamin D	Higher serum levels of vitamin D may be associated with a reduced risk	Inconsistent	
Sexual factors	Sexual factors, especially sexually transmitted infections such as HPV infection and syphilis, may be related to an increased risk	Inconsistent	
Vasectomy	Vasectomy may be associated with an increased risk	Inconsistent	
Physical activity	Long-term physical activity may be associated with a reduced risk of prostate cancer	Inconsistent	
Liver cirrhosis	Patients with liver cirrhosis may have a lower risk	Inconsistent	
Diabetes	Diabetic patients may have a lower risk	Inconsistent	
Smoking	Smoking may be associated with an increased risk	Inconsistent	

Table 2. Summary of Epidemiologic Studies of Rare, High Penetrance Genes, and Prostate Cancer

Region	Gene	Markers	Studies (Ref.), No. of cases Studied, Population	Results
1q24-25	*RNASEL* (HPC1)	E265X, R462Q, D541E, I97L	Rokman et al. (2002),[75] N=116 HPC* cases, Finns	Positive association
			Nakazato et al. (2003),[76] N=101 HPC cases, Japanese	Positive association
			Wang et al. (2002),[77] N=438 HPC cases, US Caucasians	Positive association
			Casey et al. (2002),[78] N=423 HPC cases, US subjects	Positive association
				Overall, consistent positive association
17p11	*ELAC2* (HPC2)	A541T, S217L	Rebbeck et al. (2000),[79] N = 359 cases, US subjects	Positive association
			Suarez et al. (2001),[80] N = 257 HPC cases, US Caucasians	Positive association
			Tavtigian et al. (2001),[81] N = 429 HPC cases, US Caucasians	Positive association
			Vesprini et al. (2001),[82] N = 431 cases, Canadians	No association
			Wang et al. (2001),[83] N = 446 HPC cases, US Caucasians	No association
			Xu et al. (2001),[84] N = 249 cases, 159 HPC cases, US Caucasians	No association
			Rokman et al. 2001,[85] N = 467 cases, 107 HPC cases, Finns	No association
			Meitz et al. (2002),[86] N = 432 cases, UK subjects	No association
			Adler et al. (2003),[87] N = 199 cases, Canadians	Positive association

*HPC: Hereditary prostate cancer.

Table 2 (*Continued*)

Region	Gene	Markers	Studies (Ref.), No. of cases Studied, Population	Results
			Stanford *et al.* (2003),[88] N = 591 cases, US subjects	Positive association
			Takahashi *et al.* (2003),[89] N = 98 cases (BPH controls), Japanese	Positive association
			Severi *et al.* (2003),[90] N = 825 cases, Australians	No association
			Meta-analysis: Camp and Tavtigian (2002)[91]	Association only for HPC Overall, weak, inconsistent associations
				May be associated only with HPC, not sporadic disease
xq27-28	None (HPCX)		Linkage studies	AR (also on X chromosome) unlikely to be HPCX susceptibility gene
20q13	None (HPC20)		Linkage studies	Linkage studies need further confirmation
1p36	None (CAPB)		Linkage studies	Most consistent linkage to strong family history with early onset disease
1q42.2-43	PCTA-1 (PCAP)		Linkage studies	PCTA is possible candidate gene, but no functional markers
8p22-23	MSR1	PRO3, P275A, D174Y, IVS5-59, R293X	Xu *et al.* (2003),[92] N = 301 cases, US Caucasians	Positive association
			Miller *et al.*, 2003,[93] N = 134 cases, African-Americans	Positive association

Table 2 (Continued)

Region	Gene	Markers	Studies (Ref.), No. of cases Studied, Population	Results
			Wang *et al.* (2003),[94] N = 499 cases, 438 HPC cases, US Caucasians	Null association
			Seppala *et al.* (2003),[95] N = 537 cases, Finns	Null association Overall, weak results, with larger studies showing null associations even for HPC

Rates and Patterns

Incidence

There is considerable variation in reported incidence rates of prostate cancer worldwide.[5,6] Age-adjusted prostate cancer incidence rates among African-Americans are the highest in the world (185.4 per 100,000 person-years), and rates among Caucasian-Americans are second (107.8 per 100,000 person-years) (Fig. 1). Reported rates in the Caribbean and in Brazil, where there are large populations of African descent (92–96 per 100,000 person-years), are comparable to the high rates among Caucasian-Americans. In contrast, in Central America and other parts of South America, rates are much lower (28–42 per 100,000 person-years). Rates within Europe vary almost seven-fold (from 15–100 per 100,000 person-years), with Austria having the highest reported rates. Although rates in Canada, Oceania (including Australia and New Zealand), Western Europe and Scandinavia (50–103 per 100,000 person-years) are generally not as high as the rates reported in the US, they are 2–3 times higher than rates in Eastern Europe (15–36 per 100,000 person-years). Within Asia, where the rates are the lowest, there is also considerable variation in reported incidence, with more westernized Asian countries such as Israel and the Philippines (22–47 per 100,000 person-years) showing markedly

Table 3. Summary of Epidemiologic Studies of Common, Low Penetrance Genes and Prostate Cancer

Gene	Marker	Studies (Ref.), No. of Cases Studied, Population	Results and Comments
Androgen Biosynthesis/Metabolism Pathway			
CYP17	MspA1	Lunn et al. (1999),[120] N = 108 cases, US subjects	Positive association for Caucasians, null for African-Americans
		Wadelius et al. (1999),[134] N = 178 cases, Swedish Caucasians	Positive association
		Gsur et al. (2000),[135] N = 63 cases, Austrians	Positive association
		Habuchi et al. (2000),[136] N = 252 cases, Japanese	Positive association
		Haiman et al. (2001),[137] N = 600 cases, US Caucasians	Null association
		Yamada et al. (2001),[125] N = 105 cases, Japanese	Positive association
		Kittles et al. (2001),[138] N = 71 cases, African-Americans	Positive association
		Latil et al. (2001),[110] N = 226 cases, French Caucasians	Null association
		Chang et al. (2001),[139] N = 225 cases, US Caucasians	Null association
		Stanford et al. (2002),[140] N = 596 cases, US Caucasians and African-Americans	Null association overall, positive association among Caucasians with family history
		Madigan et al. (2003),[141] N = 174 cases, Chinese	Null association
		Lin et al. (2003),[142] N = 93 cases, Taiwanese	Null association
		Nam et al. (2003),[119] N = 483 cases, Canadians	Null association
		Review: Ntais et al. (2003)[98]	Meta-analysis indicates no overall association, but A2 allele may be associated with risk in African-Americans.[98] A1 is reported to be risk allele in Asians.

Table 3 (*Continued*)

Gene	Variant	Study	Association
CYP19	TTTA repeats, N264C	Latil et al. (2001),[110] N = 226 cases, French Caucasians	Positive association
		Modugno et al. (2001),[111] N = 88 cases, US Caucasians	Positive association
		Suzuki et al. (2003),[143] N = 99 HPC* cases, Japanese	Positive association
			Overall, suggestive but mixed results — longer TTTA alleles associated with higher risk in Caucasians, but lower risk in Asians. Further investigation needed.
CYP1A1	2455A>G	Murata et al. (1998),[144] N = 115 cases, Japanese	Positive associaton
	3801T>C	Suzuki et al. (2003),[145] N = 81 HPC cases, Japanese	Positive association
	2453C>A	Chang et al. (2003),[146] N = 245 cases, US Caucasians	Positive association
CYP3A4	5' promoter variant	Rebbeck et al. (1998),[147] N = 230 cases, US Caucasians	Positive association
		Paris et al. (1999),[148] N = 174 cases, African-Americans	Positive association
		Nam et al. (2003),[119] N = 483 cases, Canadians	Null association
SRD5A2	V89L, A49T, R227Q, TA repeats	Lunn et al. 1999,[120] N = 108 cases, US Caucasians and African-Americans	Null association
		Kantoff et al. (1997),[121] N = 590 cases, US Caucasians	Null association
		Febbo et al. (1999),[122] N = 592 cases, US Caucasians	Null association
		Makridakis et al. (1999),[123] N = 388 cases, US Hispanics and African-Americans	Positive association

*HPC: Hereditary prostate cancer.

Table 3 (*Continued*)

Gene	Marker	Studies (Ref.), No. of Cases Studied, Population	Results and Comments
		Margiotti et al. (2000),[124] N = 108 cases, Italians	Positive association
		Yamada et al. (2001),[125] N = 105 cases, Japanese	Null association
		Nam et al. (2001),[126] N = 158 cases, Canadians	Positive association
		Latil et al. (2001),[110] 226 cases, French	Null association
		Mononen et al. (2001),[127] N = 449 cases, Finns	Null association
		Hsing et al. (2001),[128] N = 191 cases, Chinese	Null association
		Pearce et al. (2002),[129] N = 921 cases, US subjects	Null association
		Soderstrom et al. (2002),[130] N = 176 cases, Swedes	Null association
		Lamharzi et al. (2003),[131] N = 300 cases, US subjects	Positive association
		Chang et al. (2003),[132] N = 245 cases, 159 HPC cases, US Caucasians	Null association
		Li et al. (2003),[133] N = 302 cases, Japanese	Positive association
		Nam et al. (2003),[119] N = 483 cases, Canadians	Null association
		Review: Ntais et al. (2003)[96]	Overall, the T allele of A49T (associated with higher enzymatic activity) and shorter TA repeats may be associated with a modest increase in risk.[96] While results are mixed, the V89L marker's LL genotype, which is associated with lower serum levels of androgens, may be associated with a reduced risk. R227Q is very rare, observed only in Asians.

Table 3 (*Continued*)

AR	CAG repeats, GGN repeats	Ingles *et al.* (1997),[100] N = 57 cases, US Caucasians	Positive association
		Stanford *et al.* (1997),[101] N = 301 cases, US Caucasians	Positive association
		Giovannucci *et al.* (1997),[102] N = 587 cases, US Caucasians (and Platz *et al.* (1998),[103] N = 582 cases)	Positive association
		Correa-Cerro *et al.* (1999),[104] N = 132 cases, French and Germans	Null association
		Ekman *et al.* (1999),[105] N = 93 cases, 59 HPC cases, Swedes and Japanese	Positive association
		Edwards *et al.* (1999),[106] N = 178 cases, U.K. Caucasians	Positive association
		Hsing *et al.* (2000),[107] N = 190 cases, Chinese	Positive association
		Miller *et al.* (2001),[108] N = 140 cases, US subjects	Null association
		Beilin *et al.* (2001),[109] N = 445 cases, Australians	Null association
		Latil *et al.* (2001),[110] N = 226 cases, French	Null association
		Modugno *et al.* (2001),[111] N = 88 cases, US Caucasians	Positive association
		Chang *et al.* (2002),[112] N = 245 cases, 159 HPC cases	Positive association
		Mononen *et al.* (2002),[113] N = 449 cases, Finns	Positive association
		Gsur *et al.* (2002),[114] N = 190 cases, Austrians	Null association
		Chen *et al.* (2002),[115] N = 300 cases, US subjects	Null association
		Balic *et al.* (2002),[116] N = 82 cases, Hispanics	Positive association
		Santos *et al.* (2003),[117] N = 133 cases, Brazilians	Null association
		Huang *et al.* (2003),[118] N = 66 cases, Taiwanese	Null association
		Nam *et al.* (2003),[119] N = 483 cases, Canadians	Null association
			Although overall results are mixed, shorter CAG repeat lengths may be associated with increased prostate cancer risk.

Table 3 (*Continued*)

Gene	Marker	Studies (Ref.), No. of Cases Studied, Population	Results and Comments
HSD3B1	N367T, c7062t	Chang et al. (2002),[149] N = 245 cases, 159 HPC cases, US Caucasians	Positive association
HSD3B2	c7159g, c7474t	Chang et al. (2002),[149] N = 245 cases, 159 HPC cases, US Caucasians	Null association
HSD17B3	G289S	Margiotti et al. (2002),[150] N = 103 cases, Italians	Positive association
Growth Factors and Non-androgenic Hormone Pathways			
VDR	BsmI, TaqI, polyA, ApaI, FokI	Taylor et al. (1996),[154] N = 108 cases, US Caucasians	Positive association
		Ingles et al. (1997),[100] N = 57 cases, US Caucasians	Positive association
		Ingles et al. (1998),[155] N = 151 cases, African-Americans	Null association
		Ma et al. (1998),[156] N = 372 cases, US Caucasians	Null association
		Correa-Cerro et al. (1999),[157] N = 131 cases, Europeans	Null association
		Habuchi et al. (2000),[158] N = 222 cases, Japanese	Positive association
		Furuya et al. (1999),[159] N = 66 cases, Japanese	Null association
		Watanabe et al. (1999),[160] N = 100 cases, Japanese	Null association
		Blazer et al. (2000),[161] N = 77 cases, US Caucasians	Null association
		Chokkalingam et al. (2001),[162] N = 191 cases, Chinese	Null association
		Gsur et al. (2002),[163] N = 190 cases, Austrians	Null association
		Hamasaki et al. (2002),[164] N = 110 cases, Japanese	Positive association for aggressive disease
		Medieros et al. (2002),[165] N = 163 cases, Portugese	Positive association for late-onset disease
		Suzuki et al. (2003),[166] N = 81 HPC cases, Japanese	Null association
		Nam et al. (2003),[119] N = 483 cases, Canadians	Null association

Table 3 (*Continued*)

		Review: Ntais et al. (2003)[97]	Overall, meta-analysis[97] shows null association for all markers. 3' markers (BsmI, Taq1, ApaI and polyA) are non-functional, 5' FokI marker is functional.
INS	+1127PstI	Ho et al. (2003),[153] N = 126 cases, US subjects	Positive association
TH	−4217PstI	Ho et al. (2003),[153] N = 126 cases, US subjects	Null association
IGF-1	CA repeats	Nam et al. (2003),[119] N = 483 cases, Canadians	Positive association
IGF-2	MspI	Ho et al. (2003),[153] N = 126, US subjects	Null association
IGFBP-3	−202A/C	Wang et al. (2003),[94] N = 307 cases, Japanese	Null association
		Nam et al. (2003),[119] N = 483 cases, Canadians	Null association
Carcinogen Metabolism Pathway			
GSTT1	Deletion	Medeiros et al. (2004),[167] N = 150 cases, Portugese	Null association
		Nakazato et al. (2003),[76] N = 81 cases, Japanese	Null association
		Kidd et al. (2003),[168] N = 206 cases, Finns	Null association
		Kote-Jarai et al. (2001),[169] N = 275 cases, U.K. Caucasians	Null association
		Gsur et al. (2001),[170] N = 166 cases, Austrians	Null association
		Murata et al. (2001),[171] N = 115 cases, Japanese	Null association
		Steinhoff et al. (2000),[172] N = 91 cases, Germans	Positive association
		Autrup et al. (1999),[173] N = 153 cases, Dutch subjects	Null association
		Nam et al. (2003),[119] N = 483 cases, Canadians	Positive association
		Kelada et al. (2000),[174] N = 276 cases, US subjects	Positive association
GSTM1	Deletion	Medeiros et al. (2004),[167] N = 150 cases, Portugese	Null association
		Nakazato et al. (2003),[76] N = 81 cases, Japanese	Null association
		Kidd et al. (2003),[168] N = 206 cases, Finns	Positive association
		Kote-Jarai et al. (2001),[169] N = 275 cases, U.K. Caucasians	Null association

Table 3 (*Continued*)

Gene	Marker	Studies (Ref.), No. of Cases Studied, Population	Results and Comments
		Gsur et al. (2001),[170] N = 166 cases, Austrians	Null association
		Murata et al. (2001),[171] N = 115 cases, Japanese	Positive association
		Steinhoff et al. (2000),[172] N = 91 cases, Germans	Null association
		Autrup et al., 1999,[173] N = 153 cases, Dutch subjects	Null association
		Nam et al. (2003),[119] N = 483 cases, Canadians	Null association
		Kelada et al. (2000),[174] N = 276 cases, US subjects	Null association
GSTM3		Medeiros et al. (2004),[167] N = 150 cases, Portugese	Positive association
GSTP1	I105V	Nakazato et al. (2003),[76] N = 81 cases, Japanese	Positive association
		Kidd et al. (2003),[168] N = 206 cases, Finns	Null association
		Kote-Jarai et al. (2001),[169] N = 275 cases, U.K. Caucasians	Positive association
		Gsur et al. (2001),[170] N = 166 cases, Austrians	Positive association
		Steinhoff et al. (2000),[172] N = 91 cases, Germans	Null association
		Shepard et al. (2000),[175] N = 590 cases, US Caucasians	Null association
		Autrup et al. (1999),[173] N = 153 cases, Dutch	Null association
		Wadelius et al. (1999),[134] N = 850 subjects, Swedes and Danes	Null association
NAT2		Nam et al. (2003),[119] N = 483 cases, Canadians	Null association
		Wadelius et al. (1999),[134] N = 850 subjects, Swedes and Danes	Null association
DNA Repair Pathway			
XRCC1	R399Q, R194W, R280H	Rybicki et al. (2004),[177] N = 637 cases, US Caucasians	Null association
		van Gils et al. (2002),[178] N = 77 cases, US subjects	Positive association

Table 3 (*Continued*)

Gene	Polymorphism	Study	Association
XPD	D312N, K751Q	Rybicki et al. (2004),[177] N = 637 cases, US Caucasians	Positive association, needs further investigation
hOGG1	S326C, +11657A/G	Xu et al. (2002),[179] N = 245 cases, US Caucasians	Positive association
		Chen et al. (2003),[180] N = 84 cases, US Caucasians	Positive association
Inflammation/Angiogenesis/Cytokine Pathways			
VEGF	VEGF-1154, VEGF-460	McCarron et al. (2002),[183] N = 247 cases, U.K. Caucasians	Positive association
		Lin et al. (2003),[142] N = 96 cases, Taiwanese	Positive association
TNF-α	TNF-α-308	McCarron et al. (2002),[183] N = 247 cases, U.K. Caucasians	Null association
IL-1-β	IL-1β-511	McCarron et al. (2002),[183] N = 247 cases, U.K. Caucasians	Null association
IL-8	IL-8-251	McCarron et al. (2002),[183] N = 247 cases, U.K. Caucasians	Positive association
IL-10	IL-10-1082	McCarron et al. (2002),[183] N = 247 cases, U.K. Caucasians	Positive association
PPAR-γ	P12A	Faltoo et al. (2003),[184] N = 193 cases, Finns	Null association
TGF-β	L10P	Li et al. (2004),[181] N = 351 cases, Japanese	Positive association
COX-2	-1285A/G, -1265G/A, -899G/C, -297C/G	Panguluri et al. (2004),[182] N = 288, 264 and 184 cases, African-Americans, Nigerians, and US Caucasians	Positive association in all ethnic groups

A. W. Hsing & A. P. Chokkalingam

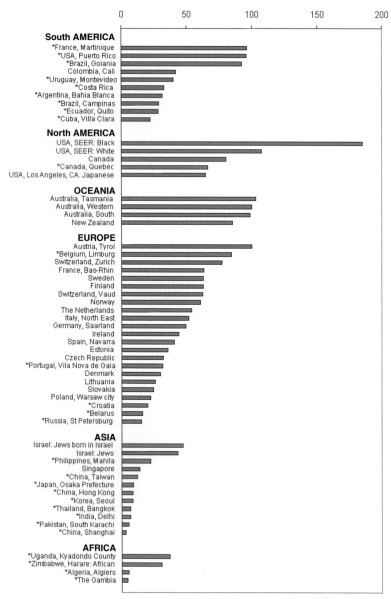

Source: Parkin DM, Whelan SL, Ferlay J, Teppo L, and Thomas DB. Cancer
Incidence in Five Continents, Vol VIII, IARC Sci Publ 155, 2003.

Fig. 1. Age-adjusted incidence rates (per 100,000 person-years) for prostate cancer in 48 countries, 1993–1997.

higher rates than Thailand, India, Pakistan and Shanghai, China (3–7 per 100,000 person-years). There are few data on incidence in Africa, with only four registries included in the IARC report.[6] The rates within the African continent vary widely, from 5–37 per 100,000 person-years. Part of the difference in incidence rates in various countries is related to the extent of prostate cancer screening, especially the use of prostate-specific antigen (PSA) testing. However, since screening is less common in developing countries, it is not likely to explain the nearly 60-fold difference in prostate cancer risk between high- and low-risk populations.

Mortality

In the US, only one in six men diagnosed with prostate cancer will eventually die from it. Nevertheless, 29,900 prostate cancer deaths are expected in 2004, making prostate cancer the second leading cause of cancer death among US men after lung cancer.[7] Age-adjusted prostate cancer mortality rates from 38 countries in 1998 are shown in Fig. 2. Overall, mortality patterns mimic those of incidence in various countries, although mortality rates show less diversity worldwide than do incidence rates, but are still higher in Western nations than in lower-risk, Asian countries (Fig. 2). Of special interest is the observation that the Caribbean nations of Barbados, the Bahamas and Trinidad and Tobago, where there are large populations of men of African descent, had the world's highest mortality rates (30.3 to 47.9 per 100,000 person-years). Mortality was higher in Scandinavian countries and parts of northern Europe than in the US (18.7–23.6 versus 14.0 per 100,000 person-years), and lowest of all in the Asian countries of South Korea, Philippines and Japan (1.6–4.4 per 100,000 person-years).

Risk Factors

Demographic Factors

Age

Over 80% of prostate tumors in the US are diagnosed among men over age 65,[8] and the incidence of prostate cancer increases exponentially

A. W. Hsing & A. P. Chokkalingam

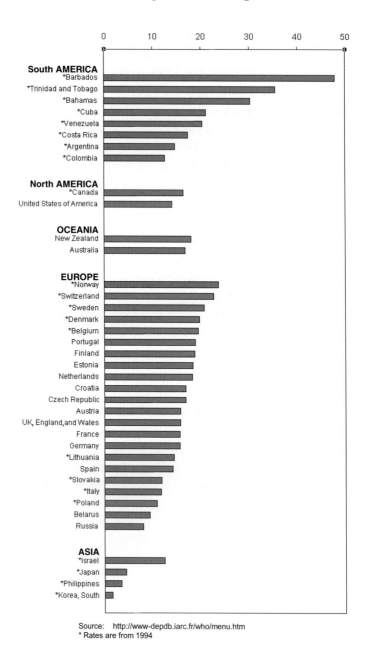

Source: http://www-depdb.iarc.fr/who/menu.htm
* Rates are from 1994

Fig. 2. Age-adjusted mortality rates (per 100,000 person-years) for prostate cancer in 38 countries, 1998.

with advancing age — an increase that is faster than that for any other malignancy (Table 1). Estimates from the Surveillance, Epidemiology, and End Results (SEER) program from 1996–2000 indicate that for US men under 65 years of age and 65 years and over, age-adjusted prostate cancer incidence rates were 56.8 and 974.7 per 100,000 person-years, respectively.[2]

Racial/Ethnic Variation

Another consistently observed but poorly understood risk factor is ethnicity. African-Americans have the highest incidence rate in the world, roughly 60 times that of the ethnic group with the world's lowest rates, in Shanghai, China[1] (Fig. 1).

Adjustment of incidence rates for prevalence of latent disease at autopsy and proportion of localized tumors among all cancers of the prostate revealed that Japanese men still experience a markedly lower incidence than Americans, indicating that the international variation cannot be explained by differences in detection alone.[9] This bolsters the results of migrant studies suggesting that ethnic factors, including genetic, lifestyle, and environmental factors, may affect prostate cancer risk and explain many of the differences in risk between high- and low-risk populations.[9,10]

Hormonal, Behavioral and Lifestyle Factors

Hormones and Growth Factors

Androgens play a key role in the development and maintenance of the prostate gland; however, the precise role of androgens in the etiology of prostate cancer is unclear. Prostate cancer is notably absent in castrated men, and laboratory studies show that administration of testosterone induces prostate cancer in rats and that androgens promote cell proliferation and inhibit prostate cell death.[11–13] However, epidemiologic data supporting a role of androgens are inconclusive.[14–16] To date, over 13 prospective studies have investigated the role of circulating androgens, and only one was able to show that men with higher serum testosterone levels have a higher risk of prostate cancer.[17] More comprehensive reviews of this topic are reported elsewhere.[14-16] Studies of genetic markers involved in the androgen pathways offer further insight into this avenue of research, and are reviewed later in this chapter.

In addition to androgens, insulin-like growth factors (IGFs), insulin and vitamin D have been implicated in prostate cancer. IGF-I and IGF-II are polypeptides that function as both tissue growth factors and endocrine hormones with mitogenic and anti-apoptotic effects on prostate epithelial cells. There are at least six known IGF binding proteins (IGFBPs) that can bind to IGFs and thus prevent activation of the IGF receptor, which mediates IGF effects. At least nine epidemiologic studies have evaluated the roles of the IGF axis in prostate cancer, and most have reported a positive association with IGF-I and an inverse association with IGFBP3.[18,19] However, the role of IGF-II is less clear.

Vitamin D is a steroid hormone obtained primarily from dermal synthesis in response to sunlight exposure. Vitamin D and its analogs have potent anti-proliferative, pro-differentiative, and pro-apoptotic effects on prostate cancer cells. In addition, vitamin D inhibits prostate tumor growth *in vivo*. In general, laboratory data are consistent and support the hypothesis that vitamin D may protect against prostate cancer. However, results from epidemiologic studies investigating serum vitamin D levels have been inconsistent.[20] The reasons for these conflicting results are unclear.

Diet

Ecologic studies have shown a strong correlation between the incidence of prostate cancer and dietary fat intake.[21] A western diet has been linked to a higher risk of prostate cancer, and it has been suggested that the western diet, high in fat, increases production and availability of both androgen and estrogen, while Asian (low-fat, high-fiber) and vegetarian diets lead to lower circulating levels of these hormones.[21]

Fat is the most studied dietary factor in relation to prostate cancer. Most epidemiologic studies have investigated the role of total, saturated, and/or animal fat. Findings from these studies suggest a possible positive association with monounsaturated, animal and saturated fats, and an inverse association with omega-3 fat. The results for polyunsaturated fat are less consistent.[22,23] Consumption of meat, particularly red meat, is also consistently linked to an increased risk of prostate cancer. However, it is unclear whether the excess risk is due to the fat content in red meat, mutagens such as heterocyclic amines that are induced during high-temperature cooking of meat products, animal proteins, or other unidentified factors.[24]

Several epidemiologic studies have also investigated whether intake of fatty fish, rich in potentially tumor-inhibitory marine fatty acids, is associated with reduced prostate cancer risk. However, a recent review of 17 studies, including eight prospective studies, found suggestive but inconsistent results, possibly due to inadequate assessment of fish intake or lack of information on specific marine fatty acids, particularly the polyunsaturated fatty acids eicosapentaenoic and docosahexaenoic acids,[25] in these studies.

Although consumption of fruits and vegetables is associated with a reduced risk of several cancers, their role in prostate cancer is less clear. The only consistent finding is an inverse association with consumption of tomatoes and tomato paste, which has been largely attributed to the antioxidant effect of lycopene.[26] Cruciferous and allium vegetables have been implicated. A recent review concluded that there is modest evidence that intake of cruciferous vegetables, including broccoli, cabbage, cauliflower, and Brussels sprouts, is inversely associated with prostate cancer risk, possibly due to their content of isothiocyanates.[27] Intake of allium vegetables, including onions, garlic, and chives, was associated with a reduced risk in a case-control study in China.[28] This protective effect may be due to the tumor inhibitory properties of organosulfur compounds.

Dietary calcium, from either dairy intake or supplements, has also been linked to prostate cancer. Because of its role in regulation of vitamin D synthesis, calcium may down-regulate vitamin D's anti-proliferative effects on prostate cancer. However, the epidemiologic evidence for calcium is as yet unclear, complicated by differences in assessment of calcium (dietary intake versus circulating levels).[29] Recent data suggest a threshold effect in that only very high calcium intake ($\geq 2000\,mg/day$) appears to be associated with disease.[30]

Chronic excess of zinc, another mineral obtained largely through dietary supplements, may be positively associated with prostate cancer risk, although *in vitro* studies demonstrating mitogenic effects of zinc on prostate cancer suggest that it may reduce risk.[31]

A large body of epidemiological evidence, including observational, case-control, cohort and randomized controlled clinical trials, supports the hypothesis that selenium may prevent prostate cancer in humans.[32] Molecular data show that selenium prevents clonal expansion of tumors by causing cell cycle arrest, promoting apoptosis, and modulating p53-dependent DNA repair mechanisms. Clinical trials have also shown that vitamin E supplementation is associated with a reduced risk of prostate cancer.[33,34] Currently a clinical trial is under way to test the chemopreventive efficacy of these two compounds.[35]

Obesity

In epidemiologic studies, overall obesity is usually measured by body mass index (weight in kg divided by the square of height in meters, kg/m^2) and abdominal obesity by the ratio of waist to hip circumference. The findings on overall obesity are mixed. However, recent data suggest that abdominal obesity may be associated with an increased risk of prostate cancer even in relatively lean men.[36,37] In addition, higher serum levels of insulin were associated with an increased risk of prostate cancer in China,[38] and higher serum levels of leptin were associated with larger tumor volume ($> 5 \ cm^3$).[39] Although the role of obesity in prostate cancer is not clearly defined, future studies should attempt to clarify it further because obesity is linked to numerous putative risk factors for prostate cancer, including high intakes of meat and fat intake, hormone metabolism, and serum level IGFs and insulin. Furthermore, the prevalence of obesity correlates with prostate cancer risk across populations. It is likely that obesity may thus provide a link between westernization and increased prostate cancer risk. With the epidemic of obesity in both developed and developing countries, the role of obesity needs to be clarified further.

Physical Activity

Physical activity may decrease levels of total and free testosterone, reduce obesity, and enhance immune function,[40] all of which may lead to protection from prostate cancer. However, perhaps due to challenges in classifying physical activity and/or identifying the age/time period at which activity may be most protective, results from numerous epidemiologic studies are equivocal.[40,41]

Occupation

Occupation is highly correlated with socioeconomic status and life-style factors. There is a large body of literature on prostate cancer and occupation, and one consistent result from these studies is that farmers and other agricultural workers have a 7–12% increased risk.[42,43] While this excess could reflect lifestyle factors such as increased intake of meat and fats, chemical exposures may also play a role. These chemicals, which have a wide variety of poorly characterized effects, may include fertilizers, solvents, pesticides and herbicides.[44] Organochlorines present in many pesticides and herbicides can affect circulating hormone levels; however the epidemiologic evidence linking specific pesticide or herbicide exposures to prostate cancer is weak. In addition to agriculture, workers in the heavy metals industry, rubber manufacturing, and newspaper printing may be at elevated risk,[42] suggesting that exposure to certain chemicals common in these work environments may increase the risk of prostate cancer.

Vasectomy

Several, but not all, studies investigating the association between vasectomy and prostate cancer risk suggest a modest positive association. The role of vasectomy remains controversial, however, since most studies are unable to exclude the possible effect of detection bias: men undergoing vasectomies are more likely to have prostate cancer detected than men who do not. Vasectomy is linked to elevations in anti-spermatozoa antibodies, decreased seminal hormone concentrations and decreased prostatic secretion.[45] Whether these conditions can influence prostate carcinogenesis needs to be clarified.

Chronic Inflammation

Evidence for chronic inflammation and prostate cancer is just emerging,[46] but an association of prostate cancer with chronic inflammation of the prostate (chronic prostatitis) has long been suspected. Inflammation is frequently found in prostate biopsy specimens obtained from both radical prostatectomy and surgical treatment for BPH,[47,48] however, epidemiologic findings have been mixed. A recent meta-analysis of 11 studies of prostatitis and prostate cancer reported an overall relative risk of 1.6.[49]

Results from pathologic and molecular surveys suggest that the earliest stages of prostate cancer may develop in lesions generally associated with chronic inflammation.[50,51] De Marzo *et al.* showed that almost all forms of focal prostatic glandular atrophy, thought to be precursors of prostatic adenocarcinoma, are proliferative, and that such proliferative inflammatory atrophy (PIA) lesions often contain inflammatory infiltrates and are frequently found adjacent to or near high-grade prostatic intraepithelial neoplasia (PIN).[50,51] Inflammation may lead to tumorigenesis by stimulating angiogenesis, enhancing cell proliferation, and damaging DNA through radical oxygen species such as nitric oxide.

Additional support for a role for chronic inflammation in prostate cancer comes from the observation that a higher intake of fish and use of aspirin and other non-steroidal anti-inflammation drugs (NSAIDs) has been associated with reduced prostate cancer risk.[52] In two large prospective studies, higher intake of fish was associated with a lower risk of total prostate cancer and metastatic prostate cancer.[53,54] Abundant in fatty fish, omega-3 fatty acids are known antagonists of arachidonic acid and suppress the production of pro-inflammatory cytokines.[55] In addition, use of anti-inflammatory agents, especially NSAIDs such as ibuprofen or aspirin, has been related to lower prostate cancer risk in epidemiologic studies,[56–58] and a recent meta-analysis of 12 of these studies concluded that aspirin use was associated with a 15% reduction in prostate cancer risk.[59] Taken together, these data suggest chronic inflammation may increase the risk of prostate cancer. However, there are few epidemiologic studies investigating this directly, possibly due to the difficulty in diagnosing chronic prostatitis and in measuring cytokine levels reliably in serum samples. This is likely to be a fruitful area for future research.

Sexually Transmitted Diseases

Chronic inflammation induced by bacterial or viral agents has been implicated as a potential underlying mechanism for the link between STDs and prostate cancer. One recent large, population-based study showed two- to three-fold increased prostate cancer risks associated with STDs, particularly syphilis and recurrent gonorrhea infections.[60] Other studies reported associations of human papillomavirus-16, -18 and -33 serology with an increased risk of prostate cancer.[61,62] In addition, epidemiological data are accumulating to suggest that sexual history may be associated with prostate cancer risk,[63] and a recent meta-analysis of 17 studies concluded that increased sexual frequency and number of partners are associated with increased prostate cancer risk.[49]

Benign Prostatic Hyperplasia

The relationship between BPH and prostate cancer is not well established. BPH is currently not considered a precursor to prostate cancer, since prostate cancer occurs mostly in the peripheral zone of the prostate and BPH is more common in the transition and periurethral zones. However, because both conditions are common in elderly men, and because they may coexist within the prostate, they appear to share risk profiles, making it difficult to elucidate the independent role, if any, of BPH in prostate cancer etiology. Detection bias also complicates investigation: excess prostate cancer risk in men who are symptomatic for BPH may be simply a reflection of the increased intensity of evaluation and medical surveillance in such patients. In addition, in most epidemiologic studies, it has been difficult to completely rule out the presence of BPH in control populations, since the prevalence of BPH is very common in elderly men. Due in part to these limitations, the epidemiologic evidence for BPH as a risk factor for prostate cancer remains weak and inconsistent,[64] with the largest study to date (over 85,000 BPH patients) showing only a marginally elevated risk of prostate cancer versus the general population (< 2% in 10 years).[65]

Other Factors

Several other risk factors, such as smoking, use of alcohol, diabetes and liver cirrhosis, have been investigated, but their roles in prostate cancer are weak or unclear based on data in the current literature.[66-68]

Genetic Factors

Family History of Cancer

Prostate cancer etiology has a hereditary component. Numerous studies have consistently reported familial aggregation of prostate cancer, showing a two- to three-fold increased risk of prostate cancer among men who have a first-degree male relative (father, brother, son) with a history of prostate cancer.[69] Recent data from a large twin study suggests that as much as 42% (95% CI 29–50%) of the risk of prostate cancer may be accounted for by genetic factors.[70] Genetic factors involved in prostate cancer include individual and combined effects of rare, highly penetrant genes, more common weakly penetrant genes and genes acting in concert with each other.

High-Penetrance Markers

Segregation and linkage analyses have shown that certain early-onset prostate cancers may be inherited in an autosomal dominant fashion,[71] and it is estimated that such hereditary prostate cancers (HPCs) due to highly penetrant genes may account for about 10% of all prostate cancer cases.[70] Several family studies are currently underway to identify hereditary prostate cancer candidate genes. However, these investigations have proven to be difficult for several reasons.[72] One is that, due to the high incidence of prostate cancer and the heterogeneity of tumors, it is possible that sporadic cases are included in HPC families, thereby reducing the statistical power to detect genes for HPC. In addition, because prostate cancer is generally diagnosed at a late age, it is often impossible to obtain DNA specimens from fathers of HPC cases, and sons of HPC cases are often too young to have developed prostate cancer. Therefore, studies of HPC families are often unable to include more than one generation. Finally, the genetic heterogeneity of prostate cancer makes it difficult to devise appropriate statistical transmission models that also account for multiple susceptibility genes, many of which may be at only moderate penetrance. Despite these challenges, seven loci have been described to date, including *HPC1, ELAC2, HPCX, HPC20, CAPB, PCAP*, and an unnamed locus at 8p22-23 (Table 2), and fine mapping has led to the identification of a number of candidate genes, including *RNASEL, ELAC2* and MSR-1.[73,74] The results of studies of these loci,[75-95] which have been extensively reviewed elsewhere,[73] have largely been mixed, with subsequent studies failing to replicate promising earlier findings. The absence of strong, consistent results for high penetrance markers strongly suggests that the heritable component of prostate cancer largely comprises effects of multiple factors, including common, weakly penetrant markers, possibly interacting with one another and with environmental factors.

Common Low-Penetrance Markers

Results of epidemiologic studies of common polymorphisms are summarized below and in Table 3 by biological pathway; several of these markers have been reviewed elsewhere.[73,96-99] In reviewing these results, it is important to note that, as with any other epidemiologic exposure, replication of findings is critical to establishing causality. This is particularly true of genetic association studies, because the recent explosion of genetic data has increased the potential for publication bias as investigators and publishers become more selective about writing up and publishing findings.

Androgen Biosynthesis and Metabolism Pathway

Because prostate cancer is an androgen-dependent tumor, it is likely that markers in genes whose gene products are involved in androgen biosynthesis and metabolism (Fig. 3) may be associated with disease. Recent epidemiologic studies have investigated the role of polymorphisms of over 10 genes involved in androgen biosynthesis, metabolism, transport, and regulation. These data are promising and accumulating at a remarkable pace but still are too sparse to support a role for any particular gene.

Results for the androgen receptor (*AR*), which is involved in androgen binding and transport, are fairly consistent, showing that shorter CAG repeat lengths are associated with increased risk in most, but not all, populations.[100-119] For the type II steroid 5α-reductase (*SRD5A2*), which converts testosterone to the more active androgen dihydrotestosterone, the results are mixed,[110,119-133] with a recent meta-analysis showing modest

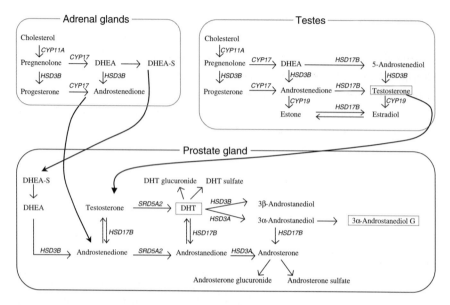

Fig. 3. Androgen biosynthesis and metabolism pathway.

risk increases associated with shorter TA repeats and the T allele of the A49T marker, but not for other studied markers.[96] Markers in several other genes, including cytochrome p450-17 (*CYP17*), cytochrome p450-19 aromatase (*CYP19*), cytochrome p450-1A1 (*CYP1A1*) and cytochrome p450-3A4 (*CYP3A4*) have shown promising initial results that often cannot be replicated.[110,111,119,120,125,134–148] Furthermore, recent initial studies of 17β-hydroxysteroid dehydrogenase 3 (*HSD17B3*) and 3β-hydroxysteroid dehydrogenase 1 (*HSD3B1*) have shown promising results,[149,150] but further study is needed to elucidate the role these may play in prostate cancer.

The totality of current data suggests that racial/ethnic variation exists in polymorphisms of genes involved in the androgen pathways.[151,152] However, their role in prostate cancer needs to be clarified further.

Growth Factor and Non-Androgenic Hormone Pathways

Due to serological evidence linking them to prostate cancer, a number of studies have explored the prostate cancer risk associated with polymorphic markers in genes involved in the insulin and insulin-like growth factor (IGF) signaling pathway. However, while the only study of the insulin gene (*INS*) has shown promising results, early studies of markers in the IGF-II and IGF binding protein-3 (IGFBP-3) genes have shown null results.[94,119,153]

Strong laboratory evidence showing chemoprotection of vitamin D against prostate cancer, in addition to suggestive but inconsistent sero-epidemiological studies, has led to numerous studies of the vitamin D receptor gene (*VDR*).[100,119,154–166] However, despite promising early studies, a recent comprehensive meta-analysis showed no overall associations and concluded that markers in the *VDR* gene are unlikely to be major genetic determinants of prostate cancer risk.[97]

Carcinogen Metabolism Pathway

Genes encoding enzymes that metabolize carcinogens and other toxins may play a role in prostate cancer. However, results from several studies of markers in different glutathione-*S*-transferases (GSTs), including *GSTT1*, *GSTP1* and *GSTM1*, have mostly been null.[76,119,134,167–175] Recent initial epidemiologic studies of other genes in these pathways, including *GSTM3* and *N*-acetyl transferase 2 (*NAT2*), have been positive but require confirmation.[134,167]

DNA Repair Pathway

The DNA repair pathway serves to prevent disruptions in DNA integrity that might otherwise lead to gene rearrangements, translocations, amplifications and deletions that may contribute to cancer development.[176] Initial reports of markers in genes encoding DNA repair enzymes, including the X-ray repair cross-complementing group (*XRCC1*), human 8-oxoguanine glycosylase I (*hOGG1*) and the xeroderma pigmentosum group D (*XPD*), show promising results.[177–180] These results, combined with strong biological plausibility, suggest that this may be a fruitful area for further research.

Chronic Inflammation Pathway

Several lines of evidence point to a role of inflammation in prostate cancer etiology, and studies of markers in the genes involved in inflammation are emerging.[46] Initial studies show positive results for transforming growth factor-β (*TGF-β*) and COX-2[181,182] and negative results for tumor necrosis factor-α-308 (*TNF-α-308*), interleukin-1β (*IL-1β*) and peroxisome proliferator-activated receptor-γ (*PPAR-γ*).[183,184] Evidence for a role of inflammation markers in prostate cancer is increasing. Given the biological plausibility of this hypothesis, this should be a fruitful area for future research.

Angiogenesis Pathways

The need for increased vasculature to support cancer growth is an area of research that is currently gaining momentum. Genetic investigations of angiogenesis in prostate cancer have thus far involved the vascular endothelial growth factor (*VEGF*) gene as well as the genes for *IL-8* and *IL-10*, and the handful of studies conducted to date have shown positive results.[142,183] These findings await further confirmation and support the notion that angiogenesis may indeed be involved in prostate cancer.

Biological Pathways Related to Dietary Factors

It is clear that genetic susceptibility to both Phase I and II enzymes (cytochrome p450) affects the association between certain dietary factors and prostate cancer risk. For example, the effect of cruciferous vegetables is related to both their high glycosinolate content and functional variations in enzymes, particularly *GSTM1* and *GSTT1*, that metabolize glycosinolates to isothiocyanates (ITCs).[27] Thus, to better assess the role of ITCs in prostate cancer, studies with both comprehensive and reliable assessment of cruciferous vegetable intake and genetic polymorphisms in *GSTM1* and *GSTT1* will be required. Moreover, genetic polymorphisms in receptors and transcription factors that interact with these compounds may contribute to variations in response to cruciferous vegetable intake. With sufficiently large sample size and careful assessment of diet and genetic factors, this important area should be investigated further.

Challenges of Studies with Common Polymorphisms

Currently, the totality of data suggests that racial/ethnic variation exists in common polymorphisms of certain genes, such as the *SRD5A2, AR*, and

ELAC2/HPC2, but few variants or genes have been firmly shown to contribute to prostate cancer susceptibility. Challenges in molecular epidemiology studies of common polymorphisms include the selection of relevant single nucleotide polymorphisms (SNPs) for genotyping and the difficulty in replicating results. The difficulty in replicating earlier findings in subsequent association studies is due, in part, to (1) the relatively small to modest effects of most common polymorphisms, ranging from 10 to 80%, (2) the relatively small sample size in most previous studies, ranging from 100 to 500 cases, and the limited power of these studies to detect a modest effect on the order of 10 to 50%, (3) the tendency of small studies to produce false positive findings, and (4) differences in study design and populations, including differences in the severity of cases. Thus, studies with large sample size (>1000 cases) are needed to clarify further the role of these polymorphic markers. In addition, it is becoming clear that a single gene or SNP alone is unlikely to explain most of the variation in prostate cancer susceptibility, thereby requiring even larger sample sizes (>3000 cases) to evaluate the effect of multiple variants.

Another challenge in epidemiologic studies investigating the role of genetic variants in complex disease (e.g., prostate cancer) is the limited ability to identify "causal SNPs" through association studies. This is partly related to two factors, (1) the difficulty in selecting biologically relevant SNPs for genotyping and (2) the inability to tease out causal SNPs from blocks of SNPs that are in high linkage disequilibrium (LD). For each gene of interest, there may be a dozen to a few hundred SNPs. The conventional approach is to choose SNPs with functional significance for genotyping. This is a difficult task in practice, given the very large pool of known SNPs and the limited information on the functional significance of many SNPs. In some studies, a haplotype-tagging approach has been used to identify informative SNPs by exploiting blocks of SNPs that are in high LD.[185–187]

Rapid progress in molecular epidemiology during the next few years is likely to hinge upon several factors, including the availability of large well-designed interdisciplinary epidemiologic studies, development of novel approaches, and statistical methods to deal with the vast amount of data, and innovative laboratory methods, such as DNA pooling[188] or whole genome scans, that permit typing multiple genetic markers at a much lower cost with higher throughput.

It is clear that prostate cancer etiology involves an intricate interplay between lifestyle and genetic factors. To fully explore the complexity of interrelationships between the numerous elements in these pathways will require large cohort studies in which blood is sampled prior to diagnosis. Such studies will be important for identifying which modifiable aspects of lifestyle (such as diet, obesity, and physical activity) can be targeted for prevention and risk reduction. To this end, studies such as the Cohort Consortium, a collaborative agreement launched in 2003 involving over 10 large, prospective cohorts with a combined total of over 7000 incident prostate cancer cases, have been organized to provide unique opportunities to evaluate the complex relationships between lifestyle and genetics in prostate cancer etiology with sufficient statistical power.

The widespread use of PSA testing in western populations has changed the characteristics of cases included in epidemiologic studies.[189] Prostate cancer cases diagnosed in the PSA era are more likely to have early lesions, which may differ in etiology from advanced lesions and more aggressive tumors. This is frequently reflected in recent epidemiologic investigations that include a large number of cases with both early and advanced lesions, which frequently show positive associations for advanced stage or more aggressive tumors but not for early stage or localized tumors. It is important that future studies include prostate tumor subclassification, such as methods of detection, markers of biological aggressiveness, and genetic changes, in order to provide more accurate risk estimates related to specific risk factors.

Summary

Epidemiologic observations provide important clues to the etiology of prostate cancer. Although the causes of prostate cancer remain unclear, there are many intriguing leads, including both environmental and genetic factors. The pathogenesis of prostate cancer reflects complex interactions between several environmental and genetic factors. With newly available tools in molecular biology and genomics, a new generation of large-scale multidisciplinary population-based studies is beginning to investigate the individual and combined effects of environmental and genetic factors. These studies are likely to provide unique information on risk factors and help identify subsets of the population that are more susceptible to prostate cancer through certain environmental insults.

References

1. Hsing AW, Tsao L, Devesa SS (2000) International trends and patterns of prostate cancer incidence and mortality. *Int J Cancer* 85:60–67.
2. Ries LAG, Eisner MP, Kosary CL, Hankey BF, Miller BA, Clegg L, Mariotto A, Fay MP, Feuer EJ, Edwards BK (eds.) (2003) *SEER Cancer Statistics Review*, 1975–2000. National Cancer Institute, Bethesda, MD.
3. Potosky AL, Kessler L, Gridley G, Brown CC, Horm JW (1990) Rise in prostatic cancer incidence associated with increased use of transurethral resection. *J Natl Cancer Inst* 82:1624–1628.
4. Potosky AL, Miller BA, Albertsen PC, Kramer BS (1995) The role of increasing detection in the rising incidence of prostate cancer. *JAMA* 273:548–552.
5. Hsing AW, Devesa SS (2001) Trends and patterns of prostate cancer: what do they suggest? *Epidemiol Rev* 23:3–13.
6. Parkin DM, Whelan SJ, Ferlay J, Teppo L, Thomas DB (eds.) (2003) *Cancer Incidence in Five Continents*, Vol VIII. IARC Press, Lyon.
7. Jemal A, Tiwari RC, Murray T, Ghafoor A, Samuels A, Ward E, Feuer EJ, Thun MJ (2004) Cancer statistics, 2004. *CA Cancer J Clin* 54:8–29.
8. Parkin DM, Pisani P, Ferlay J (1999) Global cancer statistics. *CA Cancer J Clin* 49:33–64.
9. Shimizu H, Ross RK, Bernstein L, Yatani R, Henderson BE, Mack TM (1991) Cancers of the prostate and breast among Japanese and white immigrants in Los Angeles County. *Br J Cancer* 63:963–966.
10. Cook LS, Goldoft M, Schwartz SM, Weiss NS (1999) Incidence of adenocarcinoma of the prostate in Asian immigrants to the United States and their descendants. *J Urol* 161:152–155.
11. Huggins C, Hodges CV (1941) Studies on prostatic cancer: Effect of castration, of estrogen, and of androgen injection on serum phosphatases in metastatic carcinoma of the prostate. *Cancer Res.* 1:293–297.
12. Niu Y, Xu Y, Zhang J, Bai J, Yang H, Ma T (2001) Proliferation and differentiation of prostatic stromal cells. *BJU Int* 87:386–393.
13. Noble RL (1977) The development of prostatic adenocarcinoma in Nb rats following prolonged sex hormone administration. *Cancer Res* 37:1929–1933.
14. Hsing AW (2001) Hormones and prostate cancer: what's next? *Epidemiol Rev* 23:42–58.

15. Hsing AW (1996) Hormones and prostate cancer: where do we go from here? *J Natl Cancer Inst* 88:1093–1095.

16. Eaton NE, Reeves GK, Appleby PN, Key TJ (1999) Endogenous sex hormones and prostate cancer: a quantitative review of prospective studies. *Br J Cancer* 80:930–934.

17. Gann PH, Hennekens CH, Ma J, Longcope C, Stampfer MJ (1996) Prospective study of sex hormone levels and risk of prostate cancer. *J Natl Cancer Inst* 88:1118–1126.

18. Yu H, Rohan T (2000) Role of the insulin-like growth factor family in cancer development and progression. *J Natl Cancer Inst* 92:1472–1489.

19. LeRoith D, Roberts CT Jr (2003) The insulin-like growth factor system and cancer. *Cancer Lett* 195:127–317.

20. Zhao XY, Feldman D (2001) The role of vitamin D in prostate cancer. *Steroids* 66:293–300.

21. Hill P, Wynder EL, Garbaczewski L, Garnes H, Walker AR (1979) Diet and urinary steroids in black and white North American men and black South African men. *Cancer Res* 39:5101–5105.

22. Kolonel LN, Nomura AM, Cooney RV (1999) Dietary fat and prostate cancer: current status. *J Natl Cancer Inst* 91:414–428.

23. Kolonel LN (2001) Fat, meat, and prostate cancer. *Epidemiol Rev* 23:72–81.

24. Norrish AE, Ferguson LR, Knize MG, Felton JS, Sharpe SJ, Jackson RT (1999) Heterocyclic amine content of cooked meat and risk of prostate cancer. *J Natl Cancer Inst* 91:2038–2044.

25. Terry PD, Rohan TE, Wolk A (2003) Intakes of fish and marine fatty acids and the risks of cancers of the breast and prostate and of other hormone-related cancers: a review of the epidemiologic evidence. *Am J Clin Nutr* 77:532–543.

26. Giovannucci E (1999) Nutritional factors in human cancers. *Adv Exp Med Biol* 472:29–42.

27. Kristal AR, Lampe JW (2002) Brassica vegetables and prostate cancer risk: a review of the epidemiological evidence. *Nutr Cancer* 42:1–9.

28. Hsing AW, Chokkalingam AP, Gao YT, Madigan MP, Deng J, Gridley G, Fraumeni JF, Jr (2002) Allium vegetables and risk of prostate cancer: a population-based study. *J Natl Cancer Inst* 94:1648–1651.

29. Chan JM, Giovannucci EL (2001) Dairy products, calcium, and vitamin D and risk of prostate cancer. *Epidemiol Rev* 23:87–92.

30. Rodriguez C, McCullough ML, Mondul AM, Jacobs EJ, Fakhrabadi-Shokoohi D, Giovannucci EL, Thun MJ, Calle EE (2003) Calcium, dairy products, and risk of prostate cancer in a prospective cohort of United States men. *Cancer Epidemiol Biomarkers Prev* 12:597–603.

31. Leitzmann MF, Stampfer MJ, Wu K, Colditz GA, Willett WC, Giovannucci EL (2003) Zinc supplement use and risk of prostate cancer. *J Natl Cancer Inst* 95:1004–1007.

32. Klein EA (2004) Selenium: epidemiology and basic science. *J Urol* 171: S50–53; discussion p. S53.

33. Virtamo J, Pietinen P, Huttunen JK, Korhonen P, Malila N, Virtanen MJ, Albanes D, Taylor PR, Albert P (2003) Incidence of cancer and mortality following alpha-tocopherol and beta-carotene supplementation: a post-intervention follow-up. *JAMA* 290:476–485.

34. Pak RW, Lanteri VJ, Scheuch JR, Sawczuk IS (2002) Review of vitamin E and selenium in the prevention of prostate cancer: implications of the selenium and vitamin E chemoprevention trial. *Integr Cancer Ther* 1:338–344.

35. Klein EA, Thompson IM, Lippman SM, Goodman PJ, Albanes D, Taylor PR, Coltman C (2001) SELECT: the next prostate cancer prevention trial. Selenum and Vitamin E Cancer Prevention Trial. *J Urol* 166:1311–1315.

36. Hsing AW, Deng J, Sesterhenn IA, Mostofi FK, Stanczyk FZ, Benichou J, Xie T, Gao YT (2000) Body size and prostate cancer: a population-based case-control study in China. *Cancer Epidemiol Biomarkers Prev* 9:1335–1341.

37. Hubbard JS, Rohrmann S, Landis PK, Metter EJ, Muller DC, Andres R, Carter HB, Platz EA (2004) Association of prostate cancer risk with insulin, glucose, and anthropometry in the Baltimore longitudinal study of aging. *Urology* 63:253–258.

38. Hsing AW, Chua S, Jr, Gao YT, Gentzschein E, Chang L, Deng J, Stanczyk FZ (2001) Prostate cancer risk and serum levels of insulin and leptin: a population-based study. *J Natl Cancer Inst* 93:783–789.

39. Chang S, Hursting SD, Contois JH, Strom SS, Yamamura Y, Babaian RJ, Troncoso P, Scardino PS, Wheeler TM, Amos CI, Spitz MR (2001) Leptin and prostate cancer. *Prostate* 46:62–67.

40. Lee IM, Sesso IID, Chen JJ, Paffenbarger RS, Jr (2001) Does physical activity play a role in the prevention of prostate cancer? *Epidemiol Rev* 23:132–137.

41. Lee IM (2003) Physical activity and cancer prevention — data from epidemiologic studies. *Med Sci Sports Exerc* 35:1823–1827.

42. Sharma-Wagner S, Chokkalingam AP, Malker HS, Stone BJ, McLaughlin JK, Hsing AW (2000) Occupation and prostate cancer risk in Sweden. *J Occup Environ Med* 42:517–525.

43. van der Gulden JW, Kolk JJ, Verbeek AL (1995) Work environment and prostate cancer risk. *Prostate* 27:250–257.

44. Alavanja MC, Samanic C, Dosemeci M, Lubin J, Tarone R, Lynch CF, Knott C, Thomas K, Hoppin JA, Barker J, Coble J, Sandler DP, Blair A

(2003) Use of agricultural pesticides and prostate cancer risk in the Agricultural Health Study cohort. *Am J Epidemiol* 157:800–814.

45. Bernal-Delgado E, Latour-Perez J, Pradas-Arnal F, Gomez-Lopez LI (1998) The association between vasectomy and prostate cancer: a systematic review of the literature. *Fertil Steril* 70:191–200.

46. Platz EA, De Marzo AM (2004) Epidemiology of inflammation and prostate cancer. *J Urol* 171:S36–40.

47. Nickel JC, True LD, Krieger JN, Berger RE, Boag AH, Young ID (2001) Consensus development of a histopathological classification system for chronic prostatic inflammation. *BJU Int* 87:797–805.

48. Di Silverio F, Gentile V, De Matteis A, Mariotti G, Giuseppe V, Luigi PA, Sciarra A (2003) Distribution of inflammation, pre-malignant lesions, incidental carcinoma in histologically confirmed benign prostatic hyperplasia: a retrospective analysis. *Eur Urol* 43:164–175.

49. Dennis LK, Dawson DV (2002) Meta-analysis of measures of sexual activity and prostate cancer. *Epidemiology* 13:72–79.

50. De Marzo AM, Marchi VL, Epstein JI, Nelson WG (1999) Proliferative inflammatory atrophy of the prostate: implications for prostatic carcinogenesis. *Am J Pathol* 155:1985–1992.

51. DeMarzo AM, Nelson WG, Isaacs WB, Epstein JI (2003) Pathological and molecular aspects of prostate cancer. *Lancet* 361:955–964.

52. Nelson JE, Harris RE (2000) Inverse association of prostate cancer and non-steroidal anti-inflammatory drugs (NSAIDs): results of a case-control study. *Oncol Rep* 7:169–170.

53. Terry P, Lichtenstein P, Feychting M, Ahlbom A, Wolk A (2001) Fatty fish consumption and risk of prostate cancer. *Lancet* 357:1764–1766.

54. Augustsson K, Michaud DS, Rimm EB, Leitzmann MF, Stampfer MJ, Willett WC, Giovannucci E (2003) A prospective study of intake of fish and marine fatty acids and prostate cancer. *Cancer Epidemiol Biomarkers Prev* 12:64–67.

55. Calder PC (2002) Fatty acids and gene expression related to inflammation. *Nestle Nutr Workshop Ser Clin Perform Programme* 7:19–36; discussion pp. 36–40.

56. Norrish AE, Jackson RT, McRae CU (1998) Non-steroidal anti-inflammatory drugs and prostate cancer progression. *Int J Cancer* 77:511–515.

57. Leitzmann MF, Stampfer MJ, Ma J, Chan JM, Colditz GA, Willett WC, Giovannucci E (2002) Aspirin use in relation to risk of prostate cancer. *Cancer Epidemiol Biomarkers Prev* 11:1108–1111.

58. Thun MJ, Namboodiri MM, Calle EE, Flanders WD, Heath CW, Jr (1993) Aspirin use and risk of fatal cancer. *Cancer Res* 53:1322–1327.

59. Mahmud S, Franco E, Aprikian A (2004) Prostate cancer and use of non-steroidal anti-inflammatory drugs: systematic review and meta-analysis. *Br J Cancer* 90:93–99.

60. Hayes RB, Pottern LM, Strickler H, Rabkin C, Pope V, Swanson GM, Greenberg RS, Schoenberg JB, Liff J, Schwartz AG, Hoover RN, Fraumeni JF, Jr (2000) Sexual behaviour, STDs and risks for prostate cancer. *Br J Cancer* 82:718–725.

61. Adami HO, Kuper H, Andersson SO, Bergstrom R, Dillner J (2003) Prostate cancer risk and serologic evidence of human papilloma virus infection: a population-based case-control study. *Cancer Epidemiol Biomarkers Prev* 12:872–875.

62. Rosenblatt KA, Carter JJ, Iwasaki LM, Galloway DA, Stanford JL (2003) Serologic evidence of human papillomavirus 16 and 18 infections and risk of prostate cancer. *Cancer Epidemiol Biomarkers Prev* 12:763–768.

63. Strickler HD, Goedert JJ (2001) Sexual behavior and evidence for an infectious cause of prostate cancer. *Epidemiol Rev* 23:144–151.

64. Guess HA (2001) Benign prostatic hyperplasia and prostate cancer. *Epidemiol Rev* 23:152–158.

65. Chokkalingam AP, Nyren O, Johansson JE, Gridley G, McLaughlin JK, Adami HO, Hsing AW (2003) Prostate carcinoma risk subsequent to diagnosis of benign prostatic hyperplasia: a population-based cohort study in Sweden. *Cancer* 98:1727–1734.

66. Giovannucci E (2001) Medical history and etiology of prostate cancer. *Epidemiol Rev* 23:159–162.

67. Dennis LK, Hayes RB (2001) Alcohol and prostate cancer. *Epidemiol Rev* 23:110–114.

68. Hickey K, Do KA, Green A (2001) Smoking and prostate cancer. *Epidemiol Rev* 23:115–125.

69. Stanford JL, Ostrander EA (2001) Familial prostate cancer. *Epidemiol Rev* 23:19–23.

70. Lichtenstein P, Holm NV, Verkasalo PK, Iliadou A, Kaprio J, Koskenvuo M, Pukkala E, Skytthe A, Hemminki K (2000) Environmental and heritable factors in the causation of cancer-analyses of cohorts of twins from Sweden, Denmark, and Finland. *N Engl J Med* 343:78–85.

71. Carter BS, Bova GS, Beaty TH, Steinberg GD, Childs B, Isaacs WB, Walsh PC (1993) Hereditary prostate cancer: epidemiologic and clinical features. *J Urol* 150:797–802.

72. Simard J, Dumont M, Soucy P, Labrie F (2002) Perspective: prostate cancer susceptibility genes. *Endocrinology* 143:2029–2040.
73. Schaid DJ (2004) The complex genetic epidemiology of prostate cancer. *Hum Mol Genet* 13:R103–121 (Epub 2004 Jan 28).
74. Ostrander EA, Stanford JL (2000) Genetics of prostate cancer: too many loci, too few genes. *Am J Hum Genet* 67:1367–1375 (Epub 2000 Nov 7).
75. Rokman A, Ikonen T, Seppala EH, Nupponen N, Autio V, Mononen N, Bailey-Wilson J, Trent J, Carpten J, Matikainen MP, Koivisto PA, Tammela TL, Kallioniemi OP, Schleutker J (2002) Germline alterations of the RNASEL gene, a candidate HPC1 gene at 1q25, in patients and families with prostate cancer. *Am J Hum Genet* 70:1299–1304 (Epub 2002 Apr 8).
76. Nakazato H, Suzuki K, Matsui H, Koike H, Okugi H, Ohtake N, Takei T, Nakata S, Hasumi M, Ito K, Kurokawa K, Yamanaka H (2003) Association of genetic polymorphisms of glutathione-S-transferase genes (GSTM1, GSTT1 and GSTP1) with familial prostate cancer risk in a Japanese population. *Anticancer Res* 23:2897–2902.
77. Wang L, McDonnell SK, Elkins DA, Slager SL, Christensen E, Marks AF, Cunningham JM, Peterson BJ, Jacobsen SJ, Cerhan JR, Blute ML, Schaid DJ, Thibodeau SN (2002) Analysis of the RNASEL gene in familial and sporadic prostate cancer. *Am J Hum Genet* 71:116–123 (Epub 2002 May 17).
78. Casey G, Neville PJ, Plummer SJ, Xiang Y, Krumroy LM, Klein EA, Catalona WJ, Nupponen N, Carpten JD, Trent JM, Silverman RH, Witte JS (2002) RNASEL Arg462Gln variant is implicated in up to 13% of prostate cancer cases. *Nat Genet* 32:581–583.
79. Rebbeck TR, Walker AH, Zeigler-Johnson C, Weisburg S, Martin AM, Nathanson KL, Wein AJ, Malkowicz SB (2000) Association of HPC2/ ELAC2 genotypes and prostate cancer. *Am J Hum Genet* 67:1014–1019 (Epub 2000 Sep 12).
80. Suarez BK, Gerhard DS, Lin J, Haberer B, Nguyen L, Kesterson NK, Catalona WJ (2001) Polymorphisms in the prostate cancer susceptibility gene HPC2/ELAC2 in multiplex families and healthy controls. *Cancer Res* 61:4982–4984.
81. Tavtigian SV, Simard J, Teng DH, Abtin V, Baumgard M, Beck A, Camp NJ, Carillo AR, Chen Y, Dayananth P, Desrochers M, Dumont M, Farnham JM, Frank D, Frye C, Ghaffari S, Gupte JS, Hu R, Iliev D, Janecki T, Kort EN, Laity KE, Leavitt A, Leblanc G, McArthur-Morrison J, Pederson A, Penn B, Peterson KT, Reid JE, Richards S, Schroeder M, Smith R, Snyder SC, Swedlund B, Swensen J, Thomas A, Tranchant M, Woodland AM, Labrie F,

Skolnick MH, Neuhausen S, Rommens J, Cannon-Albright LA (2001) A candidate prostate cancer susceptibility gene at chromosome 17p. *Nat Genet* 27:172–180.

82. Vesprini D, Nam RK, Trachtenberg J, Jewett MA, Tavtigian SV, Emami M, Ho M, Toi A, Narod SA (2001) HPC2 variants and screen-detected prostate cancer. *Am J Hum Genet* 68:912–917 (Epub 2001 Mar 14).

83. Wang L, McDonnell SK, Elkins DA, Slager SL, Christensen E, Marks AF, Cunningham JM, Peterson BJ, Jacobsen SJ, Cerhan JR, Blute ML, Schaid DJ, Thibodeau SN (2001) Role of HPC2/ELAC2 in hereditary prostate cancer. *Cancer Res* 61:6494–6499.

84. Xu J, Zheng SL, Carpten JD, Nupponen NN, Robbins CM, Mestre J, Moses TY, Faith DA, Kelly BD, Isaacs SD, Wiley KE, Ewing CM, Bujnovszky P, Chang B, Bailey-Wilson J, Bleecker ER, Walsh PC, Trent JM, Meyers DA, Isaacs WB (2001) Evaluation of linkage and association of HPC2/ELAC2 in patients with familial or sporadic prostate cancer. *Am J Hum Genet* 68:901–911 (Epub 2001 Mar 14).

85. Rokman A, Ikonen T, Mononen N, Autio V, Matikainen MP, Koivisto PA, Tammela TL, Kallioniemi OP, Schleutker J (2001) ELAC2/HPC2 involvement in hereditary and sporadic prostate cancer. *Cancer Res* 61:6038–6041.

86. Meitz JC, Edwards SM, Easton DF, Murkin A, Ardern-Jones A, Jackson RA, Williams S, Dearnaley DP, Stratton MR, Houlston RS, Eeles RA (2002) HPC2/ELAC2 polymorphisms and prostate cancer risk: analysis by age of onset of disease. *Br J Cancer* 87:905–908.

87. Adler D, Kanji N, Trpkov K, Fick G, Hughes RM (2003) HPC2/ELAC2 gene variants associated with incident prostate cancer. *J Hum Genet* 48:634–638 (Epub 2003 Nov 19).

88. Stanford JL, Sabacan LP, Noonan EA, Iwasaki L, Shu J, Feng Z, Ostrander EA (2003) Association of HPC2/ELAC2 polymorphisms with risk of prostate cancer in a population-based study. *Cancer Epidemiol Biomarkers Prev* 12:876–881.

89. Takahashi H, Lu W, Watanabe M, Katoh T, Furusato M, Tsukino H, Nakao H, Sudo A, Suzuki H, Akakura K, Ikemoto I, Asano K, Ito T, Wakui S, Muto T, Hano H (2003) Ser217Leu polymorphism of the HPC2/ELAC2 gene associated with prostatic cancer risk in Japanese men. *Int J Cancer* 107:224–228.

90. Severi G, Giles GG, Southey MC, Tesoriero A, Tilley W, Neufing P, Morris H, English DR, McCredie MR, Boyle P, Hopper JL (2003) ELAC2/HPC2 polymorphisms, prostate-specific antigen levels, and prostate cancer. *J Natl Cancer Inst* 95:818–824.

91. Camp NJ, Tavtigian SV (2002) Meta-analysis of associations of the Ser217Leu and Ala541Thr variants in ELAC2 (HPC2) and prostate cancer. *Am J Hum Genet* 71:1475–1478.

92. Xu J, Zheng SL, Komiya A, Mychaleckyj JC, Isaacs SD, Chang B, Turner AR, Ewing CM, Wiley KE, Hawkins GA, Bleecker ER, Walsh PC, Meyers DA, Isaacs WB (2003) Common sequence variants of the macrophage scavenger receptor 1 gene are associated with prostate cancer risk. *Am J Hum Genet* 72:208–212.

93. Miller DC, Zheng SL, Dunn RL, Sarma AV, Montie JE, Lange EM, Meyers DA, Xu J, Cooney KA (2003) Germ-line mutations of the macrophage scavenger receptor 1 gene: association with prostate cancer risk in African-American men. *Cancer Res* 63:3486–3489.

94. Wang L, Habuchi T, Tsuchiya N, Mitsumori K, Ohyama C, Sato K, Kinoshita H, Kamoto T, Nakamura A, Ogawa O, Kato T (2003) Insulin-like growth factor-binding protein-3 gene -202 A/C polymorphism is correlated with advanced disease status in prostate cancer. *Cancer Res* 63:4407–4411.

95. Seppala EH, Ikonen T, Autio V, Rokman A, Mononen N, Matikainen MP, Tammela TL, Schleutker J (2003) Germ-line alterations in MSR1 gene and prostate cancer risk. *Clin Cancer Res* 9:5252–5256.

96. Ntais C, Polycarpou A, Ioannidis JP (2003) SRD5A2 gene polymorphisms and the risk of prostate cancer: a meta-analysis. *Cancer Epidemiol Biomarkers Prev* 12:618–624.

97. Ntais C, Polycarpou A, Ioannidis JP (2003) Vitamin D receptor gene polymorphisms and risk of prostate cancer: a meta-analysis. *Cancer Epidemiol Biomarkers Prev* 12:1395–1402.

98. Ntais C, Polycarpou A, Ioannidis JP (2003) Association of the CYP17 gene polymorphism with the risk of prostate cancer: a meta-analysis. *Cancer Epidemiol Biomarkers Prev* 12:120–126.

99. Gsur A, Feik E, Madersbacher S (2004) Genetic polymorphisms and prostate cancer risk. *World J Urol* 21:414–423 (Epub 2003 Nov 26).

100. Ingles SA, Ross RK, Yu MC, Irvine RA, La Pera G, Haile RW, Coetzee GA (1997) Association of prostate cancer risk with genetic polymorphisms in vitamin D receptor and androgen receptor. *J Natl Cancer Inst* 89: 166–170.

101. Stanford JL, Just JJ, Gibbs M, Wicklund KG, Neal CL, Blumenstein BA, Ostrander EA (1997) Polymorphic repeats in the androgen receptor gene: molecular markers of prostate cancer risk. *Cancer Res* 57:1194–1198.

102. Giovannucci E, Stampfer MJ, Krithivas K, Brown M, Dahl D, Brufsky A, Talcott J, Hennekens CH, Kantoff PW (1997) The CAG repeat within the

androgen receptor gene and its relationship to prostate cancer. *Proc Natl Acad Sci USA* 94:3320–3323.

103. Platz EA, Giovannucci E, Dahl DM, Krithivas K, Hennekens CH, Brown M, Stampfer MJ, Kantoff PW (1998) The androgen receptor gene GGN microsatellite and prostate cancer risk. *Cancer Epidemiol Biomarkers Prev* 7:379–384.

104. Correa-Cerro L, Wohr G, Haussler J, Berthon P, Drelon E, Mangin P, Fournier G, Cussenot O, Kraus P, Just W, Paiss T, Cantu JM, Vogel W (1999) (CAG)nCAA and GGN repeats in the human androgen receptor gene are not associated with prostate cancer in a French-German population. *Eur J Hum Genet* 7:357–362.

105. Ekman P, Gronberg H, Matsuyama H, Kivineva M, Bergerheim US, Li C (1999) Links between genetic and environmental factors and prostate cancer risk. *Prostate* 39:262–268.

106. Edwards SM, Badzioch MD, Minter R, Hamoudi R, Collins N, Ardern-Jones A, Dowe A, Osborne S, Kelly J, Shearer R, Easton DF, Saunders GF, Dearnaley DP, Eeles RA (1999) Androgen receptor polymorphisms: association with prostate cancer risk, relapse and overall survival. *Int J Cancer* 84:458–465.

107. Hsing AW, Gao YT, Wu G, Wang X, Deng J, Chen YL, Sesterhenn IA, Mostofi FK, Benichou J, Chang C (2000) Polymorphic CAG and GGN repeat lengths in the androgen receptor gene and prostate cancer risk: a population-based case-control study in China. *Cancer Res* 60: 5111–5116.

108. Miller EA, Stanford JL, Hsu L, Noonan EA, Ostrander EA (2001) Polymorphic repeats in the androgen receptor gene in high-risk sibships. *Prostate* 48:200–205.

109. Beilin J, Harewood L, Frydenberg M, Mameghan H, Martyres RF, Farish SJ, Yue C, Deam DR, Byron KA, Zajac JD (2001) A case-control study of the androgen receptor gene CAG repeat polymorphism in Australian prostate carcinoma subjects. *Cancer* 92:941–949.

110. Latil AG, Azzouzi R, Cancel GS, Guillaume EC, Cochan-Priollet B, Berthon PL, Cussenot O (2001) Prostate carcinoma risk and allelic variants of genes involved in androgen biosynthesis and metabolism pathways. *Cancer* 92:1130–1137.

111. Modugno F, Weissfeld JL, Trump DL, Zmuda JM, Shea P, Cauley JA, Ferrell RE (2001) Allelic variants of aromatase and the androgen and estrogen receptors: toward a multigenic model of prostate cancer risk. *Clin Cancer Res* 7:3092–3096.

112. Chang BL, Zheng SL, Hawkins GA, Isaacs SD, Wiley KE, Turner A, Carpten JD, Bleecker ER, Walsh PC, Trent JM, Meyers DA, Isaacs WB, Xu J (2002) Polymorphic GGC repeats in the androgen receptor gene are associated with hereditary and sporadic prostate cancer risk. *Hum Genet* 110:122–129 (Epub 2002 Jan 23).

113. Mononen N, Ikonen T, Autio V, Rokman A, Matikainen MP, Tammela TL, Kallioniemi OP, Koivisto PA, Schleutker J (2002) Androgen receptor CAG polymorphism and prostate cancer risk. *Hum Genet* 111:166–171 (Epub 2002 Jul 3).

114. Gsur A, Preyer M, Haidinger G, Zidek T, Madersbacher S, Schatzl G, Marberger M, Vutuc C, Micksche M (2002) Polymorphic CAG repeats in the androgen receptor gene, prostate-specific antigen polymorphism and prostate cancer risk. *Carcinogenesis* 23:1647–1651.

115. Chen C, Lamharzi N, Weiss NS, Etzioni R, Dightman DA, Barnett M, DiTommaso D, Goodman G (2002) Androgen receptor polymorphisms and the incidence of prostate cancer. *Cancer Epidemiol Biomarkers Prev* 11: 1033–1040.

116. Balic I, Graham ST, Troyer DA, Higgins BA, Pollock BH, Johnson-Pais TL, Thompson IM, Leach RJ (2002) Androgen receptor length polymorphism associated with prostate cancer risk in Hispanic men. *J Urol* 168: 2245–2248.

117. Santos ML, Sarkis AS, Nishimoto IN, Nagai MA (2003) Androgen receptor CAG repeat polymorphism in prostate cancer from a Brazilian population. *Cancer Detect Prev* 27:321–326.

118. Huang SP, Chou YH, Chang WS, Wu MT, Yu CC, Wu T, Lee YH, Huang JK, Wu WJ, Huang CH (2003) Androgen receptor gene polymorphism and prostate cancer in Taiwan. *J Formos Med Assoc* 102:680–686.

119. Nam RK, Zhang WW, Trachtenberg J, Jewett MA, Emami M, Vesprini D, Chu W, Ho M, Sweet J, Evans A, Toi A, Pollak M, Narod SA (2003) Comprehensive assessment of candidate genes and serological markers for the detection of prostate cancer. *Cancer Epidemiol Biomarkers Prev* 12:1429–1437.

120. Lunn RM, Bell DA, Mohler JL, Taylor JA (1999) Prostate cancer risk and polymorphism in 17 hydroxylase (CYP17) and steroid reductase (SRD5A2). *Carcinogenesis* 20:1727–1731.

121. Kantoff PW, Febbo PG, Giovannucci E, Krithivas K, Dahl DM, Chang G, Hennekens CH, Brown M, Stampfer MJ (1997) A polymorphism of the 5 alpha-reductase gene and its association with prostate cancer: a case-control analysis. *Cancer Epidemiol Biomarkers Prev* 6:189–192.

122. Febbo PG, Kantoff PW, Platz EA, Casey D, Batter S, Giovannucci E, Hennekens CH, Stampfer MJ (1999) The V89L polymorphism in the 5alpha-reductase type 2 gene and risk of prostate cancer. *Cancer Res* 59: 5878–5881.

123. Makridakis NM, Ross RK, Pike MC, Crocitto LE, Kolonel LN, Pearce CL, Henderson BE, Reichardt JK (1999) Association of mis-sense substitution in SRD5A2 gene with prostate cancer in African-American and Hispanic men in Los Angeles, USA. *Lancet* 354:975–978.

124. Margiotti K, Sangiuolo F, De Luca A, Froio F, Pearce CL, Ricci-Barbini V, Micali F, Bonafe M, Franceschi C, Dallapiccola B, Novelli G, Reichardt JK (2000) Evidence for an association between the SRD5A2 (type II steroid 5 alpha-reductase) locus and prostate cancer in Italian patients. *Dis Markers* 16:147–150.

125. Yamada Y, Watanabe M, Murata M, Yamanaka M, Kubota Y, Ito H, Katoh T, Kawamura J, Yatani R, Shiraishi T (2001) Impact of genetic polymorphisms of 17-hydroxylase cytochrome P-450 (CYP17) and steroid 5alpha-reductase type II (SRD5A2) genes on prostate-cancer risk among the Japanese population. *Int J Cancer* 92:683–686.

126. Nam RK, Toi A, Vesprini D, Ho M, Chu W, Harvie S, Sweet J, Trachtenberg J, Jewett MA, Narod SA (2001) V89L polymorphism of type-2, 5-alpha reductase enzyme gene predicts prostate cancer presence and progression. *Urology* 57:199–204.

127. Mononen N, Ikonen T, Syrjakoski K, Matikainen MP, Schleutker J, Tammela TL, Koivisto PA, Kallioniemi OP (2001) A missense substitution A49T in the steroid 5-alpha-reductase gene (SRD5A2) is not associated with prostate cancer in Finland. *Br J Cancer* 84:1344–1347.

128. Hsing AW, Chen C, Chokkalingam AP, Gao YT, Dightman DA, Nguyen HT, Deng J, Cheng J, Sesterhenn IA, Mostofi FK, Stanczyk FZ, Reichardt JK (2001) Polymorphic markers in the SRD5A2 gene and prostate cancer risk: a population-based case-control study. *Cancer Epidemiol Biomarkers Prev* 10:1077–1082.

129. Pearce CL, Makridakis NM, Ross RK, Pike MC, Kolonel LN, Henderson BE, Reichardt JK (2002) Steroid 5-alpha reductase type II V89L substitution is not associated with risk of prostate cancer in a multiethnic population study. *Cancer Epidemiol Biomarkers Prev* 11: 417–418.

130. Soderstrom T, Wadelius M, Andersson SO, Johansson JE, Johansson S, Granath F, Rane A (2002) 5alpha-reductase 2 polymorphisms as risk factors in prostate cancer. *Pharmacogenetics* 12:307–312.

131. Lamharzi N, Johnson MM, Goodman G, Etzioni R, Weiss NS, Dightman DA, Barnett M, DiTommaso D, Chen C (2003) Polymorphic markers in the 5alpha-reductase type II gene and the incidence of prostate cancer. *Int J Cancer* 105:480–483.

132. Chang BL, Zheng SL, Isaacs SD, Turner AR, Bleecker ER, Walsh PC, Meyers DA, Isaacs WB, Xu J (2003) Evaluation of SRD5A2 sequence variants in susceptibility to hereditary and sporadic prostate cancer. *Prostate* 56:37–44.

133. Li Z, Habuchi T, Mitsumori K, Kamoto T, Kinoshitu H, Segawa T, Ogawa O, Kato T (2003) Association of V89L SRD5A2 polymorphism with prostate cancer development in a Japanese population. *J Urol* 169:2378–2381.

134. Wadelius M, Andersson AO, Johansson JE, Wadelius C, Rane E (1999) Prostate cancer associated with CYP17 genotype. *Pharmacogenetics* 9:635–639.

135. Gsur A, Bernhofer G, Hinteregger S, Haidinger G, Schatzl G, Madersbacher S, Marberger M, Vutuc C, Micksche M (2000) A polymorphism in the CYP17 gene is associated with prostate cancer risk. *Int J Cancer* 87:434–437.

136. Habuchi T, Liqing Z, Suzuki T, Sasaki R, Tsuchiya N, Tachiki H, Shimoda N, Satoh S, Sato K, Kakehi Y, Kamoto T, Ogawa O, Kato T (2000) Increased risk of prostate cancer and benign prostatic hyperplasia associated with a CYP17 gene polymorphism with a gene dosage effect. *Cancer Res* 60: 5710–5713.

137. Haiman CA, Stampfer MJ, Giovannucci E, Ma J, Decalo NE, Kantoff PW, Hunter DJ (2001) The relationship between a polymorphism in CYP17 with plasma hormone levels and prostate cancer. *Cancer Epidemiol Biomarkers Prev* 10:743–748.

138. Kittles RA, Panguluri RK, Chen W, Massac A, Ahaghotu C, Jackson A, Ukoli F, Adams-Campbell L, Isaacs W, Dunston GM (2001) Cyp17 promoter variant associated with prostate cancer aggressiveness in African Americans. *Cancer Epidemiol Biomarkers Prev* 10:943–947.

139. Chang B, Zheng SL, Isaacs SD, Wiley KE, Carpten JD, Hawkins GA, Bleecker ER, Walsh PC, Trent JM, Meyers DA, Isaacs WB, Xu J (2001) Linkage and association of CYP17 gene in hereditary and sporadic prostate cancer. *Int J Cancer* 95:354–359.

140. Stanford JL, Noonan EA, Iwasaki L, Kolb S, Chadwick RB, Feng Z, Ostrander EA (2002) A polymorphism in the CYP17 gene and risk of prostate cancer. *Cancer Epidemiol Biomarkers Prev* 11:243–247.

141. Madigan MP, Gao YT, Deng J, Pfeiffer RM, Chang BL, Zheng S, Meyers DA, Stanczyk FZ, Xu J, Hsing AW (2003) CYP17 polymorphisms

in relation to risks of prostate cancer and benign prostatic hyperplasia: a population-based study in China. *Int J Cancer* 107:271–275.

142. Lin CC, Wu HC, Tsai FJ, Chen HY, Chen WC (2003) Vascular endothelial growth factor gene-460 C/T polymorphism is a biomarker for prostate cancer. *Urology* 62:374–377.

143. Suzuki K, Nakazato H, Matsui H, Koike H, Okugi H, Ohtake N, Takei T, Nakata S, Hasumi M, Yamanaka H (2003) Association of the genetic polymorphism of the CYP19 intron 4[TTTA]n repeat with familial prostate cancer risk in a Japanese population. *Anticancer Res* 23:4941–4946.

144. Murata M, Shiraishi T, Fukutome K, Watanabe M, Nagao M, Kubota Y, Ito H, Kawamura J, Yatani R (1998) Cytochrome P4501A1 and glutathione S-transferase M1 genotypes as risk factors for prostate cancer in Japan. *Jpn J Clin Oncol* 28:657–660.

145. Suzuki K, Matsui H, Nakazato H, Koike H, Okugi H, Hasumi M, Ohtake N, Nakata S, Takei T, Hatori M, Ito K, Yamanaka H (2003) Association of the genetic polymorphism in cytochrome P450 (CYP) 1A1 with risk of familial prostate cancer in a Japanese population: a case-control study. *Cancer Lett* 195:177–183.

146. Chang BL, Zheng SL, Isaacs SD, Turner A, Hawkins GA, Wiley KE, Bleecker ER, Walsh PC, Meyers DA, Isaacs WB, Xu J (2003) Polymorphisms in the CYP1A1 gene are associated with prostate cancer risk. *Int J Cancer* 106:375–358.

147. Rebbeck TR, Jaffe JM, Walker AH, Wein AJ, Malkowicz SB (1998) Modification of clinical presentation of prostate tumors by a novel genetic variant in CYP3A4. *J Natl Cancer Inst* 90:1225–1229.

148. Paris PL, Kupelian PA, Hall JM, Williams TL, Levin H, Klein EA, Casey G, Witte JS (1999) Association between a CYP3A4 genetic variant and clinical presentation in African-American prostate cancer patients. *Cancer Epidemiol Biomarkers Prev* 8:901–905.

149. Chang BL, Zheng SL, Hawkins GA, Isaacs SD, Wiley KE, Turner A, Carpten JD, Bleecker ER, Walsh PC, Trent JM, Meyers DA, Isaacs WB, Xu J (2002) Joint effect of HSD3B1 and HSD3B2 genes is associated with hereditary and sporadic prostate cancer susceptibility. *Cancer Res* 62: 1784–1789.

150. Margiotti K, Kim E, Pearce CL, Spera E, Novelli G, Reichardt JK (2002) Association of the G289S single nucleotide polymorphism in the HSD17B3 gene with prostate cancer in Italian men. *Prostate* 53:65–68.

151. Hsing AW, Reichardt JK, Stanczyk FZ (2002) Hormones and prostate cancer: current perspectives and future directions. *Prostate* 52:213–235.

152. Ross RK, Pike MC, Coetzee GA, Reichardt JK, Yu MC, Feigelson H, Stanczyk FZ, Kolonel LN, Henderson BE (1998) Androgen metabolism and prostate cancer: establishing a model of genetic susceptibility. *Cancer Res* 58:4497–4504.

153. Ho GY, Melman A, Liu SM, Li M, Yu H, Negassa A, Burk RD, Hsing AW, Ghavamian R, Chua SC, Jr (2003) Polymorphism of the insulin gene is associated with increased prostate cancer risk. *Br J Cancer* 88:263–269.

154. Taylor JA, Hirvonen A, Watson M, Pittman G, Mohler JL, Bell DA (1996) Association of prostate cancer with vitamin D receptor gene polymorphism. *Cancer Res* 56:4108–4110.

155. Ingles SA, Coetzee GA, Ross RK, Henderson BE, Kolonel LN, Crocitto L, Wang W, Haile RW (1998) Association of prostate cancer with vitamin D receptor haplotypes in African-Americans. *Cancer Res* 58:1620–1623.

156. Ma J, Stampfer MJ, Gann PH, Hough HL, Giovannucci E, Kelsey KT, Hennekens CH, Hunter DJ (1998) Vitamin D receptor polymorphisms, circulating vitamin D metabolites, and risk of prostate cancer in United States physicians. *Cancer Epidemiol Biomarkers Prev* 7:385–390.

157. Correa-Cerro L, Berthon P, Haussler J, Bochum S, Drelon E, Mangin P, Fournier G, Paiss T, Cussenot O, Vogel W (1999) Vitamin D receptor polymorphisms as markers in prostate cancer. *Hum Genet* 105:281–287.

158. Habuchi T, Suzuki T, Sasaki R, Wang L, Sato K, Satoh S, Akao T, Tsuchiya N, Shimoda N, Wada Y, Koizumi A, Chihara J, Ogawa O, Kato T (2000) Association of vitamin D receptor gene polymorphism with prostate cancer and benign prostatic hyperplasia in a Japanese population. *Cancer Res* 60:305–308.

159. Furuya Y, Akakura K, Masai M, Ito H (1999) Vitamin D receptor gene polymorphism in Japanese patients with prostate cancer. *Endocr J* 46:467–470.

160. Watanabe M, Fukutome K, Murata M, Uemura H, Kubota Y, Kawamura J, Yatani R (1999) Significance of vitamin D receptor gene polymorphism for prostate cancer risk in Japanese. *Anticancer Res* 19:4511–4514.

161. Blazer DG, 3rd, Umbach DM, Bostick RM, Taylor JA (2000) Vitamin D receptor polymorphisms and prostate cancer. *Mol Carcinog* 27:18–23.

162. Chokkalingam AP, McGlynn KA, Gao YT, Pollak M, Deng J, Sesterhenn IA, Mostofi FK, Fraumeni JF, Jr, Hsing AW (2001) Vitamin D receptor gene polymorphisms, insulin-like growth factors, and prostate cancer risk: a population-based case-control study in China. *Cancer Res* 61:4333–4336.

163. Gsur A, Madersbacher S, Haidinger G, Schatzl G, Marberger M, Vutuc C, Micksche M (2002) Vitamin D receptor gene polymorphism and prostate cancer risk. *Prostate* 51:30–34.

164. Hamasaki T, Inatomi H, Katoh T, Ikuyama T, Matsumoto T (2002) Significance of vitamin D receptor gene polymorphism for risk and disease severity of prostate cancer and benign prostatic hyperplasia in Japanese. *Urol Int* 68:226–231.

165. Medeiros R, Morais A, Vasconcelos A, Costa S, Pinto D, Oliveira J, Lopes C (2002) The role of vitamin D receptor gene polymorphisms in the susceptibility to prostate cancer of a southern European population. *J Hum Genet* 47:413–418.

166. Suzuki K, Matsui H, Ohtake N, Nakata S, Takei T, Koike H, Nakazato H, Okugi H, Hasumi M, Fukabori Y, Kurokawa K, Yamanaka H (2003) Vitamin D receptor gene polymorphism in familial prostate cancer in a Japanese population. *Int J Urol* 10:261–266.

167. Medeiros R, Vasconcelos A, Costa S, Pinto D, Ferreira P, Lobo F, Morais A, Oliveira J, Lopes C (2004) Metabolic susceptibility genes and prostate cancer risk in a southern European population: The role of glutathione S-transferases GSTM1, GSTM3, and GSTT1 genetic polymorphisms. *Prostate* 58:414–420.

168. Kidd LC, Woodson K, Taylor PR, Albanes D, Virtamo J, Tangrea JA (2003) Polymorphisms in glutathione-S-transferase genes (GST-M1, GST-T1 and GST-P1) and susceptibility to prostate cancer among male smokers of the ATBC cancer prevention study. *Eur J Cancer Prev* 12: 317–320.

169. Kote-Jarai Z, Easton D, Edwards SM, Jefferies S, Durocher F, Jackson RA, Singh R, Ardern-Jones A, Murkin A, Dearnaley DP, Shearer R, Kirby R, Houlston R, Eeles R (2001) Relationship between glutathione S-transferase M1, P1 and T1 polymorphisms and early onset prostate cancer. *Pharmacogenetics* 11:325–330.

170. Gsur A, Haidinger G, Hinteregger S, Bernhofer G, Schatzl G, Madersbacher S, Marberger M, Vutuc C, Micksche M (2001) Polymorphisms of glutathione-S-transferase genes (GSTP1, GSTM1 and GSTT1) and prostate-cancer risk. *Int J Cancer* 95:152–155.

171. Murata M, Watanabe M, Yamanaka M, Kubota Y, Ito H, Nagao M, Katoh T, Kamataki T, Kawamura J, Yatani R, Shiraishi T (2001) Genetic polymorphisms in cytochrome P450 (CYP) 1A1, CYP1A2, CYP2E1, glutathione S-transferase (GST) M1 and GSTT1 and susceptibility to prostate cancer in the Japanese population. *Cancer Lett* 165:171–177.

172. Steinhoff C, Franke KH, Golka K, Thier R, Romer HC, Rotzel C, Ackermann R, Schulz WA (2000) Glutathione transferase isozyme genotypes in patients with prostate and bladder carcinoma. *Arch Toxicol* 74:521–526.

173. Autrup JL, Thomassen LH, Olsen JH, Wolf H, Autrup H (1999) Glutathione S-transferases as risk factors in prostate cancer. *Eur J Cancer Prev* 8: 525–532.
174. Kelada SN, Kardia SL, Walker AH, Wein AJ, Malkowicz SB, Rebbeck TR (2000) The glutathione S-transferase-mu and -theta genotypes in the etiology of prostate cancer: genotype-environment interactions with smoking. *Cancer Epidemiol Biomarkers Prev* 9:1329–1334.
175. Shepard TF, Platz EA, Kantoff PW, Nelson WG, Isaacs WB, Freije D, Febbo PG, Stampfer MJ, Giovannucci E (2000) No association between the I105V polymorphism of the glutathione S-transferase P1 gene (GSTP1) and prostate cancer risk: a prospective study. *Cancer Epidemiol Biomarkers Prev* 9:1267–1268.
176. Berwick M, Vineis P (2000) Markers of DNA repair and susceptibility to cancer in humans: an epidemiologic review. *J Natl Cancer Inst* 92: 874–897.
177. Rybicki BA, Conti DV, Moreira A, Cicek M, Casey G, Witte JS (2004) DNA repair gene XRCC1 and XPD polymorphisms and risk of prostate cancer. *Cancer Epidemiol Biomarkers Prev* 13:23–29.
178. van Gils CH, Bostick RM, Stern MC, Taylor JA (2002) Differences in base excision repair capacity may modulate the effect of dietary antioxidant intake on prostate cancer risk: an example of polymorphisms in the XRCC1 gene. *Cancer Epidemiol Biomarkers Prev* 11:1279–1284.
179. Xu J, Zheng SL, Turner A, Isaacs SD, Wiley KE, Hawkins GA, Chang BL, Bleecker ER, Walsh PC, Meyers DA, Isaacs WB (2002) Associations between hOGG1 sequence variants and prostate cancer susceptibility. *Cancer Res* 62:2253–2257.
180. Chen L, Elahi A, Pow-Sang J, Lazarus P, Park J (2003) Association between polymorphism of human oxoguanine glycosylase 1 and risk of prostate cancer. *J Urol* 170:2471–2474.
181. Li Z, Habuchi T, Tsuchiya N, Mitsumori K, Wang L, Ohyama C, Sato K, Kamoto T, Ogawa O, Kato T (2004) Increased risk of prostate cancer and benign prostatic hyperplasia associated with transforming growth factor-beta 1 gene polymorphism at codon10. *Carcinogenesis* 25:237–240 (Epub 2003 Nov 6).
182. Panguluri RC, Long LO, Chen W, Wang S, Coulibaly A, Ukoli F, Jackson A, Weinrich S, Ahaghotu C, Isaacs W, Kittles RA (2004) COX-2 gene promoter haplotypes and prostate cancer risk. *Carcinogenesis* 30:30
183. McCarron SL, Edwards S, Evans PR, Gibbs R, Dearnaley DP, Dowe A, Southgate C, Easton DF, Eeles RA, Howell WM (2002) Influence of

cytokine gene polymorphisms on the development of prostate cancer. *Cancer Res* 62:3369–3372.

184. Paltoo D, Woodson K, Taylor P, Albanes D, Virtamo J, Tangrea J (2003) Pro12Ala polymorphism in the peroxisome proliferator-activated receptor-gamma (PPAR-gamma) gene and risk of prostate cancer among men in a large cancer prevention study. *Cancer Lett* 191:67–74.

185. Loukola A, Chadha M, Penn SG, Rank D, Conti DV, Thompson D, Cicek M, Love B, Bivolarevic V, Yang Q, Jiang Y, Hanzel DK, Dains K, Paris PL, Casey G, Witte JS (2003) Comprehensive evaluation of the association between prostate cancer and genotypes/haplotypes in CYP17A1, CYP3A4, and SRD5A2. *Eur J Hum Genet* 15:15.

186. Haiman CA, Stram DO, Pike MC, Kolonel LN, Burtt NP, Altshuler D, Hirschhorn J, Henderson BE (2003) A comprehensive haplotype analysis of CYP19 and breast cancer risk: the Multiethnic Cohort. *Hum Mol Genet* 12:2679–2692.

187. Stram DO, Haiman CA, Hirschhorn J, Altshuler D, Kolonel LN, Henderson BE, Pike MC (2003) Choosing haplotype-tagging SNPS based on unphased genotype data using a preliminary sample of unrelated subjects with an example from the Multiethnic Cohort Study. *Hum Hered* 55:27–36.

188. Risch N, Teng J (1998) The relative power of family-based and case-control designs for linkage disequilibrium studies of complex human diseases I. DNA pooling. *Genome Res* 8:1273–1288.

189. Platz EA, De Marzo AM, Giovannucci E (2004) Prostate cancer association studies: pitfalls and solutions to cancer misclassification in the PSA era. *J Cell Biochem* 91:553–571.

15

PROFILING GENE EXPRESSION CHANGES IN PROSTATE CARCINOMA

Peter S. Nelson

Fred Hutchinson Cancer Research Center
Seattle, Washington, USA

Introduction

Prostate carcinogenesis represents a complex process involving a series of overlapping molecular events that occur in the transformation from a normal to a malignant cell. The accumulation of mutations and epigenetic modifications in critical genes involved in growth regulatory pathways result in sporadic cancers. This process can be accelerated with inherited predispositions resulting from the transmission of one or more of the necessary genetic alterations to successive generations. Despite great advances over the last several decades in identifying and characterizing individual molecular alterations mediating various aspects of prostate cancer growth and invasion, it is now clear that a more comprehensive approach may be required to fully understand the complex network of genes, their protein products and the various intra- and inter-cellular interactions that together comprise the neoplastic phenotype. Advances brought about by the Human Genome Project now allow for comprehensive analyses of DNA, transcripts, and proteins such that the complexities of the normal cellular machinery and the attendant perturbations in neoplasia, can at least be thoroughly identified. This knowledge provides a starting point for understanding how molecular alterations actually dysregulate cellular controls governing growth, death, invasion, and ultimately, responses to therapy.

Methods for Profiling Gene Expression Alterations

Several methods have been developed for thoroughly assessing and comparing gene expression between two or more tissues or cell types. Most approaches have centered on studies of messenger RNA (mRNA) molecules or transcripts, due to the versatility and stability offered by the conversion of mRNA into complementary DNA (cDNA) and the ability to use hybridization and amplification strategies to evaluate RNA extracted from small quantities of cells and tissues. One approach, termed *subtractive hybridization*, relies on the molecular binding of complementary nucleic acids to remove transcripts in common between tumor cells and normal cells, leaving behind for analyses those transcripts differing in abundance between the two cell states.[1] The method of *differential display* utilizes the polymerase chain reaction to amplify transcripts comprised of regions complimentary to combinations of primer sequences such that mRNAs expressed in different quantities between cells of interest can be visualized as bands following separation by polyacrylamide gel electrophoresis.[2] Several genes with altered levels in prostate carcinoma have been identified using this technique including *Hevin,*[3] *dd3,*[4] *PCGEM,*[5] and *COSVIc.*[6] The large scale partial sequencing of clones from cDNA libraries constructed from normal and neoplastic tissues generated *expressed sequence tags* (ESTs) that can be assessed to provide qualitative and quantitative data on gene expression.[7] Statistical algorithms allow for computational *in silico* comparisons of EST numbers between multiple tissue types, termed virtual Northern or Digital Differential Display comparisons.[8] Using EST profiles generated through the Cancer Genome Anatomy Project (CGAP), several genes such as *PATE,*[9] *PRAC*[10] and *GDEP*[11] have been determined to be specifically expressed in prostate epithelium, or differentially expressed between normal prostate and prostate carcinomas. An elegant enhancement of the EST approach involves the truncation of cDNAs by restriction enzymes, followed by concatenation and amplification such that multiple transcript tags can be identified and quantitated with a single sequence analysis.[12] This method, termed the Serial Analysis of Gene Expression (SAGE) has been used to profile the genes expressed by normal and neoplastic prostate tissues; identifying PMEPA1[13] and E2F4[14] as up-regulated in malignancy. While each of these approaches can provide a deep sampling of a tissue or cellular gene expression repertoire, they remain poorly suited for the analysis and comparisons of multiple different tissue samples due to the labor entailed in conducting the procedures.

The current method of choice for high-throughput comprehensive studies of gene expression involves the analyses of microarrays: wafers, chips, or slides with spatially-defined immobilized DNA fragments representing genes of interest.[15,16] This technique combines the proven chemistry of nucleic acid hybridization with advanced automation and image-analysis technology to quantitatively monitor changes in gene expression patterns. Briefly, individual cDNAs or oligonucleotides representing known or unknown genes are spotted or synthesized on a solid support such as a glass slide. Replicates are made of the arrays using high-precision robotics. Complex tissue probes are constructed with radioactive or fluorescent labels and hybridized to the arrays. Individual or groups of transcripts with differential expression signals are identified using quantitative image analysis software. This methodology allows the simultaneous assessment of expression levels of thousands of genes represented at 0.01%–0.001% abundance in a population, making it ideally suited for the identification of the numerous molecular alterations that occur in the development and progression of human cancers (see Fig. 1).

Microarray Studies of Gene Expression in Prostate Carcinoma

Microarray analysis has been used in several published studies designed to profile gene expression alterations in prostate carcinoma (Table 1). Importantly, although all of these experiments used microarrays, there are important differences that preclude a simple comparison of the reported results. These include the use of different patient samples, microarrays with different genes represented and variations in experimental and analytical approaches. Magee *et al.* used oligonucleotide arrays to characterize the expression of 4712 genes in four benign and 11 prostate cancer samples.[17] Most of the neoplastic samples represented primary tumors of various Gleason grades, though two metastatic lesions were also characterized. The samples were enriched for epithelial cells using macrodissection procedures. Analyses of the gene-expression profiles identified four genes with significant changes associated with carcinoma, including Hepsin, a type-II membrane-bound serine protease. Luo *et al.* used microarrays comprised

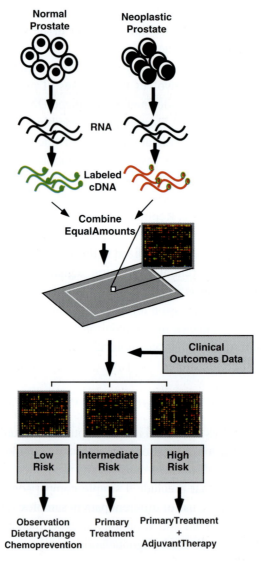

Fig. 1. Prostate cancer outcomes determined by microarray expression profiles. Messenger RNA (mRNA) is isolated separately from normal and neoplastic prostate tissues, preferably from specific microdissected cell types. RNA samples are either labeled directly with fluorescent probes or first converted to complementary cDNA followed by hybridization to microarrays of spotted or synthesized DNAs representing genes of interest. Gene expression measurements are determined by analyzing the fluorescent signal intensity for each gene on the microarray and subsequently comparing the signal levels between normal

and neoplastic cell types and neoplastic cell types representing different clinical outcomes. Expression data are correlated with known clinical outcomes to determine a profile or fingerprint capable of predicting the risk of local and distant cancer progression. Patients with a minimal risk of progression (i.e. with indolent disease) would receive no primary intervention but could be considered for dietary alteration or chemoprevention trials. Patients at intermediate risk would receive primary curative therapy such as radical prostatectomy or radiation therapy. Patients at high risk would receive primary therapy with the addition of systemic adjuvant or neoadjuvant therapy.

of 6500 spotted cDNAs to profile gene expression in nine benign prostatic hyperplasia (BPH) specimens and 16 prostate cancer samples.[18] A common reference standard was used to facilitate comparisons and clearly discernable patterns that discriminated prostate cancer and BPH was evident. The study identified 210 genes with statistically significant expression differences between the two tissue types. This study also identified Hepsin overexpression in cancer epithelium relative to benign epithelium. A study by Dhanasekaran *et al.* characterized the gene expression signatures of more than 50 normal and cancerous prostate specimens and three prostate cancer cell lines using arrays comprised of 9984 cDNAs.[19] Cohorts of genes distinguishing normal prostate, BPH, localized prostate cancer and metastatic hormone-refractory prostate cancer were identified. Examples of genes differentially-expressed between benign and neoplastic prostate tissue include *Hepsin, PIM1, IGFBP-5, DAN1, FAT, RAB5A* and *HEVIN*. This study further explored the correlation of *Hepsin* and *PIM1* protein expression using tissue microarrays comprised of 700 prostate-cancer specimens with known clinical attributes. The expression levels of *Hepsin* and *PIM1* were shown to independently correlate with cancer progression. Overall, these microarray-based studies of prostate gene expression demonstrate consistent alterations in a subset of genes that can be grouped into a cancer-associated profile. These results provide important substrates for mechanistic studies designed to evaluate their utility as diagnostic, prognostic and therapeutic targets.

Transcript Profiling and Predicting Cancer Outcomes

Despite a variety of clinical and histological parameters used to classify prostate and other cancers, patients receiving the same diagnosis can have strikingly different disease progression rates and responses to treatment.

Table 1. Studies Using Microarray Analysis to Identify Differentially Expressed Genes in Prostate Carcinoma

Tissues		# Genes Studied	# Differential Genes	Differentially-Expressed Genes: Examples	Reference
Benign	Cancer*				
1	1	588	13[a]	GSTM1	Chetcuti et al. (2001)[53]
1	1	588	15[b]	VEGF	Chaib et al. (2001)[54]
9	16	~6112	210[c]	Hepsin	Luo et al. (2001)[18]
Pool	36[20]	~9984	>200[d]	Hepsin, PIM1	Dhanasekaran (2001)[19]
4	11[3]	~4712	4[e]	Hepsin	Magee et al. (2001)[17]
9	24[1]	~8920	>400[f]	Hepsin, MIC1, FAS	Welsh et al. (2001)[55]
8	9	~6800	86[g]	Hepsin, PSMA	Stamey et al. (2001)[56]
15	15	~35,000[#]	84[h]	Hepsin, AMACR	Luo et al. (2002)[57]
9	17	~12,600	216[i]	Hepsin, AMACR	Ernst et al. (2002)[58]
3	32[9]	~12,000	>3400[j]	USP13, STK11	LaTulippe et al. (2002)[59]
50	52	~12,600	456[k]	Hepsin, Tetraspan1	Singh et al. (2002)[29]
8	28[5]	~12,600	50[l]	Hepsin, AMACR	Vanaja et al. (2003)[60]
Pool	13	6400	136[m]	Hepsin, Nectin3, CALLA	Best et al. (2003)[28]
NA	72	~46,000	266[n]	trp-p8, seladin-1, SOCS2	Henshall et al. (2003)[31]

[#]Estimated by the authors.

*Superscript indicates the number of metastatic prostate cancer samples analyzed.

[a]Differential gene expression was determined by calculating the ratios of hybridization intensities between normal and neoplastic samples following array normalization. Genes with ratios ≥ 3-fold were called differentially expressed.

[b]Differential gene expression was determined by calculating the ratios of hybridization intensities between normal and neoplastic samples following array normalization. Genes with ratios ≥ 2-fold were called differentially expressed.

[c]Differential gene expression was determined by computing the discriminative weight (w) of each gene to separate cancer from benign tissue. P values were assigned based on the (w) values of randomized data.

[d]Several approaches used: t-statistics (of prostate cancer versus benign tissue) ranked based on effect size: 200 genes reported. An analysis using fold-change identified 1520 genes with 2-fold changes between 50% of cancer samples and normal adjacent tissue and 1006 genes with 3-fold change in 75% of cancer samples compared with a normal commercial pool.

[e]Differential expression between benign and neoplastic prostate tissue; $\geq$ 3-fold change in all 11 tumors compared with four benign samples. P values were calculated by a two-tailed t-test for independent data sets of unequal size and variance.

[f]Differential expression between benign and neoplastic prostate tissue was determined by equally weighing contributions from differences in hybridization intensities, the quotient of hybridization intensities and the result of an unpaired t-test between expression levels in tumor and normal tissues.

[g]Differential expression between BPH and neoplastic prostate tissue; $p < 0.0005$ and expressed in all samples examined.

[h]Differential expression between benign and neoplastic prostate tissue; $p < 0.05$ by Student's t-test; signal intensity >500 units.

[i]Differential expression between benign and neoplastic tissue; $p < 0.05$ by Student's t-test and fold change >2.5.

[j]Differential expression between non-recurrent primary prostate cancers and metastasis; fold-difference $\geq$3-fold.

[k]Differential expression between normal versus tumor samples was determined using a variation of a signal-to-noise metric. The statistical significance of the gene expression correlations was determined by comparing the observed correlations to the results mined by comparing the observed correlations to the results derived from permutations of the class labels (normal and tumor).

[l]Differential expression between benign and cancer samples was determined by combining equally weighted contributions from differences in hybridization intensities, the quotient of the hybridization intensities, and the results of an unpaired t-test between expression levels. Selection criteria were further narrowed to a fold-change >2.35 and a $p < 0.001$ by Student's t-test.

[m]Differential expression between normal and cancer tissue was determined at the $p < 0.001$ level by a one sample t-test and Wilcoxian ranking.

[n]This report was designed to identify gene expression changes associated with disease progression. Cox proportional hazard survival analysis predicting relapse was used to evaluate each gene (probe set). Gene expression predictors of relapse at the $p < 0.01$ level were reported. A False-Discovery Rate (FDR) was calculated to be 23% (61 of the 265 findings are false positives).

A major objective in the field of oncology centers on accurate prediction of outcome and patient stratification for planned interventions such as surgery, radiation treatment and chemotherapy. Clues to tumor behavior may be found in the molecular heterogeneity within individual cancer diagnostic categories such as chromosomal translocations, deletions of tumor suppressor genes, amplifications or mutations of oncogenes, and numerous chromosomal abnormalities. Ultimately, the majority of these molecular alterations will produce changes in gene expression that manifest in phenotypic behaviors of invasion, metastasis and drug resistance.

A landmark study involving the molecular analysis of Non-Hodgkins Lymphoma (NHL) proved the hypothesis that gene expression profiles could be used to stratify cancers into clinically relevant categories. This study compared the variability in the natural history of a NHL subtype with analyses of molecular heterogeneity in the tumors as assessed by cDNA microarray fingerprints.[20] Although histologically-indistinguishable, two distinct forms of this NHL subtype were identified by expression patterns that reflected different stages of B-cell differentiation. The outcome of patients with different expression profiles was demonstrated by divergent survival curves following the best available therapy. The study concluded that a molecular classification of tumors on the basis of gene expression can identify previously undetected and clinically significant subtypes of cancer.[20] Similar studies have now been performed in other tumor types. van't Veer *et al.* used microarrays to profile genes expressed in breast cancers.[21] A classifier comprised of 70 "prognosis reporter genes" was developed that distinguished which primary tumors were destined to progress to distant metastases versus those that did not relapse. These and other studies point to an emerging use for genomics in the management of patients with neoplastic diseases.

The strongest predictive factors for prostate cancer disease progression are the Gleason score, serum PSA, and clinical stage.[22] The Gleason grading system in biopsy or prostatectomy specimens is a measure of biological aggressiveness.[22-24] Several groups have recently combined clinical stage, serum PSA level, and Gleason score to generate "nomograms" that predict pathological stage or outcomes[23,25-27] and allow prognostic estimates to be made with readily available clinical data. To identify biological correlates of the Gleason histology, Best *et al.* used microarray analysis to profile transcripts expressed in 13 high and moderate-grade prostate cancers.[28] Using permutation *t*-tests, 21 genes were found to segregate based on tumor grade (p < 0.001). Genes with this discriminatory power included tumor protein D52, BRCA1 binding protein 1 and CD69. Future studies will demonstrate the utility of these genes in delineating patient outcomes prospectively.

To date, three studies have been published with designs aimed toward independently identifying molecular signatures correlating with outcomes of relapsed disease following radical prostatectomy. Singh *et al.* used oligonucleotide microarrays to characterize the expression levels of ~12,600 transcripts in primary prostate carcinomas.[29] The study identified 456 differentially expressed genes between benign and malignant prostate tissues. A molecular classifier comprised of five genes (*ITPR3, sialyl-transferase 1, PDGFR-β, chromogranin A* and *HoxC6*) was capable of segregating primary cancers into two groups, those cancers that relapsed within four years of radical prostatectomy and those that did not recur within four years. In a second study, Ramaswamy *et al.* used microarrays to define a gene expression signature of metastasis present in multiple tumor types, including prostate cancer.[30] Comparing metastases with primary cancers identified a group of 17 genes capable of discriminating metastases from primary tumors. A subset of primary tumors was also found to contain the metastasis signature and these tumors exhibited a high likelihood of disease relapse and poor clinical outcome following primary therapy. Henshall *et al.* used microarrays comprised of 46,000 unique sequences to profile 72 cases of primary prostate carcinoma.[31] At the time of analysis, 17 patients were known to have relapsed as determined by rising PSA measurements and the expression levels of 266 genes were shown to correlate with disease relapse. This cohort included the putative calcium channel protein *trp-p8*, a transcript whose loss of expression in neoplastic tissue was strongly associated with disease relapse (p ≤ 0.001) independently of pre-treatment PSA levels.

Although both the five-gene molecular classifier defined by Singh *et al.*[21] and the 17-gene metastasis signature defined by Ramaswamy *et al.*[30] independently predicted disease relapse, no genes are shared between the two predictive cohorts. Similarly, none of the progression-associated genes identified by Henshall *et al.*[31] are included in the five-gene outcome classifier, though there may be overlaps in the biochemical pathways in which these genes participate. Of the 70 genes used to predict breast cancer progression in the van't Veer study,[21] none are shared with the five or 17-gene prostate cancer outcome predictors. Therefore, while quite provocative and statistically valid, the utility of these predictive signatures will require validation in additional independent data sets and in prospective studies.

Proteomic Approaches for Assessing Gene Expression in Prostate Carcinoma

While important information has been gained through the profiling of transcripts, it is important to keep in mind that the end-point for gene expression is the protein, as proteins represent the actual scaffolds, molecular engines and communication mechanisms utilized by cells. In addition, the development of most biomedical interventions center on protein endpoints. Large-scale efforts are underway to analyze the proteome: the total protein complement of the genome.[32] However, the proteome represents a complex dynamic entity due to the many forms of a given protein that result from alternative transcript splicing and the numerous post-translational modifications that often define functional protein states.[33,34]

A core technology developed for the global analysis of proteins involves the electrophoretic separation of proteins along two dimensions: size and charge, using polyacrylamide gels (2D-PAGE).[35] Comparisons of gel profiles from two different cell states (e.g. normal versus cancer) can identify differential protein expression or protein modifications. The identity of individual protein spots can be determined by immunodetection or by calculating the theoretical locations of known proteins based upon charge and mass. More recently, microsequencing and mass spectrometry have gained widespread use for characterizing protein spots of interest.[36,37] The 2D-PAGE technique is theoretically capable of resolving more than 10,000 proteins and peptides from complex mixtures. However, practical applications of 2D-PAGE have rarely identified more than a small percentage of proteins comprising the cellular proteome.[38] Despite this drawback, 2D-PAGE has been used to identify androgen-regulated genes in prostate epithelium[39] and prostate cancer-associated protein alterations such as NEDD8 and calponin.[40]

Mass spectrometry (MS) has evolved to become a key technology in proteomics research. The basic mass spectrometer is comprised of an ion source, a mass analyzer, and a detector to record the spectra of ion intensity versus the mass to charge ratio of proteins or peptides under analysis.[36] Currently, surface enhanced laser assisted desorption (SELDI), matrix assisted laser desorption (MALDI) and electrospray ionization (ESI) represent the preferred methods for ionizing peptides and proteins. Comparing the mass spectra of complex protein mixtures such as human serum offers the potential for identifying proteins or protein fragments that are present in different abundances and that associate with disease states.[33,41] Several reports have used SELDI mass spectrometry as a biomarker discovery method to distinguish serum profiles or fingerprints that reflect the presence of prostate carcinoma in comparison to serum protein profiles derived from normal controls.[42,43] A major drawback to these profiling approaches involves a lack of reproducible quantitative accuracy and a difficulty in positively identifying the peptides and parent proteins that account for the fingerprint differences.

Several strategies have been devised to provide MS with the ability to accurately quantitate differences in protein levels between two cellular states.[44-47] One technique employs Isotope Coded Affinity Tags (ICAT) comprised of three components: a biotin affinity tag, a linker with either eight hydrogen or eight deuterium atoms (generating a light and a heavy form of the molecule), and a SH-reactive group capable of covalently linking to cysteine residues (Fig. 2).[48] The proteins of one cell state (e.g. normal epithelium) are labeled with the light reagent and those of a second cell state (e.g. neoplastic epithelium) with the heavy reagent. Equal quantities of labeled cells are mixed and the proteins are separated, digested with a proteolytic enzyme and the resulting mixture of peptides are passed over an avidin column to isolate the cysteine labeled peptides (about 90% of proteins have cysteine residues). These can be fractionated and analyzed by tandem mass spectrometry (MS/MS). The first MS analysis gives the areas under the curves of the paired isotopic peptides (hence, their relative abundances); the second MS analysis provides a peptide fingerprint that can be used to identify the parent protein. Thus, the ICAT method dramatically increases throughput by reducing sample redundancy (only cysteine-containing peptides are assessed) and

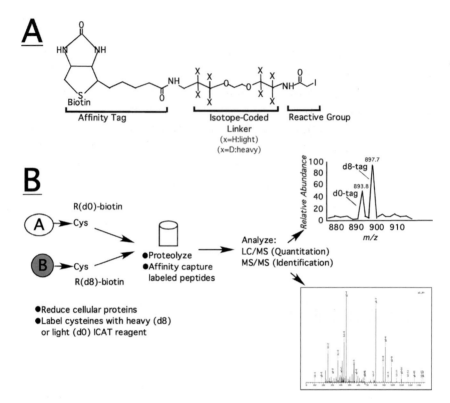

Fig . 2. Relative Quantitation of Cellular Proteins using Isotope Coded Affinity Tags (ICAT) and Mass Spectrometry. **(A)** To facilitate the quantitative analysis of proteins in complex mixtures, peptides are labeled with an isotope-coded affinity tag (ICAT) reagent that consists of three parts: an affinity tag (biotin) that is used to isolate ICAT-labeled peptides, a linker that can incorporate stable isotopes, and a reactive group with specificity toward thiol groups (cysteines [Cys]). Two forms of the reagent are made: heavy (contains eight deuteriums [d8]) and light (no deuteriums [d0]). **(B)** The strategy for ICAT-based differential protein quantitation involves separately extracting proteins from two different cell states (e.g. normal and cancer) followed by labeling each with a different (d0 or d8) ICAT reagent. The ICAT reagent covalently bonds to each cysteinyl residue in every protein. The protein mixtures are combined and proteolyzed to peptides and only ICAT-labeled peptides are isolated using the biotin tag. These peptides are separated by microcapillary high-performance liquid chromatography (LC). ICAT-labeled peptide pairs are chemically identical and easily visualized. Peptide fragments faithfully maintain the ratios of the original amounts of proteins from the two cell states. Relative peptide/protein quantification is calculated by the ratios of the d0- and d8-tagged peptide pairs. Periodic scans are devoted to fragmenting peptides and recording sequence information (tandem mass spectrum [MS/MS]). Protein identifications are made by database searches of the tandem mass spectrum.

retains sample complexity while allowing for accurate relative protein quantification.[48,49]

The ICAT approach has been used to identify secreted[50] and androgen-regulated proteins[51] expressed by prostate cancer cells. In addition to identifying genes previously not known to be regulated by androgens, comparisons of global transcript and protein abundance levels showed that for most genes (>90%), protein levels were concordant with transcript abundance. However, there were distinct outliers that indicate multiple levels of gene expression regulation (e.g. post-transcriptional, post-translational). These results suggest immediately testable hypotheses for characterizing mechanism(s) of gene expression regulation. The results also demonstrate that to *fully* delineate a gene expression profile, measurements of protein levels are necessary, since, for some genes, protein alterations would not have been predicted by transcript abundance measurements.

Conclusion and Future Directions

Gene expression profiles offer an extraordinary assessment of both the diversity and consistency of genetic alterations in prostate carcinomas. Published studies have provided the first glimpse of the potential of profiling technologies to identify individual genes that participate in neoplastic growth and to define molecular predictors of cancer behavior. However, there clearly are limitations to the approach and significant hurdles to be overcome. It is somewhat disconcerting that cohorts of genes statistically associated with disease outcome in different studies do not correlate with each other. This may be explained by the extreme heterogeneity of neoplastic prostate lesions. In addition, tissue samples used in most studies are comprised of various amounts of normal epithelium, stromal cells, inflammatory cells, blood vessels, and other constituents. While gene expression changes in these cell types may influence neoplastic transformation, growth, and invasion, the variable amounts of these cell types between different studies may make inter-study comparisons difficult. To address this problem, microdissection techniques that compare only specific cell types can be employed.[52] The ultimate endpoint of such an approach is the characterization of individual cell expression profiles within the tumor environment. Although such an approach represents a daunting task, the pace of biotechnological advances do not rule out single-cell analysis using high-speed flow cytometers and nanotechnology in the near future. Finally, a major factor that could influence the outcomes of tumors with identical gene expression profiles centers on variables within the host. Most expression profiling studies have focused on defining molecular determinants within tumor tissue. However, host characteristics involving immune response, dietary factors and the hormone milieu may influence tumor cell proliferation, invasion and metastasis. In the future, we will likely gain important additional knowledge of tumor behavior and response to therapy through the integration of profiles reflecting both tumor and host gene expression.

Acknowledgments

Peter Nelson is supported by a Scholar Award from the Damon-Runyon Cancer Research Foundation.

References

1. Diatchenko L, Lau YF, Campbell AP, *et al.* (1996) Suppression subtractive hybridization: a method for generating differentially regulated or tissue-specific cDNA probes and libraries. *Proc Natl Acad Sci USA* 93:6025–6030.
2. Liang P, Pardee AB (1992) Differential display of eukaryotic messenger RNA by means of the polymerase chain reaction. *Science* 257:967–971.
3. Nelson PS, Plymate SR, Wang K, *et al.* (1998) Hevin, an antiadhesive extracellular matrix protein, is down-regulated in metastatic prostate adenocarcinoma. *Cancer Res* 58:232–236.
4. Bussemakers MJ, van Bokhoven A, Verhaegh GW, *et al.* (1999) DD3: a new prostate-specific gene, highly overexpressed in prostate cancer. *Cancer Res* 59:5975–5979.
5. Srikantan V, Zou Z, Petrovics G, *et al.* (2000) PCGEM1, a prostate-specific gene, is overexpressed in prostate cancer. *Proc Natl Acad Sci USA* 97: 12216–12221.
6. Wang FL, Wang Y, Wong WK, *et al.* (1996) Two differentially expressed genes in normal and human prostate tissue and in carcinoma. *Cancer Res* 56:3634–3637.
7. Nelson PS, Ng WL, Schummer M, *et al.* (1998) An expressed-sequence-tag database of the human prostate: sequence analysis of 1168 cDNA clones [In Process Citation]. *Genomics* 47:12–25.

8. Scheurle D, DeYoung MP, Binninger DM, Page H, Jahanzeb M, Narayanan R (2000) Cancer gene discovery using digital differential display [In Process Citation]. *Cancer Res* 60:4037–4043.

9. Bera TK, Maitra R, Iavarone C, *et al.* (2002) PATE, a gene expressed in prostate cancer, normal prostate, and testis, identified by a functional genomic approach. *Proc Natl Acad Sci USA* 99:3058–3063.

10. Liu XF, Olsson P, Wolfgang CD, *et al.* (2001) PRAC: A novel small nuclear protein that is specifically expressed in human prostate and colon. *Prostate* 47:125–131.

11. Olsson P, Bera TK, Essand M, *et al.* (2001) GDEP, a new gene differentially expressed in normal prostate and prostate cancer. *Prostate* 48:231–241.

12. Velculescu VE, Zhang L, Vogelstein B, Kinzler KW (1995) Serial analysis of gene expression. *Science* 270:384–387.

13. Xu LL, Shanmugam N, Segawa T, *et al.* (2000) A novel androgen-regulated gene, PMEPA1, located on chromosome 20q13 exhibits high level expression in prostate [In Process Citation]. *Genomics* 66:257–263.

14. Waghray A, Schober M, Feroze F, Yao F, Virgin J, Chen YQ (2001) Identification of differentially expressed genes by serial analysis of gene expression in human prostate cancer. *Cancer Res* 61:4283–4286.

15. Schena M, Shalon D, Davis RW, Brown PO (1995) Quantitative monitoring of gene expression patterns with a complementary DNA microarray. *Science* 270:467–470.

16. DeRisi J, Penland L, Brown PO, *et al.* (1996) Use of a cDNA microarray to analyse gene expression patterns in human cancer. *Nature Genet* 14:457–460.

17. Magee JA, Araki T, Patil S, *et al.* (2001) Expression profiling reveals Hepsin overexpression in prostate cancer. *Cancer Res* 61:5692–5696.

18. Luo J, Duggan DJ, Chen Y, *et al.* (2001) Human prostate cancer and benign prostatic hyperplasia: molecular dissection by gene expression profiling. *Cancer Res* 61:4683–4688.

19. Dhanasekaran SM, Barrette TR, Ghosh D, *et al.* (2001) Delineation of prognostic biomarkers in prostate cancer. *Nature* 412:822–826.

20. Alizadeh AA, Eisen MB, Davis RE, *et al.* (2000) Distinct types of diffuse large B-cell lymphoma identified by gene expression profiling. *Nature* 403:503–511.

21. van 't Veer LJ, Dai H, van de Vijver MJ, *et al.* (2002) Gene expression profiling predicts clinical outcome of breast cancer. *Nature* 415:530–536.

22. Partin AW, Yoo J, Carter HB, *et al.* (1993) The use of prostate specific antigen, clinical stage and Gleason score to predict pathological stage in men with localized prostate cancer [see comments]. *J Urol* 150:110–114.

23. Partin AW, Kattan MW, Subong EN, *et al.* (1997) Combination of prostate-specific antigen, clinical stage, and Gleason score to predict pathological stage of localized prostate cancer. A multi-institutional update. *JAMA* 277:1445–1451.
24. Stamey TA, McNeal JE, Yemoto CM, Sigal BM, Johnstone IM (1999) Biological determinants of cancer progression in men with prostate cancer. *JAMA* 281:1395–1400.
25. Kattan MW, Stapleton AM, Wheeler TM, Scardino PT (1997) Evaluation of a nomogram used to predict the pathologic stage of clinically localized prostate carcinoma. *Cancer* 79:528–537.
26. Kattan MW, Eastham JA, Stapleton AM, Wheeler TM, Scardino PT (1998) A preoperative nomogram for disease recurrence following radical prostatectomy for prostate cancer. *J Natl Cancer Inst* 90:766–771.
27. Kattan MW, Wheeler TM, Scardino PT (1999) Postoperative nomogram for disease recurrence after radical prostatectomy for prostate cancer. *J Clin Oncol* 17:1499–1507.
28. Best CJ, Leiva IM, Chuaqui RF, *et al.* (2003) Molecular differentiation of high- and moderate-grade human prostate cancer by cDNA microarray analysis. *Diagn Mol Pathol* 12:63–70.
29. Singh D, Febbo PG, Ross K, *et al.* (2002) Gene expression correlates of clinical prostate cancer behavior. *Cancer Cell* 1:203–209.
30. Ramaswamy S, Ross KN, Lander ES, Golub TR (2003) A molecular signature of metastasis in primary solid tumors. *Nat Genet* 33:49–54.
31. Henshall SM, Afar DE, Hiller J, *et al.* (2003) Survival analysis of genome-wide gene expression profiles of prostate cancers identifies new prognostic targets of disease relapse. *Cancer Res* 63:4196–4203.
32. Humphery-Smith I, Blackstock W (1997) Proteome analysis: genomics via the output rather than the input code. *J Protein Chem* 16:537–544.
33. Corthals GL, Nelson PS (2001) Large-scale proteomics and its future impact on medicine. *Pharmacogenomics J* 1:15–19.
34. Martin DB, Nelson PS (2001) From genomics to proteomics: techniques and applications in cancer research. *Trends Cell Biol* 11:S60–65.
35. O'Farrell PH (1975) High resolution two-dimensional electrophoresis of proteins. *J Biol Chem* 250:4007–4021.
36. Corthals G, Gygi SP, Aebersold R, Patterson SD (1999) Identification of proteins by mass spectrometry. In: Rabilloud T, ed. *Proteome Research: 2D Gel Electrophoresis and Detection Methods.* Springer, New York, pp. 197–232.
37. Yates JR, 3rd (1998) Database searching using mass spectrometry data. *Electrophoresis* 19:893–900.

38. Gygi SP, Corthals GL, Zhang Y, Rochon Y, Aebersold R (2000) Evaluation of two-dimensional gel electrophoresis-based proteome analysis technology. *Proc Natl Acad Sci USA* 97:9390–9395.

39. Waghray A, Feroze F, Schober MS, *et al.* (2001) Identification of androgen-regulated genes in the prostate cancer cell line LNCaP by serial analysis of gene expression and proteomic analysis. *Proteomics* 1: 1327–1338.

40. Meehan KL, Holland JW, Dawkins HJ (2002) Proteomic analysis of normal and malignant prostate tissue to identify novel proteins lost in cancer. *Prostate* 50:54–63.

41. Issaq HJ, Veenstra TD, Conrads TP, Felschow D (2002) The SELDI-TOF MS approach to proteomics: protein profiling and biomarker identification. *Biochem Biophys Res Commun* 292:587–592.

42. Qu Y, Adam BL, Yasui Y, *et al.* (2002) Boosted decision tree analysis of surface-enhanced laser desorption/ionization mass spectral serum profiles discriminates prostate cancer from noncancer patients. *Clin Chem* 48: 1835–1843.

43. Petricoin EF, 3rd, Ornstein DK, Paweletz CP, *et al.* (2002) Serum proteomic patterns for detection of prostate cancer. *J Natl Cancer Inst* 94: 1576–1578.

44. Olsen JV, Andersen JR, Nielsen PA, *et al.* (2003) Hystag — a novel proteomic quantification tool applied to differential display analysis of membrane proteins from distinct areas of mouse brain. *Mol Cell Proteom* 10:10.

45. Espina V, Mehta AI, Winters ME, *et al.* (2003) Protein microarrays: molecular profiling technologies for clinical specimens. *Proteomics* 3:2091–2100.

46. Grubb RL, Calvert VS, Wulkuhle JD, *et al.* (2003) Signal pathway profiling of prostate cancer using reverse phase protein arrays. *Proteomics* 3: 2142–2146.

47. Haab BB, Dunham MJ, Brown PO (2001) Protein microarrays for highly parallel detection and quantitation of specific proteins and antibodies in complex solutions. *Genome Biol* 2:RESEARCH0004,

48. Gygi SP, Rist B, Gerber SA, Turecek F, Gelb MH, Aebersold R (1999) Quantitative analysis of complex protein mixtures using isotope-coded affinity tags. *Nat Biotechnol* 17:994–999.

49. Han DK, Eng J, Zhou H, Aebersold R (2001) Quantitative profiling of differentiation-induced microsomal proteins using isotope-coded affinity tags and mass spectrometry. *Nat Biotechnol* 19:946–951.

50. Martin DB, Gifford DR, Wright ME, Keller A, Yi E, Goodlett DR, Aebersold R, Nelson PS (2004) Quantitative proteomic analysis of proteins released by neoplastic prostate epithelium. *Cancer Res* 64:347–355.

51. Wright ME, Eng J, Sherman J, *et al.* (2003) Identification of androgen-coregulated protein networks from the microsomes of human prostate cancer cells. *Genome Biol* 5:R4.

52. Emmert-Buck MR, Bonner RF, Smith PD, *et al.* (1996) Laser capture microdissection [see comments]. *Science* 274:998–1001.

53. Chetcuti A, Margan S, Mann S, *et al.* (2001) Identification of differentially expressed genes in organ-confined prostate cancer by gene expression array. *Prostate* 47:132–140.

54. Chaib H, Cockrell EK, Rubin MA, Macoska JA (2001) Profiling and verification of gene expression patterns in normal and malignant human prostate tissues by cDNA microarray analysis. *Neoplasia* 3:43–52.

55. Welsh JB, Sapinoso LM, Su AI, *et al.* (2001) Analysis of gene expression identifies candidate markers and pharmacological targets in prostate cancer. *Cancer Res* 61:5974–5978.

56. Stamey TA, Warrington JA, Caldwell MC, *et al.* (2001) Molecular genetic profiling of Gleason grade 4/5 prostate cancers compared to benign prostatic hyperplasia. *J Urol* 166:2171–2177.

57. Luo JH, Yu YP, Cieply K, *et al.* (2002) Gene expression analysis of prostate cancers. *Mol Carcinog* 33:25–35.

58. Ernst T, Hergenhahn M, Kenzelmann M, *et al.* (2002) Decrease and gain of gene expression are equally discriminatory markers for prostate carcinoma: a gene expression analysis on total and microdissected prostate tissue. *Am J Pathol* 160:2169–2180.

59. LaTulippe E, Satagopan J, Smith A, *et al.* (2002) Comprehensive gene expression analysis of prostate cancer reveals distinct transcriptional programs associated with metastatic disease. *Cancer Res* 62:4499–4506.

60. Vanaja DK, Cheville JC, Iturria SJ, Young CY (2003) Transcriptional silencing of zinc finger protein 185 identified by expression profiling is associated with prostate cancer progression. *Cancer Res* 63:3877–3882.

16

STUDY OF ANDROGEN–ANDROGEN RECEPTOR ROLES IN PROSTATE CANCER USING MICE LACKING FUNCTIONAL PROSTATE ANDROGEN RECEPTOR

Chun-Te Wu, Shuyuan Yeh, Qingquan Xu, Zhiming Yang,
Philip Chang, Yueh-Chiang Hu and Chawnshang Chang

George H. Whipple Lab for Cancer Research
Departments of Urology, Pathology and Radiation Oncology, and
the Cancer Center, University of Rochester
Rochester, New York 14642, USA

Introduction

Prostate cancer is an androgen-dependent disease and a leading cause of cancer mortality in men. The vast majority of prostate cancers express the androgen receptor (AR), have androgen-dependent growth, initially respond to androgen ablation therapy, but eventually become androgen-independent (hormone refractory stage).[1] The mechanisms for transition of tumors from androgen-dependent to androgen-independent are generally explained by clonal selection, adaption, alternative pathways of signal transduction and aberrant AR signaling.[2–4] The AR is now known to participate in tumor progression through three mechanisms: expression, development of point mutations, and ligand-independent activation via coregulators.[5] Histological and epidemiological data have indicated the role of AR mutations and poly-Q polymorphisms in the anti-androgen withdrawal syndrome and prostate cancer susceptibility.[6] The AR point mutation T877A is common in the hormone-refractory prostate cancer.[7] *In vitro* studies have indicated the transactivation of this mutated AR can be induced by the anti-androgen, flutamide, in human prostate cancer LNCaP cells, which contain the mutant T877A (tyrptophen to alanine) AR.[8]

The involvement of this mutation in the transition to hormone-refractory stage and the anti-androgen withdrawal syndrome, remains controversial. Alleles of the CAG repeat in the first exon of the human AR gene have been shown to be associated with the risk of prostate cancer. Even in low-risk Asian populations that are favored by higher median CAG repeat lengths, a shorter CAG repeat length influences prostate cancer risk.[9] Animal models without functional AR in the prostate provide excellent tools to investigate the AR role in normal prostate development, prostate cancer carcinogenesis, progression, metastasis and transition to hormone-refractory. It is hoped that continuing research on AR expression and function in prostate cancer will provide new therapeutic strategies.

Generation of Androgen Receptor Knockout (ARKO) Mice

The AR, a member of the nuclear receptor superfamily, was first cloned in 1988.[10–11] It contains an N-terminal transactivation domain (NTD), a central DNA-binding domain (DBD) and a C-terminal ligand-binding domain (LBD). To generate ARKO mice, a cre-lox strategy for conditional KO is necessary. The cre-lox system utilizes the expression of P1 phage cre recombinase (Cre) to catalyze the excision of DNA located between flanking lox sites in exon 2 of the DBD.[12] We generated two separate lines of transgenic mice to carry the Cre and the homozygous floxed AR genes in both X chromosomes, as illustrated in Fig. 1. The generation of ar/Y-ACTB/Cre male mice in F3 resulted in total ARKO in all of the cells. Phenotype analyses showed that ARKO male mice have a low body weight and the external genitalia was ambiguous or appeared feminized, had a microphallic penis, and the urethra showed hypospadia. The scrotum is poorly developed and all vas deferens, epididymis, seminal vesicle and prostate are agenetic. Testes are small in size and cryptorchid in the low abdominal area close to the internal inguinal ring. This study indicated that disruption of AR gene in early embryonic stage had great impact in the development of normal prostate.[12] However, the systemic effects of lower androgen level in the total ARKO mice should be further explored.

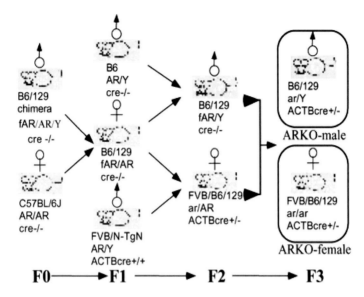

Fig. 1. Generation of ARKO female mice by mating among floxed AR (fAR) founders and cre founders. The chimera founder is B6/129 mosaic strain. The mating of the founder with the B6 female created female mice heterozygous with fAR. The following F2 generation resulted in fAR male mice. The mating between the heterozygous fAR female and the homozygous FVB/N-TgN ACTB cre male that carry Cre under β-actin promoter created a heterozygous KO of AR female carrying the Cre. The mating between the fAR male and the heterozygous ARKO female carrying the Cre generated the homozygous ARKO Cre⁺ female mice with a 1:8 ratio.

Prostate Development and Carcinogenesis in Prostate-Specific ARKO Mice

The cre-lox ARKO mouse model provides a much-needed *in vivo* animal model system to study androgen functions in the selective androgen target tissues in male mice. In this regard, it is of paramount importance to derive a cre recombinant transgenic animal system with robust expression of a biologically active Cre protein in a prostate epithelial cell-specific manner. We selected a rat probasin (PB) promoter to drive expression of the Cre gene.[13] The AR gene was gradually deleted during the adolescence stage when increased androgen levels activated the probasin promoter expression. Specific ARKO in prostate epithelium was evidenced by genotyping, RT-PCR and immunohistochemistry (IHC). Hormonal studies revealed normal serum testosterone levels in prostate-specific ARKO as compared to wild-type (WT) mice. The growth of urogenital organs other than prostate remained unchanged after the prostate epithelium no longer has a functional AR, however the size and weight of prostate glands were slightly decreased. The secretion proteins, probasin and prostatic secretory protein 94 (PSP94), were dramatically decreased in prostate-specific ARKO mice. When androgen ablation by castration was induced at 12 weeks old, both WT and prostate-specific ARKO mice showed dramatic regression of prostate and seminal vesicle growth. This model implies that the AR plays specific roles in epithelium and in stromal development. By crossing male probasin-cre mice to flox AR TRAMP female mice, the prostate-specific ARKO TRAMP mice were generated. This model will add more clues about the role of AR in the prostate cancer carcinogenesis and progression.

TRAMP Mice Lacking the Endogenous AR but Carrying the T877A Mutated Transgene

In a subgroup of patients with endocrine therapy-resistant prostate cancers, amino acid substitutions in the AR LBD have been found, which result in a broadened ligand response spectrum. The most common substitution in these cancers was T877A, which was first also described in the LNCaP prostate cancer cell line. The T877A substitution renders the AR responsive to natural low-affinity ligands and anti-androgens, such as flutamide. This mutation is believed to contribute to the prostate cancer progression and its transition to the hormone-refractory stage as well as the anti-androgen withdrawal syndrome.

By crossing the T877A transgene knock-in male mice with our ARKO female mice, we are in the process of generating ARKO male mice expressing prostate T877A AR transgene only. This will enable us to compare the effects of mutated AR and WT AR on the development of prostate gland. Further crossing female ARKO mice with T877A transgene male TRAMP mice will generate TRAMP mice which only express T877A mutated AR in the prostate. By these strategies, we can continue to explore the AR mutation on prostate cancer carcinogenesis and compare the tumor initiation and progression in the TRAMP mice with two different AR expressions.

ARKO Mice with AR-97Q and AR-24Q Transgene Expression

Despite the substantial public health impact of prostate cancer, little is known about its etiology. The generally accepted risk factors for the development of prostate cancer are advanced age, familial predisposition and perhaps ethnicity. The exon 1 of the AR contains several polymorphic repeats; the most variable is a polymorphic CAG repeat, which encodes a polyglutamine (poly-Q) chain. The range of CAG repeat lengths is from 14 to 35 repeats in man and may vary somewhat with ethnicity and race. Because the length of the polymorphic CAG trinucleotide repeat is inversely correlated with the transactivation function of the AR *in vitro*, it has been proposed that men with shorter repeats will be at higher risk for prostate cancer.[14] Several previous studies have shown that shorter CAG repeat length in AR NTD is associated with the occurrence of more aggressive prostate cancer, earlier age of onset and likelihood of recurrence.[15] However, one small study in a European population failed to support the association between CAG repeat length and prostate cancer risk.[16] The role of CAG repeats in prostate needs to be determined more clearly. By crossing AR-97Q and AR-24Q transgene male mice with our ARKO female mice, we are generating the ARKO mice carrying only 97-Q and 24-Q transgenic AR to compare the effects of different poly-Q lengths on the development of the prostate gland. Further crossing to TRAMP mice will create ARKO TRAMP mice with different poly-Q AR transgenes. By studying the differences in carcinogenesis and tumor progression in these mice, we will determine the effect of poly-Q lengths on the prostate cancer *in vivo*.

Inducible ARKO and ARKO TRAMP Mice

The normal prostate development depends on the androgen-AR signaling. In the total ARKO model, agenesis of prostate revealed that AR plays a critical role in the embryonic development of prostate. The prostate-specific ARKO model using probasin-cre lox strategy had nearly normal prostate growth after adolescence. These two models suggested the time-specific role of AR in the development of prostate. What is the role of AR between embryonic and adolescence? The time-specific role of AR in the normal prostate development can also be elucidated by the study of the inducible ARKO mice. The method uses an interferon-responsive promoter to control the expression of Cre recombinase. Here, Cre was used to delete a segment of the AR gene flanked by loxP recombinase recognition sites. Deletion was complete in liver and nearly complete in lymphocytes within a few days, whereas partial deletion was obtained in other tissues. Crossing the flox-AR female mice with Mx-1-inducible Cre male mice[17] will generate interferon-inducible ARKO mice. Our preliminary data (Xu and Chang, unpublished data), showed the efficiency of deletion of AR gene in prostate tissue was about 20% using the intraperitoneal injection of pI-pC. Some modifications can be made to improve the percentage of AR deletion, such as multiple injections and intra-prostate injection. Yet the partial deletion of AR in prostate may be sufficient for gene inactivation and result in easily detectable phenotypes. By crossing TRAMP male mice with flox-AR-cre-MX-1 female mice, the inducible ARKO TRAMP mice can be generated. As in Fig. 2, induction of IFN in 5-week-old inducible ARKO TRAMP mice resulted in a prostate tumor in one out of three mice, while all three mice without the induction of IFN had prominent prostate tumors at 20-week-old. If the AR gene was inducibly knocked out in 20-week-old mice, all the mice in WT AR and inducible ARKO groups grew prostate cancer, but the tumor size was smaller in the ARKO group. This model indicated that AR deletion in TRAMP mice might inhibit carcinogenesis at an earlier stage and delay cancer progression at a late stage. Further study is necessary to confirm the results of the preliminary observations and to explore the actual role of AR in prostate cancer carcinogenesis and progression.

ARKO Human Prostate Cancer CWR22R Cells

The advantage of using gene targeting in human somatic cells is that it provides a tool to study the roles of the signaling of interest in human cells instead of ARKO animal model. For this purpose, we attempted to disrupt AR signaling in human androgen-refractory prostate cancer cells in order

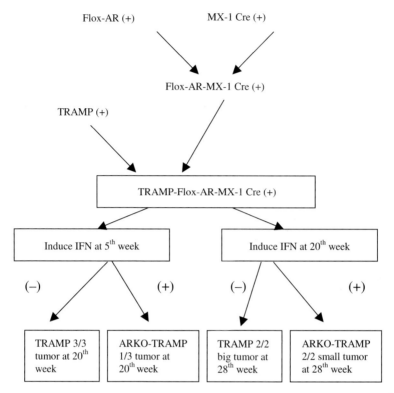

Fig. 2. Model for development of inducible ARKO-TRAMP mice.

to investigate the biological importance of AR signaling in those prostate cancers. Human prostate cancer CWR22R cells were transfected with the AR targeting vector using Superfect transfection kit (Qiagen) and selected with 400 μg/ml neomycin reagent.[18] The genotypes of the surviving clones were detected by Southern blotting using a DNA probe containing the 5′-UTR sequences of the AR gene. The untargeted and targeted loci produced approximately 9.0-kb and 3.46-kb bands, respectively. AR expression was reduced in those heterozygous clones compared to that in the parental CWR22R cells[19] confirming that one of the AR genes is targeted by homologous recombination. Therefore, this method provides a promising result and indicates that it is possible that we could target AR genes in any other cell lines of interest. Efforts to obtain homologous AR-null CWR22R cells failed after extensive screening, although homologous

AR-null MCF cells were successfully established. This suggests that AR is an essential survival factor in prostate cancer cells. The essential role of AR in androgen-refractory prostate cancer has been depicted in many other studies.[20,21] In order to knockout both AR genes, we are trying to stably transfect the tetracycline-inducible AR construct into heterozygous CWR22R cells and then target the second allele of AR in the cells. We believe this will provide a powerful tool for us to manipulate AR expression in the prostate cancer studies.

Conclusion

Although AR plays the pivot role in prostate development and prostate cancer carcinogenesis and progression, several aspects of AR function in the prostate are still not clear due to lack of appropriate animal models. One advantage of creating the floxed AR mice is to provide a base to generate tissue-specific ARKO in the prostate. Combined with different Cre-recombinases, a time-specific role of AR can also be studied by using the inducible Mx-1 mice. Based on the ARKO mice, other mutated genes can be tested as a combination of transgenic and knockout mice, such as T877A and poly-Q ARKO mice. Continued expansion of our knowledge of AR action in prostate cancer will contribute to more effective therapies. It is likely that in the future, AR ablation with a target to degenerate and/or eliminate AR protein, rather than androgen ablation to block androgen binding to the AR, will become the treatment of choice for advanced prostate cancer and hormone-refractory prostate cancer.

References

1. van der Kwast TH, Schalken J, Ruizeveld de Winter JA, van Vronnhoven CCJ, Mulder E, Boersma W, Trapman J (1991) Androgen receptors in endocrine therapy resistant human prostate cancer. *Int J Cancer* 48:189–193.
2. Visakorpi T (1999) New pieces to the prostate cancer puzzle. *Nat Med* 5:264–265.
3. Gelmann E (2002) Molecular biology of the androgen receptor. *J Clin Oncol* 20:3001–3015.
4. Suzuki H, Ueda T, Ichikawa T, Ito H (2003) Androgen receptor involvement in the progression of prostate cancer. *Endocr Relat Cancer* 10:209–216.

5. Miyamoto H, Yeh S, Wilding G, Chang C (1998) Promotion of agonist activity of anti-androgens by the androgen receptor coactivator, ARA70, in human prostate DU145 cells. *Proc Natl Acad Sci USA* 95:7379–7384.

6. Wang Q, Udayakumar TS, Vasaitis TS, Brodie AM, Fondell JD (2004) Mechanistic relationship between androgen receptor polyglutamine tract truncation and androgen-dependent transcriptional hyperactivity in prostate cancer cells. *J Biol Chem* 279:17319–17328.

7. Gaddipati JP, McLeod DG, Heidenberg HB, Sesterhenn IA, Finger MJ, Moul JW, Srivastava S (1994) Frequent detection of codon 877 mutation in the androgen receptor gene in advanced prostate cancer. *Cancer Res* 54:2861–2864.

8. Veldscholte J, Ris-Stalpers C, Kuiper G, Jenster G, Berrevoets C, Claassen E, van Rooij HCJ, Trapman AO, Brinkmann AO, Mulder E (1990) A mutation in the ligand binding domain of the androgen receptor of human LNCaP cells affects steroid binding characteristics and response to anti-androgens. *Biochem Biophys Res Commun* 173:534–540.

9. Hsing AW, Gao YT, Wu G, Wang X, Deng J, Chen YL, Sesterhenn IA, Mostofi FK, Benichou J, Chang C (2000) Polymorphic CAG and GGN repeat lengths in the androgen receptor and prostate cancer risk: a population-based case control study in China. *Cancer Res* 60:5111–5116.

10. Chang C, Kokontis J, Liao S (1988) Molecular cloning of human and rat complementary DNA encoding androgen receptors. *Science* 240:324–326.

11. Lubahn DB, Joseph DR, Sullivan PM, Willard HF, French FS, Wilson EM (1988) Cloning of human androgen receptor complementary DNA and localization to the X chromosome. *Science* 240:327–330.

12. Yeh S, Tsai MY, Xu Q, Mu XM, Lardy H, Huang KE, Lin H, Yeh SD, Altuwaijri S, Zhou X, Xing L, Gan L, Chang C (2002) Generation and characterization of androgen receptor knockout (ARKO) mice: an *in vivo* model for the study of androgen functions in selective tissue. *Proc Natl Acad Sci USA* 99:13498–13503.

13. Wu X, Wu J, Huang J, Powell WC, Zhang J, Matusik RJ, Sangiorgi FO, Maxson RE, Sucov HM, Roy-Burman P (2001) Generation of a prostate epithelial cell-specific Cre transgenic mouse model for tissue-specific gene ablation. *Mech Dev* 101:61–69.

14. Irvine RA, Yu MC, Ross RK, Coetzee GA (1995) The CAG and GGC microsatellites of the androgen receptor gene are in linkage disequilibrium in men with prostate cancer. *Cancer Res* 55:1937–1940.

15. Nam RK, Elhaji Y, Krahn MD (2000) Significance of the CAG repeat polymorphism of the androgen receptor gene in prostate cancer progression. *J Urol* 164:672–676.

16. Correa-Cerro L, Wohr G, Haussler J (1999) (CAG)nCAA and GGN repeats in the human androgen receptor gene are not associated with prostate cancer in a French-German population. *Eur J Hum Genet* 7:357–362.
17. Kuhn R, Schwenk F, Aguet M, Rajewsky K (1995) Inducible gene targeting in mice. *Science* 269:1427–1429.
18. Yeh S, Hu YC, Wang PH, Xie C, Xu Q, Tsai MY, Dong Z, Wang RS, Lee TH, Chang C (2003) Abnormal mammary gland development and growth retardation in female mice and MCF7 breast cancer cells lacking androgen receptor. *J Exp Med* 198:1899–1908.
19. Bao BY, Hu YC, Ting HJ, Lee YF (2004) Androgen signaling is required for the vitamin D-mediated growth inhibition in human prostate cancer cells. *Oncogene* 23:3350–3360.
20. Zegarra-Moro OL, Schmidt LJ, Huang H, Tindall DJ (2002) Disruption of androgen receptor function inhibits proliferation of androgen-refractory prostate cancer cells. *Cancer Res* 62:1008–1013.
21. Chen CD, Welsbie DS, Tran C, Baek SH, Chen R, Vessella R, Rosenfeld MG, Sawyers CL (2004) Molecular determinants of resistance to anti-androgen therapy. *Nat Med* 10:33–39.

17

CAPTURING SIGNAL ANOMALIES OF HUMAN PROSTATE CANCER INTO MOUSE MODELS

Hong Wu

Department of Molecular and Medical Pharmacology
University of California Los Angeles School of Medicine
Los Angeles, California 90095, USA

Ani Khodavirdi[*] and Pradip Roy-Burman[*,†]

[*]Department of Pathology and
[†]Department of Biochemistry and Molecular Biology
Keck School of Medicine
University of Southern California, Los Angeles
California 90033, USA

Introduction

Prostatic adenocarcinoma, the most common malignant visceral neoplasm of men, displays extensive phenotypic heterogeneity, both morphologically and genetically, and is typically also admixed with non-cancerous cells within the glands.[1,2] The disease is further confounded by the presence of multiple malignant foci in a majority of cancerous glands.[3] Such complexities have hindered progress in elucidating the clinical course and the molecular parameters for the development of prostate cancer. Some evidence for molecular anomalies has been documented, albeit in a fragmentary manner. In terms of the genesis of the disease, it is recognized that the most likely primary precursor of human prostate cancer is the histopathological lesion known as intraepithelial neoplasia (PIN). PIN lesions could be described as a low grade (LG) or high grade (HG), and it is widely perceived that HGPIN is a precursor of prostatic adenocarcinoma.[4–7] Since the initial growth of prostate tumor or cancer is dependent on androgens, hormone therapy in the form of medical or surgical castration constitutes a common approach for systemic treatment. However, over a period of time, most cancers will develop androgen-independence, thereby making the continued androgen deprivation therapy ineffective.[8–10] While the mechanisms that drive the genesis of subclinical, microscopic PIN lesions, their progression to invasive cancer and androgen independence remain largely unknown and evidence collected in recent years point to certain molecular aberrations that pave the path of disease progression. For example, anomalies in specific signaling molecules, including extracellular growth factors, protein tyrosine kinase cell surface receptors, intracellular transcription factors, nuclear receptors and their ligands, growth suppressors, cell cycle regulators, and others, have been indicated in some prostate carcinomas.

Some of these issues have been well described in a number of recent reviews.[2,11–16] There is currently a strong focus on the genetic alterations or aberrations in gene expression that are frequently encountered in human prostate cancer in the design of mouse models. The goal is to recapture the pathophysiologic characteristics of the human disease in a "natural" manner in immuno-competent mice to facilitate exploration of the molecular mechanism underlying prostate cancer as well as for development or testing of new targeted therapies. The strategies, however, are logical extensions of the earlier successful efforts to derive transgenic mouse models with prostate-specific expression of viral oncogenes.[17–21] The present report only considers the mouse models that have been engineered to depict one or more genetic defects seen in human prostate cancer.

Another important issue to note at the onset is that, although both men and mice harbor functionally equivalent prostate glands, there are similarities as well as differences in the anatomy and histology of the prostate in the two species. Similar epithelial cell types, namely, secretory, basal, and neuroendocrine are found in both mouse and human prostate, although their proportions vary. While human prostate has a robust fibromuscular stroma, the mouse contains a modest stromal component. Anatomically, the human prostate gland is a single alobular structure with central, peripheral, and transitional zones. In contrast, the mouse prostate is composed of four paired lobes, namely, anterior (AP), dorsal (DP), lateral (LP), and ventral (VP) prostate. Since DP and LP share a ductal system, they are often dissected together and referred to as the dorsolateral prostate (DLP). The mouse DLP is perceived to be most similar to the human peripheral zone in which the majority of clinically diagnosed prostate cancers are found. The mouse VP does not appear to have a human homologue and the human transitional zone does not have a murine homologue. The transitional zone constitutes a site where human nodular hyperplasia (BPH) is commonly seen. The mouse AP is analogous to the human central zone, which only infrequently represents a site of neoplasia in humans. A summary of the comparative aspects of anatomy, histology, and pathology of the human and mouse prostates can be found in a recent review article.[16]

Cell Surface Signaling Molecules

Signaling interactions between various extracellular growth factors and the corresponding cell surface receptors converge to determine the fate of the cell with respect to proliferation, survival, or death. In this context, dysregulation of several growth factors or their receptors has been implicated in prostate tumorigenesis. A number of transgenic mouse lines have been produced in which genes that are known to be overexpressed in human prostate cancer are targets. All of the models reviewed here, however, concern usage of a robust prostate-specific promoter to drive the expression of the transgene, and thus exclude those which were based on promoters that are not sufficiently prostate specific. For example, the survival factor, insulin-like growth factor 1 (IGF1), which is generally overexpressed in human prostate and which may potentially be a good tumor marker in prostate cancer,[22] was a target in a transgenic line. Its expression in the mouse tissues was designed by using the bovine keratin 5 promoter.[23] These mice develop squamous papillomas, some of which progress to carcinomas of the skin. The increased IGF1 levels also lead to pathologic changes in the prostate and in other male accessory glands of these animals.[24] The severity of the lesions in the prostate ranges from PIN to carcinoma *in situ* as well as tumors with neuroendocrine differentiation.

Fibroblast Growth Factors (FGFs)

The FGF family of heparin-binding proteins is intercellular signaling molecules of which at least 23 different members (FGF1–FGF23) have been identified to date. FGF proteins are generally secreted and their effects are mediated by a complex system of FGF receptor (FGFR) tyrosine kinases, either through autocrine or paracrine mechanisms, or both.[25,26] While dysregulation of several FGFs has been described in prostate development and tumorigenesis,[27,28] two members, FGF7 and FGF8, have been further pursued through mouse modeling experiments.

Alternative splicing of the mouse *fgf8* mRNA gives rise to eight potential protein isoforms that vary in their amino termini.[29,30] In humans, however, only four isoforms (FGF8a, FGF8b, FGF8e and FGF8f) are predicted due to a blocked reading frame in an exon of the human gene. Of the four possible isoforms, FGF8b has been demonstrated to possess the most transforming and tumorigenic potential.[31–33] While expression of FGF8b appears to represent the primary species in prostatic epithelial cell lines or malignant epithelium, its expression is practically undetected in the stromal component of prostate cancer.[29,31,34,35] Increased expression of FGF8b in prostatic lesions beginning from PIN to adenocarcinoma and its persistence in androgen-independent disease has been described.[34,35] The overexpression of FGF8b in prostate cancer cells has been shown to increase proliferative and invasive properties of the affected cells directly, and proliferation of prostatic stromal cells indirectly.[36] Consistent with these results, antisense down-regulation of *FGF8* mRNA reduces the growth rate, inhibits clonogenic activity, and decreases *in vivo* tumorigenicity of prostate tumor cells.[37] Recent demonstrations that FGF8 expression in prostate cancer is, at least in part, regulated by the androgen receptor at the transcriptional level,[38] and that FGF8b is angiogenic[39] further enhance the biological relevance of this factor in prostate cancer.

To assess the effects of FGF8b overexpression in the normal prostate secretory epithelium, transgenic mice were produced by using an improved rat probasin gene promoter.[40] This promoter, ARR2PB, has been found to confer a high level of reporter transgene expression specifically in the prostatic luminal epithelium and is strongly regulated by androgens.[41,42] Prostatic hyperplasia appears in the LP and VP in some FGF8b transgenic animals as early as 2 to 3 months, and in DP and AP between 6 to 16 months. LGPIN lesions manifest from 5 to 7 months. One hundred percent of the mice display multi-focal prostatic epithelial hyperplasia during the first 14 months, with 35% also having areas of LGPIN. In subsequent months (15 to 24 months) the profile changes to a higher incidence of LGPIN (66%) along with HGPIN (51%). Occasionally, HGPIN lesions resemble the histopathology of human prostatic carcinoma *in situ.* Figure 1 represents the progression pattern in the FGF8b transgenics. Like HGPIN, stromal proliferation and appearance of papillary hyperplasia with atypia, display a delayed pattern Together, these findings suggest that FGF8b is an etiological factor in prostate tumorigenesis. The stochastic pattern of disease progression from hyperplasia to carcinoma *in situ* also implies that hyperplasia initiated by the FGF8b mitogen is conducive to the manifestation of other genetic lesions, which may represent the rate-limiting factors responsible for a temporal progression and the severity of the lesions. Additionally, the delayed development of stromal hypercellularity in the prostate of these mice mimics the results of the epithelial-stromal cocultures *in vitro*,[36] invoking an indirect effect of FGF8b signaling in the epithelial cells on the stromal cells. Thus, besides being

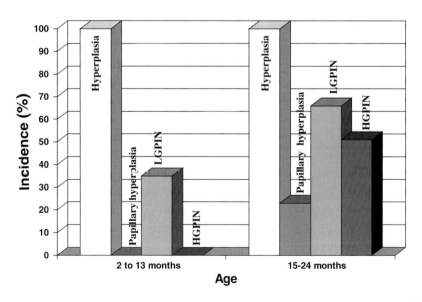

Fig. 1. Temporal incidence of appearance of prostatic lesions in FGF8b transgenic mice.[40]

an initiation factor, FGF8b is likely to act as a progression factor in the prostate disease. The reported properties of FGF8b, such as induction of tumorigenic and invasive activity to weakly tumorigenic prostate carcinoma cells or the ability to induce angiogenesis,[36,39] are noteworthy in this regard.

While FGF8 is produced in the prostate epithelium, FGF7 (keratinocyte growth factor, KGF) is made by the stroma and plays a role as a mediator of stromal-epithelial interactions in the prostate development.[43-45] It is also reported that a switch in the spatial pattern of FGF7 expression may occur in clinical prostate cancer such that cancer cells, rather than stromal cells, display stronger expression.[46] The cognate receptor for FGF7 is FGFR2 isoform b, which is normally found on the epithelium. It is also interesting to note that during prostate cancer progression, FGFR2 may switch from isoform b to isoform c in the rat Dunning tumor system.[26,47] Thus, it is possible that changes in FGF7 and its receptors may be linked to malignancy or gain of independence from stromal control. To convert FGF7 from a paracrine to autocrine factor, transgenic mice were produced in which the minimal rat probasin promoter was used to target FGF7 expression directly to the prostatic epithelium.[48] After one year of age, most of these mice develop prostatic epithelial hyperplasia, which, however, does not progress to dysplasia or tumors. These results imply that while FGF7 misexpression in the prostate could be a contributing factor, at least, in the induction of proliferation of the epithelial cells, the primary role of FGF7 may actually rest on its paracrine signaling in prostate biology and disease.

Fibroblast Growth Factor Receptors (FGFRs)

The role of FGFR signaling axis, focusing on FGFR1 and FGFR2, has been evaluated in the prostate of several transgenic mouse models. Considering that growth factor receptors like FGFRs[49] are naturally activated by oligomerization, a chemically induced dimerization technology was cleverly employed to achieve temporal control of FGFR expression.[50] Transgenic mice generated for this study had ARR2PB driven expression of either ligand-inducible FGFR1 or FGFR2. Examination of the prostates of these animals indicates that while activation of FGFR1 triggers hyperplasia followed by PIN lesions, such activation of FGFR2 does not elicit any observable changes even after 12 weeks of treatment with the inducer. All mice with the FGFR1 transgene show PIN in virtually every acinus when treated for 12 weeks with the inducer, and by timed removal of this extra FGFR1 signaling, the investigators show that induced hyperplasia is reversible until intraductal vascularization occurs. After that stage, however, it appears that hyperplastic cells become independent of FGFR1 signaling.

Depression of the FGFR2 signaling in the prostate was approached by targeting expression of a dominant negative, truncated FGFR2 form by using the minimal rat probasin promoter.[48] As with the overexpression of FGFR2 in the prostate, interference of signaling by the dominant negative mutant also does not yield gross changes in the prostate except that the size is smaller than the littermate controls. However, blocking of FGFR2 appears to lead to some histological changes, such as disorganization of the prostatic ducts and areas of hyperplastic stroma. Additionally, a trend in the emergence of epithelial-neuroendocrine transition is noted in the prostate gland of these mice.

In other studies, a potential cooperation between ectopic FGFR1 and down-regulation of FGFR2 in the induction of PIN lesions in the mouse prostate was examined.[51,52] Both probasin minimal promoter and the stronger ARR2PB promoters were used in developing separate lines of mice with either low or high expression of a constitutively active FGFR1 mutant in the prostate. While low levels of expression lead to LGPIN lesions only when the mice become older than 18 months, increased expressions dramatically accelerate PIN development. HGPIN is detected in the ARR2PB driven transgenic mice within 8 months. The results indicate a correlation between the FGFR1 expression level and the development or progression of PIN lesions. Studies of bigenic mice with repressed FGFR2 via dominant negative mutant and either low or higher expression of the constitutively active FGFR1 also led to interesting results. While a combination of depressed FGFR2 and low level of FGFR1 appears to contribute to preneoplastic lesions in the prostate, expression of the dominant negative form of FGFR2 does not display any measurable synergy with high expression of FGFR1. The combination of low FGFR1 and dominant negative FGFR2 also synergistically increase the population of neuroendocrine cells in the prostate.

Together, these different models highlight the physiological differences between FGFR1 and FGFR2 receptor functions in the prostate epithelium. Similar to what is described for FGF8 and FGF7 transgenic mice, these studies underscore the specificity and potency of the individual players as well as their dose-dependent effects in FGF-FGFR signaling, which could potentially be exploited for targeted intervention of prostate tumorigenesis.

Intracellular Signaling Molecules

A number of transgenic mouse lines have been produced in which a single gene encoding an intracellular signaling molecule is overexpressed or disrupted in the prostate epithelium. The design to increase expression concerns genes that are known to be overexpressed in human prostate cancer. Similarly, the targets of inactivation are those genes each of whose function is diminished or abolished in human prostate cancer. While the first approach is straightforward transgenic development, the latter invokes bigenics, particularly when conventional knockout is unproductive because of embryonic lethality or premature death. The powerful approach of conditional, cell-type, and tissue-specific deletion of genes, through the commonly referred Cre-loxP recombination, has been productive. Although three reports have recently appeared describing alternative prostate-specific Cre systems,[42,53,54] the power and utility of the PB-Cre4 line[42] has been fully documented.

Androgen Receptor (AR)

AR is expressed in normal prostate in the secretory epithelial cells at high levels and in a subset of smooth muscle cells.[55,56] All phases of prostate tumorigenesis ranging from preneoplastic lesions to androgen-dependent adenocarcinoma to androgen-independent disease require the activity of this nuclear receptor.[9,10,15] The failure of androgen ablation therapy and development of "androgen-resistant" prostate cancer is thought to be, at least partly, due to hypersensitized AR signaling, either by gain-of-function mutations or through increased AR levels, that operates in the absence of optimal levels of the ligand.[10,15,57] To assess the effects of AR overexpression in the normal prostate secretory epithelium, a transgenic mouse line was produced by using the minimal PB promoter to drive a murine AR transgene expression.[58]

Although the effect of AR overexpression in the model is not significant up to one year of age, with further aging focal areas of VP and DLP begin to display PIN lesions. Interestingly, hyperplasia is not prominent in the prostate of these animals, which may be a consequence of simultaneous increase in the rate of apoptosis. Since PIN lesions are focal and increased with age, it is suggested that a balanced increase in proliferation and apoptosis may be a conducive factor for secondary genetic or epigenetic events that lead to dysplasia.

Homeobox Transcription Factor, NKX3.1

NKX3.1, which displays prostate-specific expression, is a candidate tumor suppressor in its properties. *NKX3.1* gene is mapped in a chromosomal region (8p21), which is found to undergo allelic deletion in about 80% of prostate cancers.[59] Unlike the conventional inactivation of the remaining allele of a tumor suppressor gene by mutation, epigenetic modifications, yet to be clearly understood, may be involved in loss of NKX3.1 protein expression in prostate cancer.[60,61] Both conventional and conditional knockouts of the *Nkx3.1* gene in mice were attempted to define the role of NKX3.1 in prostate tumorigenesis.[53,62–64] All models point to this homeobox transcription factor as a regulator of ductal branching and secretory activity of the glandular epithelium, and when lost, as a factor in the development of LGPIN by one year of age, largely in AP. Mice with further aging up to two years reveal progression of lesions but not beyond HGPIN.[62] To extend the "life" of these lesions, when tissue recombination/transplantation approach[65] was used, the lesions did progress to a more advanced stage of PIN, but did not convert to invasive cancer.[66] The results implied that other secondary events for progression might not manifest in the *Nkx3.1* knockout model. However, studies of both homozygous and heterozygous mutants clearly indicated that not only null status, but also reduced NKX3.1 expression, may be directly related to initiation of preneoplastic lesions in the prostate, a point which is clinically very relevant.[62,67]

Retinoid Receptor, RXRα

There has been long term interest in retinoids and prostate biology.[68] Actions of retinoids are largely mediated by their nuclear receptors comprising retinoic acid receptor (RAR) and retinoid X receptor (RXR) families. The physiological consequences of RARs and RXRs inactivation have been investigated via conventional knockout technology.[69] Considering that the active retinoid receptor is mostly a heterodimer of one RAR and one RXR,[70] it was noteworthy that RARγ null mutant mice develop squamous metaplasia of the prostate.[71] Since mice lacking both RXRβ and RXRγ are normal in terms of prostate morphology and function,[72] the critical RXR in prostate biology appears to be RXRα. The human chromosomal region, 9q34.3, in which *RXRα* gene is mapped, is characterized by a high rate of recombination,[73] and, the incidence of loss of heterozygosity at this locus has been reported to be 20% in prostate cancer.[74] In a recent study, it was demonstrated that the nuclear expression of RXRα is generally down-regulated in human prostate cancer cell lines and specimens, and that manipulated overexpression of just RXRα subtype in prostate cancer cells can significantly induce cell death by apoptosis.[75,76]

Since conventional disruption of the RXRα gene is embryonic lethal, the PB-Cre4/loxP system was used to inactivate *RXRα* alleles in the mouse prostate.[77] Developmentally, prostatic branching is increased from the loss of RXRα function. Histopathologically, homozygous *RXRα*-deficient prostates show multifocal hyperplasia as early as 4 months of age. Lesions, which are like LGPINs, are detected after 5 months. Subsequently, beginning at about 10 months of age, HGPINs develop in some animals, and could be present in any of the lobes. Similar to homozygous mice, the monoallelic mice appear to develop hyperplasia, LGPIN, and HGPIN in a temporal fashion, except that incidence is substantially delayed by several months (Fig. 2). Thus, it appears that, like NKX3.1, haploinsufficiency of RXRα could be a factor in prostate disease, the reduced production or delayed accumulation of which might promote a positive environment for proliferation and, perhaps following other secondary events, transformation to preneoplastic lesions. All in all, results from the model underscore that a major component of retinoid

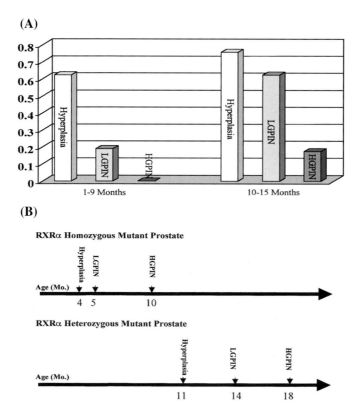

Fig. 2. Incidence and onset of prostate lesions in mice with monoallelic or biallelic inactivation of RXRα in the prostate epithelium. (**A**) Homozygous mutant prostate displays LGPIN after 5 months, while HGPIN begin to appear after 10 months. (**B**) The heterozygous mutant mice also develop similar phenotypes, but in a delayed manner, implying a dose effect.[77]

action in the prostate is mediated by a retinoid receptor, RXRα, the inactivation of which in the prostatic epithelium leads to early stage neoplastic disease.

Cell Cycle Inhibitor p27Kip1 and Its Regulator SKP2

Protein ubiquitinylation for proteolysis of regulatory proteins in the cell is a complex process involving a series of components, both invariable and variable, which is targeted towards a specific protein. A ubiquitin E3 ligase, the SCF SKP2 complex, consisting of SKP1, Cull, Rbx1, and the F-box protein SKP2, and mediates the polyubiquitination of the CDK inhibitor p27Kip1.[78–80] In this complex SKP2 serves as a substrate-targeting subunit that binds to the phosphorylated p27. Based on the knowledge of inverse relationship between the levels of SKP2 and p27, and by the general observation that low or lack of p27 expression may be associated with human cancers including prostate cancer,[81–83] transgenic mouse lines were generated that express SKP2 under the control of the ARR2PB promoter in the prostate epithelium.[84] Overexpression of SKP2 down-regulates p27 and is associated with incidences of epithelial hyperplasia and dysplasia up to HGPIN in both VP and DLP glands. It is likely that SKP2 acts, at least partly, as an oncoprotein in the mouse prostate through induction of ubiquitin-dependent degradation of p27. There appear to be other mechanisms in play which, however, remain to be defined. For instance, although hyperplasia and dysplasia are prominent by 3 to 7 months of age in SKP2 transgenic mice, only hyperplasia, but not dysplasia, develops in p27-deficient mice at the advanced age of 14 months.[83,85] One possibility could be a consequence of differences in the mouse strains used, but potentially more intriguing would be a relationship to differential levels of p27. The p27 protein, besides being a major CDK inhibitor in the cell cycle, may also function in the assembly of the cyclin D/CDK4 or CDK6 complex.[86] It is thought that if SKP2 expression fails to completely abolish p27 levels, as in p27 null mice, the residual p27 may be critical in sustaining the assembly role.[84] Still another possibility could be that SKP2 might promote earlier onset of hyperplasia and subsequent progression to dysplastic lesions by not only targeting p27, but perhaps other cell cycle regulators for proteolysis.

c-MYC Transcription Factor

c-MYC has been widely implicated in various human cancers.[87] Involvement of c-MYC in the multi-step tumorigenesis was first demonstrated in Burkitt's lymphoma in which the translocation from chromosome 8 to chromosome 14 results in deregulated c-MYC expression. Increased c-*MYC* gene copy number has been described in a significant portion of human prostate cancers[88,89] and overexpression of c-*MYC* mRNA is detected in several prostate cancers.[90] To address the role of c-MYC in the prostate, transgenic mice were generated in which the transgene is expressed from two different strength prostate epithelium-specific promoters, namely minimal PB and ARR2PB.[91] Several interesting observations were made from the examination of these two model systems, designated Lo-Myc and Hi-Myc, respectively.

Multifocal proliferative lesions and dysplasia develop in both Lo-Myc and Hi-Myc mice mostly in VP and DLP. The PIN lesions appear to progress to invasive adenocarcinomas by 3 to 6 months in the Hi-Myc mice and by 10 to 12 months in the Lo-Myc mice. These results imply a dose effect of c-MYC in the rate of disease progression. Invasion noted to date is mostly local as determined from the penetration through the fibromuscular layer, and in some cancers, with detection of foci indicative of lymphovascular invasion. On the molecular level, c-MYC is known to normally regulate early cell growth and proliferation. In certain contexts, c-MYC also induces apoptosis, and, in fact, in *c-myc* transgenic models, both proliferation and apoptosis are evident, although it appears that proliferation may outpace apoptosis to some extent.[91] It is also noteworthy that c-MYC levels are increased in the prostate after castration.[92] Furthermore, a recent study describes that overexpression of c-MYC may lead to defects in double-strand DNA break repair and induction of chromosome translocations, suggesting that c-MYC may serve as a "dominant mutator" to accelerate tumor development.[93]

Microarray-based expression profiling of the *c-myc* transgenics has led to identification of some signature gene activities, which are shared between human and mouse prostate cancers. For example, while NKX3.1 protein is detected in PINs at variable levels, it is not detected in the prostate tumor in the transgenics. Another gene, *pim*1, whose serine/threonine kinase product is known to cooperate with c-MYC in murine lymphomagenesis, is also overexpressed in tumors in the *c-myc* transgenic mice. Interestingly, PIM1 expression is increased in a subset of human prostate cancers that also display poor clinical outcome.[94]

Protein Kinase AKT and Master Tumor Suppressor PTEN

The cellular proto-oncogene c-*Akt* was originally identified as a homologue of the viral oncogene v-*Akt*.[95] AKT is a protein kinase whose activity is positively regulated by PI3-kinase.[96] Activated AKT, in turn, controls multiple signaling pathways, including cell survival and cell proliferation. Phosphatase and tensin homologue detected on chromosome 10 (*PTEN*) is a tumor suppressor gene, which is most frequently mutated or deleted in various human cancers. Germ line mutations in the *PTEN* gene are associated with Cowden Syndrome and related diseases in which patients develop hyperplastic lesions (harmatomas) in multiple organs with increased risks of malignant transformation.[97,98] *PTEN* alteration is strongly implicated in prostate cancer development. Its deletions and/or mutations are found in 30% of primary prostate cancers[97,99] and 63% of metastatic prostate cancers,[100] placing *PTEN* aberrations among the most common genetic alterations reported in human prostate cancers. The major function of PTEN relies on its lipid phosphatase activity that antagonizes the PI3K/AKT pathway.[101–103] Loss of PTEN function results in accumulation of PIP3 and activation of its downstream effectors including AKT/PKB.[42,104,105] As a serine/threonine protein kinase, AKT functions by phosphorylating key intermediate signaling molecules, such as glycogen synthase kinase 3, BAD, caspase 9, IκB, and others leading to increased cell metabolism, cell growth, and cell survival.[102,106,107]

To determine whether AKT activation is sufficient for the transformation of normal prostatic epithelial cells, a transgenic mouse line, with the use of a probasin promoter driving the expression of a constitutively activated form of *Akt*, was generated.[108] These animals develop hyperplastic/dysplastic lesions, which do not progress further, and the longevity of the animals is compromised apparently related to a bladder outlet obstruction. Analyses of gene expression profiles in the VP of this transgenic line led to some interesting findings that have relevance to human prostate tumorigenesis. For example, the up-regulated genes include prostate stem cell antigen (PSCA), which is expressed in prostate ductal tips during prostate development,[109] osteocalcin (or gla protein), which is overexpressed in prostate cancer,[110,111] and angiogenin-3 and other family members which induce angiogenesis.

To directly assess the role of prostate-specific *Pten* deletion, mice harboring floxed alleles of *Pten* were crossed with the PB-Cre4 line.[42,112,113] In another study, Cre/loxP strategy involving PB-Cre4[42] or PB-Cre,[54] was used to define the effect of *Pten* deletion in the prostate.[114] A "hypomorphic" strain of mice was also developed which exhibits only 25%–35% of PTEN compared to heterozygous *Pten* alleles (50%) and wild-type (100%).[114] Several exciting sets of information have been derived from these new models. In homozygous *Pten* null prostates,[113] multifocal hyperplasia is evident starting from DLP and VP from 4 weeks and later reaching AP. These mice develop PIN at 6 weeks and prostatic adenocarcinoma at 9 weeks. The latency of PIN formation is shorter than heterozygous animals that display these lesions from 8 to 10 months. While heterozygous mice of this strain progress only up to HGPIN in their late life, mice with homozygous *Pten* deletion display invasive adenocarcinoma as early as 9 weeks. Practically all lobes are involved, and from 15 weeks, there is evidence for the cancer cell invasion into lymph and blood vessel systems. Some of the cancer cells appear to survive in the circulation, as seeding into distant sites such as subcapsular sinus of lymph nodes and the lung is evident. The metastatic tumor cells remain AR positive and null for PTEN immunostaining. The progression of the disease in this conditional *Pten* null mouse strain is depicted in Fig. 3.

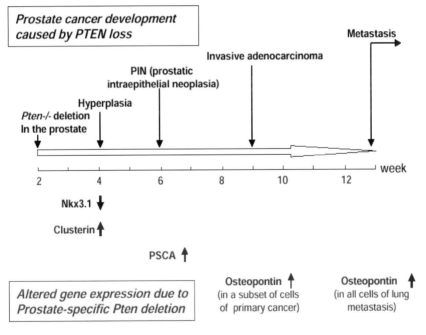

Fig. 3. A summary of onset and progression of prostate cancer development in mice with homozygous *Pten* deletion in the prostate epithelium.[113]

Androgen ablation in these mice reveals that the cancer cells do respond to the treatment, as there is a significant reduction of prostate volume. However, even though the survival of *Pten* null prostate cancer cells appears to be androgen-dependent, their proliferation is not sensitive to androgen withdrawal. This property of androgen-independent growth observed in this model is likely to contribute to formation of hormone-resistant cancer.

Although the mixed genetic backgrounds of the mouse strains used in different laboratories do limit direct correlation of the results, it is clear that the activity of PTEN is critical in suppression of prostate tumorigenesis. Inclusion of the hypomorphic *Pten* allele in the work of Trotman *et al.*[114] underscores the point that PTEN dose dictates cancer progression in the prostate. Furthermore, this study also illustrates that qualitative morphological changes are a function of the number of cells suffering complete *Pten* inactivation as well as the strength of Cre expression.

As expected, in all *Pten* null prostate mouse lines, the AKT is activated. AKT-activated prostate epithelial cells are also larger than the wild type or heterozygous control cells, consistent with the role of PTEN in controlling cell size.[115,116] While AKT activation is likely to be an important mechanism in this model, there must be other PTEN-directed signaling pathways that allow progression to invasive prostate cancer, since disease progression stops at dysplasia with AKT activation alone. In this regard, interesting clues are emerging from the global assessment of molecular changes caused by homozygous *Pten* deletion in the prostate, including changes in levels of factors like NKX3.1, PSCA, clusterin and osteoponin.[113]

Collaboration Between Signaling Molecules

Since carcinogenesis is a multi-step process involving a number of genetic changes or aberrations, successive development of increasingly complex mouse models with respect to these aberrations should be important in critical analysis of the disease progression. To date, only a few models have been developed incorporating up to two gene functions in a single system for prostate tumorigenesis, although most of them may lack the desired degree of tissue specificity. As the field is still at an early stage, only two examples are described below.

NKX3.1 and PTEN

The conventional knockout mice for *Nkx3.1* and *Pten* alleles were cross-bred to examine progression of prostatic lesions. The latency of PIN development in the NKX3.1 insufficiency background is reduced by half in the *Nkx3.1* +/−; *Pten* +/− mice.[67] Furthermore, evidence is obtained for the loss of NKX3.1 protein as well as the loss of the second allele of *Pten* in focal areas of tumors formed in the prostate of these compound mutants carrying each of the two genes as heterozygous alleles. The malignant potential of the pre-invasive lesions from the compound mice have further been investigated using a serial tissue recombination/transplantation assay or as a consequence of aging beyond one year of life.[117] Such prolonged observation or propagation appears conducive to the development of invasive adenocarcinoma, which is also frequently accompanied by metastases to lymph nodes. These results are quite consistent with the observations made with the conditional inactivation of *Pten* alleles in the prostate, in which there is also concomitant disease in NKX3.1 protein levels.[113]

p27Kip1 and PTEN

Since loss of p27 and PTEN is a frequent observation in human prostate cancer, one approach was to attempt concomitant inactivation of one *Pten* allele and one or both p27 alleles.[85] p27 is a downstream target of the PTEN controlled signaling pathway. Activated AKT phosphorylates the forkhead transcription factors, such as AFX, FKHR, and FKHR-L1, which, in turn, act to reduce p27 mRNA and protein levels, leading to accelerated G1-S cell cycle transition.[105,118,119] PTEN and PI3K pathways also regulate p27 protein stability. For example, PTEN deficiency in embryonic stem (ES) cells causes a decrease of p27 levels and concomitant increase of SKP2, a key component of the SCF SKP2 ubiquitin E3 ligase complex as described above.

While most of the *Pten* +/− heterozygous mice die within eight months from massive lympho-splenomegaly, long-term survivors develop a spectrum of epithelial tumors with propensities for those of adrenal, endometrial, and thyroid tissues. They also manifest a high incidence of

PIN after nine months.[85,120] Mice null for *p27* alleles do not display enhanced spontaneous tumors.[121,122] In this regard, it is noteworthy that when *Pten* +/− mice are produced in the background of *p27* null genotype, the compound mutants develop prostate carcinoma within 3 months postnatally with complete penetrance along with tumors of various other histological origins.[85] The prostate cancer is formed in DLP and AP, but not in VP, and is described to be locally invasive as rupture of the basal membrane of the epithelium is frequently seen. These results testify to a cooperative role of PTEN and p27 in tumor progression in epithelial tissues including the prostate.

Summary and Conclusions

Evidence has been collected to demonstrate that dysregulated expression of endogenous genes in the mouse prostate can lead to stages of prostate tumorigenesis. Transgenic mouse models that represent robust and tissue-specific activation of FGF8b, FGFR1, or SKP2 in the prostatic secretory epithelium, and those that address genome-wide knockout of a target gene, such as *Nkx3.1* or conditional prostate-specific gene inactivation, such as RXRalpha, display a stochastic pattern of increasing degree of phenotypic abnormalities of lesions, beginning with epithelial hyperplasia followed by presentations of preneoplastic lesions. Other types of modeling, like overexpression of a strong proto-oncogene c-*myc* or disruption of the master tumor suppressor gene *Pten*, in the prostate epithelium, lead to the rapid development of invasive adenocarcinoma of the prostate with 100% penetrance. Evidence is accumulating to suggest that some of prostate cancer models, such as *Pten* null prostate, further progress to distant metastases in lung and lymph nodes, and possibly also to the bones for which more compelling data remain to be derived. While the adenocarcinomas in the advanced disease models respond to androgen ablation through increased apoptosis, the *Pten* null prostate cancer cells do appear to survive and eventually proliferate. With time, it is expected that the ability to proliferate under the condition of androgen deprivation may actually lead to development of hormone refractory prostate cancer as it happens in humans after prolonged hormone therapy.

The models generated to date are beginning to shed light into the molecular features of the disease. Global assessment of molecular changes in the advanced disease models has already identified key genes known to be relevant to prostate cancer. The preneoplastic disease models are being similarly scrutinized to identify molecular expression changes that are associated with progression from one early step to the next in time. Revelations of new molecular targets will likely contribute to the current theme of compound mutants to recapture the pathologic characteristics of the human disease to a fuller extent. In this regard, it would be important to increase focus on the models that favor the genesis and progression of the tumor in the DLP so as to increase relevance to the pathology that is frequently seen in the peripheral zone of the human prostate.

It is predicted that the next generation mouse models of prostate cancer, which are founded on prostate-specific, regulatable expression of appropriate proto-oncogenes in combination with conditional as well as temporal inactivation of relevant tumor suppressor or metastasis suppressor genes, will be forthcoming not too far in the future. These models will be of further value if simultaneously engineered with the power for noninvasive quantitation of tumor burden, its spread or colonization to distant sites. This capability is reflected in the recent successful generation of a reporter mouse that facilitates visualization of spontaneous tumor development via *in vivo* bioluminescence imaging.[123] Potentially, any Cre/loxP models for prostate cancer can be combined with this reporter line to make them amenable to longitudinal monitoring of tumor growth. Thus, the future complex models mimicking the sporadic prostate cancer and equipped with new approaches to follow the disease progression are anticipated to compliment the current models to a great extent. All of these will contribute to new insights into the pathogenesis of this common disease as well as for initiating the essential preclinical tests for therapeutic or chemopreventive regimens.

Acknowledgments

The research concerning modeling human prostate cancer in mice is primarily supported by NIH grant R01CA59705 (to P.R-B), and grants

U01CA98013 and DOD PC991538 (to H.W.). The authors thank Leslie Wauke for secretarial assistance in the preparation of this manuscript.

References

1. Roy-Burman P, Zheng J, Miller GJ (1997) Molecular heterogeneity in prostate cancer: can TP53 mutation unravel tumorigenesis? *Mol Med Today* 3:476–482.
2. DeMarzo AM, Nelson WG, Isaacs WB, Epstein JI (2003) Pathological and molecular aspects of prostate cancer. *Lancet* 361:955–964.
3. Miller GJ, Cygan JM (1994) Morphology of prostate cancer: the effects of multifocality on histological grade, tumor volume and capsule penetration. *J Urol* 152:1709–1713.
4. McNeal JE, Villers A, Redwine EA, Freiha FS, Stamey TA (1991) Microcarcinoma in the prostate: its association with duct-acinar dysplasia. *Hum Pathol* 22:644–652.
5. Haggman MJ, Macoska JA, Wojno KJ, Oesterling JE (1997) The relationship between prostatic intraepithelial neoplasia and prostate cancer: critical issues. *J Urol* 158:12–22.
6. Isaacs W, De Marzo A, Nelson WG (2002) Focus on prostate cancer. *Cancer Cell* 2:113–116.
7. Park JH, Walls JE, Galvez JJ, *et al.* (2002) Prostatic intraepithelial neoplasia in genetically engineered mice. *Am J Pathol* 161:727–735.
8. Pilat MJ, Kamradt JM, Pienta KJ (1998) Hormone resistance in prostate cancer. *Cancer Metastasis Rev* 17:373–381.
9. Feldman BJ, Feldman D (2001) The development of androgen-independent prostate cancer. *Nat Rev Cancer* 1:34–45.
10. Taplin ME, Balk SP (2004) Androgen receptor: a key molecule in the progression of prostate cancer to hormone independence. *J Cell Biochem* 91:483–490.
11. Abate-Shen C, Shen MM (2000) Molecular genetics of prostate cancer. *Genes Dev* 14:2410–2434.
12. Elo JP, Visakorpi T (2001) Molecular genetics of prostate cancer. *Ann Med* 33:130–141.
13. Gao AC, Isaacs JT (2000) The molecular basis of prostate carcinogenesis. In: Coleman WB, Tsongalis GJ, eds. *Molecular Basis of Human Cancer*. The Humana Press Inc., Totowa, NJ, pp. 365–379.

14. Powell WC, Cardiff RD, Cohen MB, Miller GJ, Roy-Burman P (2003) Mouse strains for prostate tumorigenesis based on genes altered in human prostate cancer. *Curr Drug Targets* 4:263–279.
15. Litvinov IV, De Marzo AM, Isaacs JT (2003) Is the Achilles' heel for prostate cancer therapy a gain of function in androgen receptor signaling? *J Clin Endocrinol Metab* 88:2972–2982.
16. Roy-Burman P, Wu H, Powell WC, Hagenkord J, Cohen MB (2004) Genetically defined mouse models that mimic natural aspects of human prostate cancer development. *Endocr Relat Cancer* 11:225–254.
17. Greenberg NM, DeMayo F, Finegold MJ, *et al.* (1995) Prostate cancer in a transgenic mouse. *Proc Natl Acad Sci USA* 92:3439–3443.
18. Gingrich JR, Barrios RJ, Kattan MW, Nahm HS, Finegold MJ, Greenberg NM (1997) Androgen-independent prostate cancer progression in the TRAMP model. *Cancer Res* 57:4687–4691.
19. Kasper S, Sheppard PC, Yan Y, *et al.* (1998) Development, progression, and androgen-dependence of prostate tumors in probasin-large T antigen transgenic mice: a model for prostate cancer. *Lab Invest* 78:i–xv.
20. Masumori N, Thomas TZ, Chaurand P, *et al.* (2001) A probasin-large T antigen transgenic mouse line develops prostate adenocarcinoma and neuroendocrine carcinoma with metastatic potential. *Cancer Res* 61:2239–2249.
21. Winter SF, Cooper AB, Greenberg NM (2003) Models of metastatic prostate cancer: a transgenic perspective. *Prostate Cancer Prostatic Dis* 6:204–211.
22. Woodson K, Tangrea JA, Pollak M, *et al.* (2003) Serum insulin-like growth factor I: tumor marker or etiologic factor? A prospective study of prostate cancer among Finnish men. *Cancer Res* 63:3991–3994.
23. DiGiovanni J, Bol DK, Wilker E, *et al.* (2000) Constitutive expression of insulin-like growth factor-1 in epidermal basal cells of transgenic mice leads to spontaneous tumor promotion. *Cancer Res* 60:1561–1570.
24. DiGiovanni J, Kiguchi K, Frijhoff A, *et al.* (2000) Deregulated expression of insulin-like growth factor 1 in prostate epithelium leads to neoplasia in transgenic mice. *Proc Natl Acad Sci USA* 97:3455–3460.
25. Wilkie AO, Morriss-Kay GM, Jones EY, Heath JK (1995) Functions of fibroblast growth factors and their receptors. *Curr Biol* 5:5000–5007.
26. McKeehan WL, Wang F, Kan M (1998) The heparan sulfate-fibroblast growth factor family: diversity of structure and function. *Prog Nucleic Acid Res Mol Biol* 59:135–176.
27. Djakiew D (2000) Dysregulated expression of growth factors and their receptors in the development of prostate cancer. *Prostate* 42:150–160.

28. Thomson AA (2001) Role of androgens and fibroblast growth factors in pro-static development. *Reproduction* 121:187–195.

29. Tanaka A, Furuya A, Yamasaki M, *et al.* (1998) High frequency of fibroblast growth factor (FGF) 8 expression in clinical prostate cancers and breast tissues, immunohistochemically demonstrated by a newly established neutralizing monoclonal antibody against FGF 8. *Cancer Res* 58:2053–2056.

30. Gemel J, Gorry M, Ehrlich GD, MacArthur CA (1996) Structure and sequence of human FGF8. *Genomics* 35:253–257.

31. Ghosh AK, Shankar DB, Shackleford GM, *et al.* (1996) Molecular cloning and characterization of human FGF8 alternative messenger RNA forms. *Cell Growth Differ* 7:1425–1434.

32. MacArthur CA, Lawshe A, Shankar DB, Heikinheimo M, Shackleford GM (1995) FGF-8 isoforms differ in NIH3T3 cell transforming potential. *Cell Growth Differ* 6:817–825.

33. Daphna-Iken D, Shankar DB, Lawshe A, Ornitz DM, Shackleford GM, MacArthur CA (1998) MMTV-Fgf8 transgenic mice develop mammary and salivary gland neoplasia and ovarian stromal hyperplasia. *Oncogene* 17: 2711–2717.

34. Dorkin TJ, Robinson MC, Marsh C, Bjartell A, Neal DE, Leung HY (1999) FGF8 over-expression in prostate cancer is associated with decreased patient survival and persists in androgen independent disease. *Oncogene* 18: 2755–2761.

35. Valve EM, Nevalainen MT, Nurmi MJ, Laato MK, Martikainen PM, Harkonen PL (2001) Increased expression of FGF-8 isoforms and FGF receptors in human premalignant prostatic intraepithelial neoplasia lesions and prostate cancer. *Lab Invest* 81:815–826.

36. Song Z, Powell WC, Kasahara N, van Bokhoven A, Miller GJ, Roy-Burman P (2000) The effect of fibroblast growth factor 8, isoform b, on the biology of prostate carcinoma cells and their interaction with stromal cells. *Cancer Res* 60:6730–6736.

37. Rudra-Ganguly N, Zheng J, Hoang AT, Roy-Burman P (1998) Downregulation of human FGF8 activity by antisense constructs in murine fibroblastic and human prostatic carcinoma cell systems. *Oncogene* 16:1487–1492.

38. Gnanapragasam VJ, Robson CN, Neal DE, Leung HY (2002) Regulation of FGF8 expression by the androgen receptor in human prostate cancer. *Oncogene* 21:5069–8500.

39. Mattila MM, Ruohola JK, Valve EM, Tasanen MJ, Seppanen JA, Harkonen PL (2001) FGF-8b increases angiogenic capacity and tumor growth of androgen-regulated S115 breast cancer cells. *Oncogene* 20:2791–2804.

40. Song Z, Wu X, Powell WC, *et al.* (2002) Fibroblast growth factor 8 isoform B overexpression in prostate epithelium: a new mouse model for prostatic intraepithelial neoplasia. *Cancer Res* 62:5096–5105.

41. Zhang J, Thomas TZ, Kasper S, Matusik RJ (2000) A small composite probasin promoter confers high levels of prostate-specific gene expression through regulation by androgens and glucocorticoids *in vitro* and *in vivo*. *Endocrinology* 141:4698–4710.

42. Wu X, Wu J, Huang J, *et al.* (2001) Generation of a prostate epithelial cell-specific Cre transgenic mouse model for tissue-specific gene ablation. *Mech Dev* 101:61–69.

43. Leung HY, Mehta P, Gray LB, Collins AT, Robson CN, Neal DE (1997) Keratinocyte growth factor expression in hormone insensitive prostate cancer. *Oncogene* 15:1115–1120.

44. Matsubara A, Yasumoto H, Usui T (1999) Hormone refractory prostate cancer and fibroblast growth factor receptor. *Breast Cancer* 6:320–324.

45. Sugimura Y, Foster BA, Hom YK, *et al.* (1996) Keratinocyte growth factor (KGF) can replace testosterone in the ductal branching morphogenesis of the rat ventral prostate. *Int J Dev Biol* 40:941–951.

46. McGarvey TW, Stearns ME (1995) Keratinocyte growth factor and receptor mRNA expression in benign and malignant human prostate. *Exp Mol Pathol* 63:52–62.

47. Yan G, Fukabori Y, McBride G, Nikolaropolous S, McKeehan WL (1993) Exon switching and activation of stromal and embryonic fibroblast growth factor (FGF)-FGF receptor genes in prostate epithelial cells accompany stromal independence and malignancy. *Mol Cell Biol* 13: 4513–4522.

48. Foster BA, Evangelou A, Gingrich JR, Kaplan PJ, DeMayo F, Greenberg NM (2002) Enforced expression of FGF-7 promotes epithelial hyperplasia whereas a dominant negative FGFR2iiib promotes the emergence of neuro-endocrine phenotype in prostate glands of transgenic mice. *Differentiation* 70:624–632.

49. Schlessinger J, Plotnikov AN, Ibrahimi OA, *et al.* (2000) Crystal structure of a ternary FGF-FGFR-heparin complex reveals a dual role for heparin in FGFR binding and dimerization. *Mol Cell* 6:743–750.

50. Freeman KW, Gangula RD, Welm BE, *et al.* (2003) Conditional activation of fibroblast growth factor receptor (FGFR) 1, but not FGFR2, in prostate cancer cells leads to increased osteopontin induction, extracellular signal-regulated kinase activation, and *in vivo* proliferation. *Cancer Res* 63: 6237–6243.

51. Jin C, McKeehan K, Guo W, *et al.* (2003) Cooperation between ectopic FGFR1 and depression of FGFR2 in induction of prostatic intraepithelial neoplasia in the mouse prostate. *Cancer Res* 63:8784–8790.

52. Wang F, McKeehan K, Yu C, Ittmann M, McKeehan WL (2004) Chronic activity of ectopic type 1 fibroblast growth factor receptor tyrosine kinase in prostate epithelium results in hyperplasia accompanied by intraepithelial neoplasia. *Prostate* 58:1–12.

53. Abdulkadir SA, Magee JA, Peters TJ, *et al.* (2002) Conditional loss of Nkx3.1 in adult mice induces prostatic intraepithelial neoplasia. *Mol Cell Biol* 22:1495–1503.

54. Maddison LA, Nahm H, DeMayo F, Greenberg NM (2000) Prostate specific expression of Cre recombinase in transgenic mice. *Genesis* 26: 154–156.

55. Cussenot O, Berthon P, Cochand-Priollet B, Maitland NJ, Le Duc A (1994) Immunocytochemical comparison of cultured normal epithelial prostatic cells with prostatic tissue sections. *Exp Cell Res* 214:83–92.

56. Leav I, McNeal JE, Kwan PW, Komminoth P, Merk FB (1996) Androgen receptor expression in prostatic dysplasia (prostatic intraepithelial neoplasia) in the human prostate: an immunohistochemical and in situ hybridization study. *Prostate* 29:137–145.

57. Chen CD, Welsbie DS, Tran C, *et al.* (2004) Molecular determinants of resistance to antiandrogen therapy. *Nat Med* 10:33–39.

58. Stanbrough M, Leav I, Kwan PW, Bubley GJ, Balk SP (2001) Prostatic intraepithelial neoplasia in mice expressing an androgen receptor transgene in prostate epithelium. *Proc Natl Acad Sci USA* 98:10823–10828.

59. Dong JT (2001) Chromosomal deletions and tumor suppressor genes in prostate cancer. *Cancer Metastasis Rev* 20:173–193.

60. Voeller HJ, Augustus M, Madike V, Bova GS, Carter KC, Gelmann EP (1997) Coding region of NKX3.1, a prostate-specific homeobox gene on 8p21, is not mutated in human prostate cancers. *Cancer Res* 57:4455–4559.

61. Bowen C, Bubendorf L, Voeller HJ, *et al.* (2000) Loss of NKX3.1 expression in human prostate cancers correlates with tumor progression. *Cancer Res* 60:6111–6115.

62. Bhatia-Gaur R, Donjacour AA, Sciavolino PJ, *et al.* (1999) Roles for Nkx3.1 in prostate development and cancer. *Genes Dev* 13:966–977.

63. Schneider A, Brand T, Zweigerdt R, Arnold H (2000) Targeted disruption of the Nkx3.1 gene in mice results in morphogenetic defects of minor salivary glands: parallels to glandular duct morphogenesis in prostate. *Mech Dev* 95: 163–174.

64. Tanaka M, Komuro I, Inagaki H, Jenkins NA, Copeland NG, Izumo S (2000) Nkx3.1, a murine homolog of *Drosophila* bagpipe, regulates epithelial ductal branching and proliferation of the prostate and palatine glands. *Dev Dyn* 219:248–260.

65. Cunha GR, Hayward SW, Wang YZ (2002) Role of stroma in carcinogenesis of the prostate. *Differentiation* 70:473–485.

66. Kim MJ, Bhatia-Gaur R, Banach-Petrosky WA, *et al.* (2002) Nkx3.1 mutant mice recapitulate early stages of prostate carcinogenesis. *Cancer Res* 62: 2999–3004.

67. Kim MJ, Cardiff RD, Desai N, *et al.* (2002) Cooperativity of Nkx3.1 and Pten loss of function in a mouse model of prostate carcinogenesis. *Proc Natl Acad Sci USA* 99:2884–2889.

68. Peehl DM, Feldman D (2003) The role of vitamin D and retinoids in controlling prostate cancer progression. *Endocr Relat Cancer* 10:131–140.

69. Chambon P (1996) A decade of molecular biology of retinoic acid receptors. *FASEB J* 10:940–954.

70. Mangelsdorf DJ, Umesone K, Evans RM (1994) The retinoid receptors. In: Sporn MB and Goodman DS, eds. *The Retinoids*. Raven Press, New York, pp. 319–349.

71. Lohnes D, Kastner P, Dierich A, Mark M, LeMeur M, Chambon P (1993) Function of retinoic acid receptor gamma in the mouse. *Cell* 73:643–658.

72. Krezel W, Dupe V, Mark M, Dierich A, Kastner P, Chambon P (1996) RXR gamma null mice are apparently normal and compound RXR alpha $+/-/$ RXR beta $-/-/$RXR gamma $-/-$ mutant mice are viable. *Proc Natl Acad Sci USA* 93:9010–9014.

73. Almasan A, Mangelsdorf DJ, Ong ES, Wahl GM, Evans RM (1994) Chromosomal localization of the human retinoid X receptors. *Genomics* 20: 397–403.

74. Ruijter E, van de Kaa C, Miller G, Ruiter D, Debruyne F, Schalken J (1999) Molecular genetics and epidemiology of prostate carcinoma. *Endocr Rev* 20:22–45.

75. Zhong C, Yang S, Huang J, Cohen MB, Roy-Burman P (2003) Aberration in the expression of the retinoid receptor, RXRalpha, in prostate cancer. *Cancer Biol Ther* 2:179–184.

76. Pandey KK, Batra SK (2003) RXRalpha: a novel target for prostate cancer. *Cancer Biol Ther* 2:185–186.

77. Huang J, Powell WC, Khodavirdi AC, *et al.* (2002) Prostatic intraepithelial neoplasia in mice with conditional disruption of the retinoid X receptor alpha allele in the prostate epithelium. *Cancer Res* 62:4812–4819.

78. Tsvetkov LM, Yeh KH, Lee SJ, Sun H, Zhang H (1999) p27(Kip1) ubiquiti-
    nation and degradation is regulated by the SCF(Skp2) complex through
    phosphorylated Thr187 in p27. *Curr Biol* 9:661–664.

79. Carrano AC, Eytan E, Hershko A, Pagano M (1999) SKP2 is required for
    ubiquitin-mediated degradation of the CDK inhibitor p27. *Nat Cell Biol*
    1:193–199.

80. Sutterluty H, Chatelain E, Marti A, *et al.* (1999) p45SKP2 promotes p27Kip1
    degradation and induces S phase in quiescent cells. *Nat Cell Biol* 1:207–214.

81. Slingerland J, Pagano M (2000) Regulation of the cdk inhibitor p27 and its
    deregulation in cancer. *J Cell Physiol* 183:10–17.

82. Lloyd RV, Erickson LA, Jin L, *et al.* (1999) p27kip1: a multifunctional
    cyclin-dependent kinase inhibitor with prognostic significance in human
    cancers. *Am J Pathol* 154:313–323.

83. Cordon-Cardo C, Koff A, Drobnjak M, *et al.* (1998) Distinct altered patterns
    of p27KIP1 gene expression in benign prostatic hyperplasia and prostatic
    carcinoma. *J Natl Cancer Inst* 90:1284–1291.

84. Shim EH, Johnson L, Noh HL, *et al.* (2003) Expression of the F-box protein
    SKP2 induces hyperplasia, dysplasia, and low-grade carcinoma in the mouse
    prostate. *Cancer Res* 63:1583–1588.

85. Di Cristofano A, De Acetis M, Koff A, Cordon-Cardo C, Pandolfi PP (2001)
    Pten and p27KIP1 cooperate in prostate cancer tumor suppression in the
    mouse. *Nat Genet* 27:222–224.

86. Cheng M, Olivier P, Diehl JA, *et al.* (1999) The p21(Cip1) and p27(Kip1)
    CDK 'inhibitors' are essential activators of cyclin D-dependent kinases in
    murine fibroblasts. *EMBO J* 18:1571–1583.

87. Nesbit CE, Tersak JM, Prochownik EV (1999) MYC oncogenes and human
    neoplastic disease. *Oncogene* 18:3004–3016.

88. Jenkins RB, Qian J, Lieber MM, Bostwick DG (1997) Detection of c-myc
    oncogene amplification and chromosomal anomalies in metastatic prostatic
    carcinoma by fluorescence *in situ* hybridization. *Cancer Res* 57:524–531.

89. Qian J, Jenkins RB, Bostwick DG (1997) Detection of chromosomal anom-
    alies and c-myc gene amplification in the cribriform pattern of prostatic
    intraepithelial neoplasia and carcinoma by fluorescence *in situ* hybridization.
    Mod Pathol 10:1113–1119.

90. Latil A, Vidaud D, Valeri A, *et al.* (2000) htert expression correlates with
    MYC over-expression in human prostate cancer. *Int J Cancer* 89:172–176.

91. Ellwood-Yen K, Graeber TG, Wongvipat J, *et al.* (2003) Myc-driven murine
    prostate cancer shares molecular features with human prostate tumors.
    Cancer Cell 4:223–238.

92. Lim K, Park C, Kim YK, *et al.* (2000) Association of castration-dependent early induction of c-myc expression with a cell proliferation of the ventral prostate gland in rat. *Exp Mol Med* 32:216–221.

93. Karlsson A, Deb-Basu D, Cherry A, Turner S, Ford J, Felsher DW (2003) Defective double-strand DNA break repair and chromosomal translocations by MYC overexpression. *Proc Natl Acad Sci USA* 100:9974–9979.

94. Dhanasekaran SM, Barrette TR, Ghosh D, *et al.* (2001) Delineation of prognostic biomarkers in prostate cancer. *Nature* 412:822–826.

95. Staal SP, Hartley JW, Rowe WP (1977) Isolation of transforming murine leukemia viruses from mice with a high incidence of spontaneous lymphoma. *Proc Natl Acad Sci USA* 74:3065–3067.

96. Franke TF, Kaplan DR, Cantley LC, Toker A (1997) Direct regulation of the Akt proto-oncogene product by phosphatidylinositol-3,4-bisphosphate. *Science* 275:665–668.

97. Dahia PL (2000) PTEN, a unique tumor suppressor gene. *Endocr Relat Cancer* 7:115–129.

98. Liaw D, Marsh DJ, Li J, *et al.* (1997) Germline mutations of the PTEN gene in Cowden disease, an inherited breast and thyroid cancer syndrome. *Nat Genet* 16:64–67.

99. Sellers WR, and Sawyers CL (2002) *Somatic Genetics of Prostate Cancer: Oncogenes and Tumor Suppressors.* Lippincott Williams & Wilkins, Philadelphia.

100. Suzuki H, Freije D, Nusskern DR, *et al.* (1998) Interfocal heterogeneity of PTEN/MMAC1 gene alterations in multiple metastatic prostate cancer tissues. *Cancer Res* 58:204–209.

101. Cantley LC, Neel BG (1999) New insights into tumor suppression: PTEN suppresses tumor formation by restraining the phosphoinositide 3-kinase/AKT pathway. *Proc Natl Acad Sci USA* 96:4240–4245.

102. Di Cristofano A, Pandolfi PP (2000) The multiple roles of PTEN in tumor suppression. *Cell* 100:387–390.

103. Maehama T, Taylor GS, Dixon JE (2001) PTEN and myotubularin: novel phosphoinositide phosphatases. *Annu Rev Biochem* 70:247–279.

104. Stambolic V, Suzuki A, de la Pompa JL, *et al.* (1998) Negative regulation of PKB/Akt-dependent cell survival by the tumor suppressor PTEN. *Cell* 95:29–39.

105. Sun H, Lesche R, Li DM, *et al.* (1999) PTEN modulates cell cycle progression and cell survival by regulating phosphatidylinositol 3,4,5,-trisphosphate and Akt/protein kinase B signaling pathway. *Proc Natl Acad Sci USA* 96: 6199–6204.

106. Hanahan D, Weinberg RA (2000) The hallmarks of cancer. *Cell* 100:57–70.
107. Vivanco I, Sawyers CL (2002) The phosphatidylinositol 3-Kinase AKT pathway in human cancer. *Nat Rev Cancer* 2:489–501.
108. Majumder PK, Yeh JJ, George DJ, *et al.* (2003) Prostate intraepithelial neoplasia induced by prostate restricted Akt activation: the MPAKT model. *Proc Natl Acad Sci USA* 100:7841–7846.
109. Reiter RE, Gu Z, Watabe T, *et al.* (1998) Prostate stem cell antigen: a cell surface marker overexpressed in prostate cancer. *Proc Natl Acad Sci USA* 95:1735–1740.
110. Levedakou EN, Strohmeyer TG, Effert PJ, Liu ET (1992) Expression of the matrix Gla protein in urogenital malignancies. *Int J Cancer* 52:534–537.
111. Coleman RE, Mashiter G, Fogelman I, *et al.* (1988) Osteocalcin: a potential marker of metastatic bone disease and response to treatment. *Eur J Cancer Clin Oncol* 24:1211–1217.
112. Lesche R, Groszer M, Gao J, *et al.* (2002) Cre/loxP-mediated inactivation of the murine Pten tumor suppressor gene. *Genesis* 32:148–149.
113. Wang S, Gao J, Lei Q, *et al.* (2003) Prostate-specific deletion of the murine Pten tumor suppressor gene leads to metastatic prostate cancer. *Cancer Cell* 4:209–221.
114. Trotman LC, Niki M, Dotan ZA, *et al.* (2003) Pten dose dictates cancer progression in the prostate. *PLoS Biol* 1:385–396.
115. Backman S, Stambolic V, Mak T (2002) PTEN function in mammalian cell size regulation. *Curr Opin Neurobiol* 12:516–522.
116. Groszer M, Erickson R, Scripture-Adams DD, *et al.* (2001) Negative regulation of neural stem/progenitor cell proliferation by the Pten tumor suppressor gene *in vivo*. *Science* 294:2186–2189.
117. Abate-Shen C, Banach-Petrosky WA, Sun X, *et al.* (2003) Nkx3.1; Pten mutant mice develop invasive prostate adenocarcinoma and lymph node metastases. *Cancer Res* 63:3886–3890.
118. Medema RH, Kops GJ, Bos JL, Burgering BM (2000) AFX-like Forkhead transcription factors mediate cell-cycle regulation by Ras and PKB through p27kip1. *Nature* 404:782–787.
119. Stiles B, Gilman V, Khanzenzon N, *et al.* (2002) Essential role of AKT-1/protein kinase B alpha in PTEN-controlled tumorigenesis. *Mol Cell Biol* 22:3842–3851.
120. Di Cristofano A, Kotsi P, Peng YF, Cordon-Cardo C, Elkon KB, Pandolfi PP (1999) Impaired Fas response and autoimmunity in Pten+/− mice. *Science* 285:2122–2125.

121. Kiyokawa H, Kineman RD, Manova-Todorova KO, *et al.* (1996) Enhanced growth of mice lacking the cyclin-dependent kinase inhibitor function of p27(Kip1). *Cell* 85:721–732.

122. Nakayama K, Ishida N, Shirane M, *et al.* (1996) Mice lacking p27(Kip1) display increased body size, multiple organ hyperplasia, retinal dysplasia, and pituitary tumors. *Cell* 85:707–720.

123. Lyons SK, Meuwissen R, Krimpenfort P, Berns A (2003) The generation of a conditional reporter that enables bioluminescence imaging of Cre/loxP-dependent tumorigenesis in mice. *Cancer Res* 63:7042–7046.

INDEX